T0342365

Tissue and Cell Donation

Tissue and Cell Donation

AN ESSENTIAL GUIDE

EDITED BY

Ruth M. Warwick, MB, ChB, FRCP, FRCPath
Consultant Specialist for Tissue Services, NHSBT
Tissue Services
Edgware, Middlesex, UK

Deirdre Fehily, PhD
Inspector and Technical Consultant, Tissues and Cells
National Transplant Centre
Rome, Italy

Scott A. Brubaker, CTBS
Chief Policy Officer, American Association of Tissue Banks
McLean, Virginia, USA

Ted Eastlund, MD
Associate Medical Director
LifeNet Health
Virginia Beach, Virginia, USA

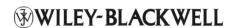

A John Wiley & Sons, Ltd., Publication

Library of Congress Cataloging-in-Publication Data
Tissue and cell donation : an essential guide / edited by Ruth M. Warwick . . . [et al.].
 p. ; cm.
 Includes bibliographical references.
 ISBN 978-1-4051-6322-4
 1. Tissue banks–Social aspects. 2. Human cell culture–Social aspects. I. Warwick, Ruth M. II. Title.
 [DNLM: 1. Tissue and Organ Procurement–ethics. 2. Tissue and Organ Procurement–organization & administration. 3. Biological Specimen Banks–ethics. 4. Biological Specimen Banks–organization & administration. WO 660 T6148 2009]
 RD127.T568 2009
 362.17'83–dc22

 2008052029

ISBN: 978-1-4051-6322-4

A catalogue record for this book is available from the British Library.

Set in 9.25 on 12 pt Meridien by SNP Best-set Typesetter Ltd., Hong Kong
Printed & bound in Singapore by Fabulous Printers Pte Ltd

1 2009

Contents

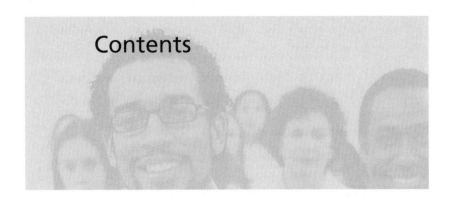

Contributors

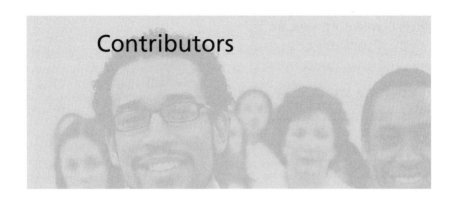

Hamid Reza Aghayan, MD
Managing Director, Iranian Tissue Bank
Tehran University of Medical Sciences
Tehran, Iran

Pamela Albert, RN, BSN, CPTC
Director, Donor Family Services
New England Organ Bank
Newton, Massachusetts, USA

Martha W. Anderson, BA
Executive Vice President, Donor Services
Musculoskeletal Transplant Foundation
Edison, New Jersey, USA

Li Baoxing
Shanxi Provincial Tissue Bank
Taiyuan, Shanxi Province, China

Muhammed Cassim, FRCS
Medical Director
Sri Lanka Eye Donation Society
Dr Hudson Silva Eye Donation Headquarters
Colombo, Sri Lanka

Jeremy Chapman, OAM, MD, MB, BChir, FRACP, FRCP
Clinical Professor and University of Sydney Director
Acute Interventional Medicine
Westmead Hospital
Westmead, New South Wales, Australia

Alessandro Nanni Costa, MD
Director
Italian National Transplant Centre
Rome, Italy

Robin Cowherd, CT, MPA, BA
Director, Donor Family Services
LifeNet Health
Virginia Beach, Virginia, USA

Lisa Dinhofer, MA, CT, CTBS
KoDen, LLC™, Consultant
Hood College, Adjunct, Frederick, Maryland, USA

Arieh Eldad, MD
Professor of Plastic Surgery (Retired)
Hebrew University School of Medicine
Jerusalem, Israel

Sarah Franklin, MA, PhD
Professor of Social Studies of Biomedicine
London School of Economics and Political Science
London, UK

Danielle B. Freedman, MB, BS, FRCPath
Medical Director
Luton & Dunstable Hospital NHS Foundation Trust
Luton, UK

Sally Gordon, RN, BA
National Executive Officer
Australian Bone Marrow Donor Registry
Sydney, New South Wales, Australia

Paolo Grossi, MD, PhD
Professor of Infectious Diseases
University of Insubria, Varese, Italy;
Infectious Disease Expert Advisor to the Italian National Transplant Centre
Rome, Italy

Patricia Hewitt, MB, ChB, FRCP, FRCPath
NBS Consultant Specialist in Transfusion Microbiology
NHS Blood and Transplant
London, UK

Sharon R. Kaufman, PhD
Professor, Medical Anthropology
Department of Anthropology, History and Social Medicine
Department of Social and Behavioral Sciences
University of California
San Francisco, California, USA

Ján Koller, MD
Associate Professor of Surgery
Teaching Department of Burns and Reconstructive Surgery
University Hospital Bratislava, Ruzinov Hospital
Bratislava, Slovakia

George McCann, MD, CTBS
Licensed Embalmer and Funeral Director
Education Director
Musculoskeletal Transplant Foundation (MTF)
Edison, New Jersey, USA

Riva Miller, BA
Systemic Psychotherapist (individual, couple, and family)
Haemophilia Centre Royal Free Hospital
London, UK;
Consultant, National Blood and Tissue Service
London, UK

Blanca Miranda, MD, PhD
Director of Transplant Services Foundation and the Transplant Coordination
Unit Hospital Clinic
Barcelona, Spain

Chris Moore, BSc, MB, BS
Associate Specialist in Transfusion Microbiology
NHS Blood and Transplant
London, UK

Aziz Nather, FRCS
Associate Professor and Senior Consultant
Department of Orthopaedic Surgery
Yong Loo Lin School of Medicine
National University of Singapore and National University Hospital
Singapore

Jane Pearson, RN
Assistant Director – Nursing
NHS Blood and Transplant
NBS Leeds
Bridle Path
Seacroft, Leeds, UK

Naomi Pfeffer
Professor of Social and Historical Studies of Medicine
Department of Applied Social Sciences
London Metropolitan University
London, UK

Diego Ponzin, MD
Medical Director
Fondazione Banca degli Occhi del Veneto
Venice, Italy

Eliana Porta, MD
Lead Inspector, Tissues and Cells
Italian National Transplant Centre
Rome, Italy

William Randell, BA(Open), RGN
Clinical Risk Manager
Luton & Dunstable Hospital NHS Foundation Trust
Luton, UK

Annette Rid, MD
Assistant Professor
Institute of Biomedical Ethics, Centre for Ethics
University of Zurich
Zurich, Switzerland

Jacinto Sánchez-Ibáñez, MD
Director, Regional Transplant Coordination Office
Galicia, A Coruña, Spain

David M. Smith, MD
Medical Director and Chief Executive Officer
Community Blood Center Community Tissue Services
Dayton, Ohio, USA

Michael Strong, MT(ASCP), PhD
Formerly
Northwest Tissue Center/Puget Sound Blood Center
Seattle, Washington, USA

Elaine Swanson, DCR, BSc(Hons) Health Sciences
Clinical Quality and NICE Guidance Manager
Luton & Dunstable Hospital NHS Foundation Trust
Luton, UK

Esteve Trias, MD
Medical Director
Processing Facilities, Transplant Services Foundation
Barcelona, Spain

Dorothy E. Vawter, PhD
Associate Director
Minnesota Center for Health Care Ethics
St. Paul, Minnesota, USA

Charles V. Wetli, MD
Formerly
Chief Medical Examiner and Director of Forensic Sciences (retired)
Suffolk County Government, Happauge, New York, USA;
Clinical Professor of Pathology (retired)
State University of New York
Stony Brook, New York, USA

Christopher Womack, MB, BS, FRCPath
Pathologist
Histologix Ltd
Nottingham, UK

Foreword

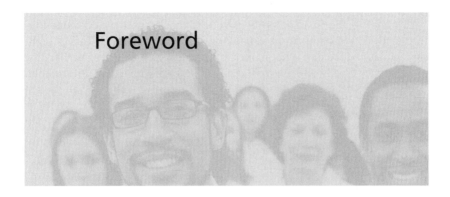

Transplantation of human tissues and cells has become increasingly frequent and successful in recent years, not just with respect to the number of implanted grafts but also in the number of therapeutic indications. Each year, all around the world, thousands of patients receive transplants of tissue and cells of human origin. These transplants are made up firstly of 'traditional transplants', the therapeutic value of which has been recognized for decades (corneas, skin, blood vessels, heart valves, hematopoietic cells, bone marrow, etc.) and secondly of biotechnological advances which are currently undergoing rapid development (cell culture, tissue engineering).

There is a general agreement that the use in medicine of products of human origin demands that the quality and safety of the whole process of tissue and cell donation, procurement, testing, processing, preservation, storage, and distribution be ensured in order to prevent the transmission of diseases. In fact, this has been the focus of the EU Tissue and Cell Directives, now in the implementation phase, and of similar regulations in other parts of the world. However, these kinds of therapies also involve specific considerations related to the origin of the transplant material: respect for the donor's consent, anonymity, and non-remuneration for the donor.

As Arthur Caplan testified before the US Congress . . . 'what is truly distinctive about transplantation is not technology or cost, but ethics. This is the only area in medicine which cannot exist without the participation of the public. It is the individual citizen who, while alive, or after death, makes organs and tissues available for transplantation. If there were no gift of organs or tissues, transplantation would come to a grinding halt'. Both aspects – technical quality standards and ethics – are and should always be strictly linked in order to assure a solid foundation for a transplant system and the best opportunities and results for the patients.

This book is the first comprehensive text that focuses on the donation-related aspects of tissue and cell banking and transplantation. That is probably its main value and what makes it attractive. In a field that is changing so rapidly, it is really difficult to find all the necessary up to date information written by a selected global group of experts from five continents presented in a very didactic way. I am sure that this volume will be really useful in meeting the training needs of professionals working in the field of human tissue and cell donation.

My sincere congratulations to the editors for this important initiative, and to all the authors for a job well done for the benefit of many patients.

Rafael Matesanz, MD, PhD
National Transplant Coordinator
Spanish National Transplant Organization (ONT)
Madrid, Spain

Preface

The banking of human tissues and cells has many facets and involves professionals with a wide range of skills and knowledge. They include experts with training in medical, technical, scientific, psychological, and communications fields. This book focuses on the human dimension – the many aspects of donation in cell and tissue banking. The issues raised are relevant on a global stage. Tissue banks and procurement agencies, and the professionals who work within them, are the guardians of the altruistic gifts that donors and their families have entrusted to them for the benefit of others, to save and improve lives. The donations range from bone marrow, cord blood, femoral head bone, and amniotic membrane from living donors to many types of tissue from deceased donors including corneas, heart valves, skin, bone, and tendons. These donations have enabled the development of a field of health care that is often scientifically and technically sophisticated, which represents a success story for the hundreds of thousands of patients who have regained sight or mobility, had pain alleviated, or even had their lives saved by tissue or cell transplantation. The application of "business management" models and, in some cases, for-profit processing and supply to hospitals has created an element of commercialism that can sit awkwardly with the donor or the donor family's motivation.

The primary obligations of the professionals involved are to ensure that donors and their families are well informed and are not coerced, and that donated tissues and cells are distributed fairly, on the basis of clinical priority, are affordable, and are not wasted. Clinical effectiveness and recipient safety must, at the same time, be maximized. In some circumstances, the protection of donor autonomy can conflict with the public good, creating a tension between the approach that focuses on achieving a free and unfettered decision by the donor, as highlighted in Chapter 4, as opposed to the approach that allows for the recipients' needs to be a significant factor in the donor consent model, as demonstrated in Chapter 2. It is an acceptable practice to give a suggested direction of response when taking consent for a therapeutic procedure such as cancer surgery or liver biopsy; it is appropriate to tell the patient how critically important this procedure is, as long as the risks and alternatives are described. For research consent, on the other hand, any promotion of the potential benefits to others would be seen as unacceptable coercion as these are actually unknown. In the donation context, a delicate balance must be achieved between describing the potential benefits to recipients and highlighting any risk, inconvenience, or undesirable outcome for the donor or the donor family. In the end, donation organizations and tissue and cell banks must reflect donor interests and protect their confidentiality while doing no harm to either the donor or the recipient. Special consideration is needed in dealing with donations used for commercial or financial gain or those used for research or education rather than for patient care.

The agreed professional requirements for the safety and quality of tissues and cells for transplantation have increased steadily over time and are reflected in the development of increasingly stringent regulations. Establishing a detailed donor history and conducting reliable and appropriate tests are critical aspects of minimizing risk of disease transmission to the recipient. Donor suitability determination has become complex, involving longer and more difficult interviews by trained specialists and sophisticated testing protocols. This means that many donations cannot be used for the purpose for which they were intended; tissue and cell banks and donation organizations must have policies in place for evaluating the significance of donor and donation findings, for communicating this information where relevant, and for disposing of untransplantable tissues and cells in an appropriate way.

The editors of this book have grappled with these challenges on a day-to-day basis over many years. We have worked in our own organizations to develop policies and practices that aim to strike a balance between the sometimes competing demands of meeting the clinical need for donated tissues and cells, while ensuring the ethical treatment of donors and donor families and the safety of recipients. During these years, we have accumulated experiences that have changed our ways of looking at the issues and, sometimes, of looking at the world! But, very importantly, we have also participated as part of a wide network of colleagues around the globe who are debating and managing the same challenges, often in different economic or social contexts. Many of them have drawn on their practical knowledge and experience to contribute to the chapters of this book and we are very grateful to them.

We hope that, by sharing what has been learned by this large group of experts from many countries, we have provided an educational tool that will allow practitioners to establish optimal policies and practices for tissue and cell donation. The issues are often difficult and sensitive, but we can learn from history and from the experiences of others so that mistakes are not repeated and there is continuous improvement in the quality of our services to donors and to the patients they want to help.

Ruth M. Warwick, MB, ChB, FRCP, FRCPath
Deirdre Fehily, PhD
Scott A. Brubaker, CTBS
Ted Eastlund, MD

1 Histories of Tissue Banking

Naomi Pfeffer

Department of Applied Social Sciences, London Metropolitan University,
London, UK

The health of a boy who had suffered a deep burn to his lap deteriorated to
such an extent that it was feared he would not survive. As a last resort,
James Barrett Brown (1899–1971), a pioneering and influential American
plastic and reconstructive surgeon, covered the wound with skin taken from
the child's mother. The grafts "took" initially but after three weeks had been
completely absorbed. Nonetheless, the child's health recovered and the
wound was much improved [1]. Mother and child were fortunate in this
instance: from the mid-1930s, when surgeons began following Brown's lead
in using skin as a biologic dressing, more often than not, a mother recovering from surgery to remove her skin would be mourning the death of her
severely burned child.

Skin taken from family members was the first choice in homografting[1]
because surgeons believed it would be better tolerated than the skin of
strangers, and also because anxious relatives were more likely to agree to
undergo the painful procedure. However, skin occasionally was recovered
from friends especially where the patient's burn covered a large area. Harold
Gillies (1882–1960), a surgeon famous for his pioneering plastic reconstruction of soldiers horribly wounded during the First World War, described how
factory hands offered their skin to dress the burns of a colleague who had
fallen into a vat of boiling water. As a result, as Gillies put it, the patient
became "the proud possessor of a part of the legs of Lucy and Annie, and
so on, all the way up his legs" [2].

---

[1] Homograft and allograft describe a graft of tissue from another person. Autograft is a graft
using the patient's own tissue.

Tissue and Cell Donation: An Essential Guide. Edited by Ruth M. Warwick, Deirdre Fehily,
Scott A. Brubaker, Ted Eastlund. © 2009 Blackwell Publishing, ISBN: 978-14051-6322-4.

A 22-year-old man's severely inflamed corneas reduced his sight to such an extent that he was unable to count fingers held up close to either eye and needed help to find his way about. In 1930, at Guy's Hospital, London, Tudor Thomas (1893–1976), the Welsh ophthalmic surgeon who pioneered keratoplasty (corneal grafting) in Britain, grafted onto his patient's left eye the cornea of another patient, a 42-year-old man whose eye had had to be removed as a result of a perforating injury. Two years after the operation, the young man could count fingers on a hand held up three feet away from him [3].

Tudor Thomas was following in the footsteps of Eduard Zirm (1863–1944), who, in December 1905, in a hospital in Olomouc (now in Moravia in the Czech Republic), had performed the first human-to-human corneal transplant to "take". The "donor" was Karl Brauer, an 11-year-old boy, a patient of Zirm's, whose eye had had to be removed because it had been penetrated by a fragment of iron. The recipient was Alois Golgar, a day laborer, another of Zirm's patients, who had been blinded in both eyes by a splash of the lime he had been using to whitewash a chicken hut. Golgar regained and retained some sight in one eye until his death some two-and-a-half years later.

Prehistory

The prehistoric age of human tissue banking began around the turn of the 20th century. It was characterized by the "direct method," which required physicians and surgeons to redistribute tissue among patients or to solicit grafting material from a patient's family and friends and sometimes from strangers. The direct method is responsible for the creation of a new category of person called a donor; it forged novel relations among both doctors, and patients. Its drawbacks emerged rapidly during the experimental phase of blood transfusion, one of the first therapeutic applications of human tissue (blood is liquid tissue), in which donor and recipient were connected arm to arm in order to prevent blood from coming into contact with air and clotting. The method placed considerable physical demands on the donor and was unreliable: doctors were unable to predict if a "donor-on-the-hoof" would belong to the same blood group as their patient.

Doctors in the first decade of the 20th century found that blood collected in a solution of citrate and glucose did not clot and kept for several days if it is stored in an ice box. However, it was not until the Spanish Civil War (1936–1939), when doctors on both sides were confronted by casualties on a mass scale, that the extended shelf life was exploited to separate donor and recipient in both time and space – the indirect approach. Civilians were recruited as donors and their blood groups identified. Blood collected in a solution of citrate and glucose was dispatched in heat-insulated wood or canvas boxes, with thick cord linings, to field hospitals near the front line [4]. Its history was recorded on standardized forms.

Bernard Fantus is reputed to be the first person to have adapted the indirect method of blood transfusion to a peacetime context. In 1937, he established a facility at the Cook County Hospital in Chicago. Blood was collected in a flask containing a small amount of sodium citrate; the flask was sealed and stored in a refrigerator. Fantus called the facility the Blood Preservation Laboratory, but given the system of deposits and withdrawals, he soon came up with "blood bank," a snappier name that immediately became part of the popular vocabulary [5].

Around this time, the indirect method began to be adapted to other kinds of human tissue. The first one was what would now be called an eye bank and was established in Odessa by Vladimir Petrovich Filatov (1875–1956), the Soviet Union's premier ophthalmologist. Filatov, in 1929, had declared war on corneal blindness and had invited its victims throughout the USSR to come to his clinic for treatment. They turned up in droves. When hospital mortuaries in and around his clinic in Odessa proved unable to satisfy the demand for cadaver eyes, Filatov arranged for eyes to be collected in the Sklifosovsky Institute, Moscow's central hospital for accidents and emergencies [6]. Many people died there. It was the city's central trauma hospital and had thousands of beds and dozens of operating theaters. Filatov designed a convenient method of packaging eyes for safe transport known as moist storage, which consists of a widemouthed container usually made out of glass with some sort of device for securing the eye in its base and which is filled with an appropriate storage medium [7]. The containers were placed in a small ice-filled thermos jug, which was fitted into a box marked with a red cross and sent by rail. The eyes reached Filatov's operating theater in Odessa some 500 miles away within the time allowed.

Histories of tissue banking

This chapter is called "histories of tissue banking" because no two tissue banks are identical. Some of the variation can be attributed to the type of tissue handled, but differences between banks handling the same body parts can only be explained by where, when, and by whom the banks were established and developed. Each bank has favored certain techniques over others and has established unique relationships with its sponsors, the state, the market, the healthcare system, doctors, donors and their kin, and recipients.

This brief and partial survey offers some snapshots illustrative of the history of banks of tissue recovered mostly from what are now called "non-heart-beating donors" within hours following death.[2] However, whereas blood banks rapidly replaced the direct method of blood collection, it has taken around 50 years for tissue banks to monopolize the recovery and supply of human tissue largely because surgeons could easily accumulate "stashes," that is, personal collections of human material recovered in either the operating theater or the mortuary.

Early experimental grafts mostly involved tissue taken from living people known to the doctor or the patient. Tissue was seldom recovered from a corpse, and then only by a bold surgeon confronted by a desperate situation. Doctors were acutely aware of the speed at which bacteria proliferate in the corpse and were understandably fearful of the medical consequences of grafting cadaver material into a living patient. It had taken considerable courage on the part of Filatov to begin grafting corneas recovered from corpses. As he put it, "I must confess that I undertook the operation with some trepidation since there were those who warned me of the danger of 'cadaver infection', 'cadaver toxin', etc." [8].

Another reason people were reluctant to recover tissue from the cadaver is that it necessitates intervening in powerful and carefully orchestrated rituals staged around death and disposal of the corpse and which speak of solicitude for the dead person and sympathy for the grieving relatives and friends. These rituals, which are observed in some form or other everywhere, also manage the liminal period between death and disposal, a period during which the corpse suffers from categorical ambiguity, a dangerous condition marked by competing claims of custodianship [9]. The competition is widely understood as a battle between death and living people reluctant to relinquish their ties with the person embodied in the corpse. Tissue banking is responsible for introducing a radical and dehumanizing claim: it seeks custodianship of the corpse in order to dismantle it into exchangeable and transplantable parts.

Tissue banks, confronted by written and unwritten rules that police the proper performance of these rituals, have placed as much importance on "cultural work" as on "organizational work" [10]. "Organizational work" is shorthand for the technical and administrative tasks involved in recovering, processing, storing, and distributing human tissue and includes practical arrangements for gaining custodianship of the corpse. "Cultural work" includes the development of official and quasi-official policies around the custodianship of the corpse and creating opportunities to give by fostering

---

[2] "Non-heart-beating donors" are people whose death is confirmed by absence of vital signs such as heartbeat and respiration. "Brain death" is controversial and is defined by signs of irremediable damage to the brain stem. It was introduced in 1968 by an ad hoc committee convened by the Harvard Medical School. It has been deployed mostly to facilitate the recovery of solid organs during the warm ischemic time. See M. Lock, *Twice Dead: Organ Transplants and the Reinvention of Death* (Berkeley: University of California Press, 2002).

habits of the heart and generating accounts of what giving means. Cultural work, which seeks legitimation by the state, is political. It seeks a high public profile, whereas organizational work has been undertaken mostly out of public sight for reasons of expediency, discretion, and taste.

Organizational work

Recovering tissue in the prehistory of tissue banks was a craft skill involving surgical instruments. James Barrett Brown, for example, used a very sharp knife of the amputation variety to cut thick, split-skin grafts. He was very adept and could vary the depth of cut according to the site. As he put it, "with some practice the thickness can be easily graduated with free-hand-cutting, and the thickness of the graft should depend on the relative full-thickness of the skin of the area . . . The essential thing is that it be cut thick, but not too thick, to prevent the donor site from healing promptly" [11].

Nowadays, tissue banks produce and distribute consistent, standardized interchangeable body parts, which can be employed uniformly across various institutional and even international boundaries [12]. Yet, in its infancy, tissue banking had been confronted by resounding proof that everyone is unique. Peter Medawar (1915–1987), a British scientist, in the 1940s and 1950s, established that rejection of "foreign" grafting material is an immunological response acquired during pregnancy. His biological "laws" of transplantation earned him (and Sir Macfarlane Burnett) a Nobel Prize in 1960. Medawar identified what he called a spectrum of affinities, with autografts at one end and a gross disparity between the donor and the recipient at the other. Research and clinical experience has allowed the various bodily tissues to be arrayed along the spectrum with corneas, which were found to be immunologically privileged, placed toward the autograft end, and skin, which is exquisitely susceptible to rejection, at the other. The spectrum has influenced the product "niches" into which various bodily tissues fall so that corneas are normally treated as universal replacement products, whereas unprocessed skin serves as a temporary biological wound dressing.

Tools capable of producing a uniform "product" out of nonstandardized human bodies were invented spasmodically. Von Hippel (1867–1939), a doctor working in Heidelberg, led the way by designing a trephine, a mechanized clockwork instrument with saw-like edges – like a tiny cookie cutter – which can cut identical disks about the size of a shirt button out of both source and recipient eyes. He used it for the first time in 1887 in an operation to replace a young girl's corneas with those of a rabbit. The first dermatome, a calibrated device for removing skin in a uniform, predetermined thickness, was designed in 1937 by Earl C. Padgett Senior. The Reese dermatome, developed during the Second World War, was a refinement, which allowed even better results. Harry Brown, a young American surgeon, conceived of the idea of an electric dermatome while being held captive in a Japanese prisoner-of-war camp.

Calibrated tools can be and are used successfully by a suitably trained lay person. The United States Navy Tissue Bank offered four-month-long courses in tissue recovery – "bone bank school" – to navy corpsmen [13]. The bank had been opened in June 1949 in the Naval Hospital, Bethesda, Maryland, the flagship of navy medicine, which treats sailors and their families. (Military medicine in the United States is socialized medicine: health care paid for out of taxation is provided free at the point of delivery according to the patient's need.) The bank was the brainchild of George Hyatt, an orthopedic surgeon investigating bone preservation. Hyatt had found salvaging bone removed during surgery on "clean" orthopedic cases a time-consuming method of collection, which also provided scant material for his research. Cadavers were the answer: the bank's motto was *Ex Morte Vita* – from death comes life. Dead bodies deteriorate rapidly and the time allowed for tissue recovery is brief. And the moment of death is notoriously unpredictable. Hyatt organized a round-the-clock rota of four or five trained technicians ready to recover tissue when a suitable patient died in the Naval Hospital. Dismantling a cadaver into up to 125 grafts of all types took 12–14 hours and involved 5 hampers of linen, 50 gowns, 400 towels, 200 sheets, and a host of miscellaneous material including 500 wrappers [14]. As a mark of respect for the dead person, talking was prohibited and hand signals were used for communication.

In the 1970s, American funeral directors and licensed embalmers were identified as people well placed to enucleate eyes from corpses. They are often the first professionals to arrive at the deathbed; they know how to manage the corpse's liminal state, and they undergo training in anatomy and surgical techniques at an embalming school. However, many legal jurisdictions stipulated that enucleation, a surgical procedure, must be performed by a licensed medical practitioner. Lay organizations, especially chapters of Lions Clubs International, lobbied state senators to change the law and, when they succeeded, offered training courses to lay people.

Expansion of tissue banking

Tissue banks are often lay rather than medical operations. Their workforce, both paid and volunteer, occupies a lower – and cheaper – rung of the occupational hierarchy than that of solid organ recovery, which is the province of transplant surgeons, medical elite. Lay people, particularly in the United States, have actively promoted and supported tissue banks with both cash and kind. As members of lay organizations, they have raised funds to build facilities and buy equipment, and they have sometimes volunteered to recover tissue, complete paperwork, manage finances, or ferry tissue from donor to recipient. Often, organizations have championed a particular body part. Lions favored eyes because their grand endeavor is sight conservation and improving the quality of life of people with impaired sight, whereas adoption of skin banks by the Ancient Arabic Order of the Nobles of the Mystic Shrine – Shriners – grew out of their hospitals, which provide free orthopedic and burn care to needy children (toddlers in peacetime are the chief victims of drastic burns). British lay organizations, working within the framework of the National Health Service (NHS), have made a smaller but occasionally significant contribution to tissue banking. The Iris Fund, for example, a London-based charity devoted to medical research into the prevention of blindness, is responsible for the passage of the Corneal Tissue Act in 1986, which allowed lay enucleation. Since it was placed on the statute book, over 300 lay people have been trained in eye recovery.

War, both hot and cold, drove the expansion of tissue banking. Modern weaponry exploits heat to wreak physical havoc on the sentient tissue of the human body. There were burns caused by incinerating materials (such as napalm and phosphorous munitions), flash burns, flame burns, contact burns from hot objects on the battlefield, and scalds from steam or hot fluids (sailors were especially susceptible to these). New weapons were developed during the Second World War such as the American-made bazooka – a warhead propelled by a rocket – that could inflict both multiple, penetrating wounds and deep burns caused by small particles of burning material [15]. Modern medicine has found ways of increasing the chances of survival of appalling injury through better control of shock. As a result, the call to arms demands bravery in the face of weaponry and fortitude in the drawn-out painful process of bodily reconstruction, which often involves the incorporation of foreign tissue [16].

Medawar's early investigations into what he called "the body's exquisite powers of discrimination" were his contribution to the war effort during the Second World War. He had begun directing his energies toward understanding the science of skin grafting after witnessing a Royal Air Force bomber burst into flames and crash into the garden of his neighbor in north Oxford. The crew was badly burned [17]. Likewise, the Navy Tissue Bank was established in 1949 as a research facility investigating how cadaver tissue might be transformed into stable medical consumables that can be used in hospitals close to the battlefield. It promoted freeze-drying, lyophilization, or drying by sublimation, because freeze-dried tissue retains its original form, is easy to store, "keeps" at room temperature, can be stockpiled in preparation for mass casualties, and, like instant coffee, is easily reconstituted by immersion in a suitable fluid. The technique had been developed by Earl Flosdorf, who, during the 1930s, in his laboratory at the University of Pennsylvania's School of Medicine, had experimented with freeze-drying of human blood.

Flosdorf, during the Second World War, had transformed what he called a "laboratory curiosity" into a reliable supply of blood plasma organized by the American Red Cross to treat American troops injured in battle overseas. Shortly afterwards, he succeeded in applying the technique to the production of penicillin on an industrial scale [18]. When the Navy Tissue Bank opened, he collaborated with Hyatt in experiments on freeze-drying bones, skin, dura mater, arteries, and other human tissues incorporated in the restoration of servicemen injured on the battlefield.

The bank created a stockpile of freeze-dried tissue ready for use in the event of a situation that would produce mass casualties. Nuclear warfare, during the Cold War, was an everyday possibility, but the estimated scale of civilian casualties was well beyond the scope of medical facilities that would be up and running in the aftermath. The bank's preparedness for service is suggested by photographs of shelves holding row upon row of small glass jars containing freeze-dried tissue, which illustrate articles describing its work. It found plenty of opportunities for testing the performance of its products close to the battlefield in the Korean War (1950–1953). The high casualty rate of the latter years of the Vietnam War (1959–1975) depleted the bank's stock of tissue to such an extent that a second recovery facility had to be opened at the Naval Hospital, San Diego.

The United States, in the aftermath of the Vietnam War, entered a new era of isolationism and antimilitary politics. Stockpiles of freeze-dried human tissue were no longer necessary, and the bank turned its attention to organ and bone marrow transplantation. Nonetheless, its impact on tissue banking in the United States was considerable. The bank, during the brief interlude of peace that separated the Korean and Vietnam Wars, had stimulated civilian demand for tissue by distributing its products to surgeons who were prepared to test them out on their patients. New uses for tissues were identified, and training in procedures involving human tissue products began to be incorporated in the medical curriculum.

The Navy Tissue Bank's alumni of trained technicians, on their return to civilian life, used their expertise in recovery techniques to either gain employment or set up their own tissue bank. Tissue banking in the United States, during the 1970s, developed into a cottage industry made up of surgeons' stashes, "casual" small-scale efforts at local hospitals, a few large formal banks attached to major medical centers, and some independent outfits operating within a region [19]. They all fell outside the frameworks regulating licensed medical practitioners, pharmaceuticals, biologicals, and medical consumables. In contrast, at this stage very few tissue banks had been established in the United Kingdom, where policy makers, fearful of the consequences of adverse publicity on public trust in the NHS, encouraged surgeons to rely on stashes [20]. Associates of the Navy Tissue Bank, worried by the haphazard and unregulated spread of tissue banking, were responsible for the founding in 1976 of the American Association of Tissue Banks

(AATB). The AATB is a not-for-profit organization committed to ensuring the safety and quality of the supply of human tissue through establishing standards, training, peer review, and accreditation [21]. Membership and adherence to guidelines is voluntary, but the evolution of their standards has become the basis for tissue regulations in the United States and elsewhere.

Fear of cadaver toxin had virtually disappeared. The general rule was to exclude people known to have had an infectious disease, malignancy, or autoimmune disease at the time of death. A history of malaria, syphilis, viral hepatitis, tuberculosis, or death associated with an overdose or poisoning were also grounds for exclusion. However, criteria were rather vague, and there was little in the way of a formal system of oversight. The AATB encouraged the production of safe and usable tissue among its members by tightening up the criteria of donor suitability and establishing standards for training of personnel and adequacy of facilities.

Cultural work

Doctors at the Sklifosovsky Institute, Moscow, were the first to recover cadaver tissue on a significant scale, when, during the 1920s, they began experimenting with transfusions of cadaver blood [22]. The cultural work that confronted them was light. They practiced medicine inside a totalitarian regime, which struggled to protect and prolong human life while simultaneously demonstrating a wanton disregard toward it [23]. The Soviet state under Stalin's dictatorship established a nationwide system of hospitals and clinics where health care was provided free at the point of delivery to all its citizens – who, at the same time, were being murdered or starved to death in millions.

In the United States, between the two World Wars, capital punishment was the principal source of fresh cadaver tissue. R. Townley Paton (1901–1984), a New York ophthalmologist with a flourishing and fashionable private practice, during the 1930s, honed his grafting skills by transplanting onto his patients' eyes corneas recovered from the eyes of men executed in the electric chair in Sing Sing Prison. A priest sought the agreement of the condemned men, Paton witnessed their death, enucleated their eyes, and, if their corneas were not used that day, stored them in his kitchen refrigerator. His son recalled how this method of storage almost led to the loss of the family cook, who was horrified to find containers filled with eyeballs on the shelf next to the milk bottle [24].

Adverse publicity put a stop to Paton treating executed men as a source of corneas (but did not lead to the abolition of the death penalty). Paton, in 1944, opened the Eye-Bank for Sight Restoration, America's first eye bank. The name capitalized on the popularity of blood banks during the war.

But New York state regulators initially refused to incorporate a not-for-profit organization called a bank on the grounds that it might mislead members of the public into thinking it engaged in financial transactions. They acquiesced when Paton agreed to hyphenate its name.

In direct donation, living donors are immediately rewarded by knowing the identity of whom they are helping and how their tissue is used. In the infancy of tissue banking, it took an effort of imagination to conjure up the reasons why during one's life one should pledge parts of one's corpse to strangers. The J. Walter Thompson Advertising Agency, the world's first and then leading advertising agency, advised the Eye-Bank on how to persuade the general public to volunteer. It faced a considerable task: Americans had to be introduced to the radical new idea that their bodies are made up of interchangeable body parts, and that eyes can "outlive" their current "owner" and restore the sight of hitherto blind strangers. The approach it pioneered, and which has been copied many times since, hid the messy thick reality of enucleation behind euphemisms with religious overtones. The Eye-Bank's first promotional leaflet compares eye donation with divine gifts: "God gave man sight at birth, and man now has sight in his gift to give to another" [25]. Put another way, sentiments associated with the "gift of sight" are, like Mother's Day cards and Easter eggs, a marketing innovation, one which encourages donation of tissue without any reference to how or from whom it is typically recovered.

The Eye-Bank provided would-be donors with cards, small enough to fit into a purse or wallet, on which they could record their pledge. Pledge cards, but not Madison Avenue marketing techniques, were adopted by Archibald McIndoe (1900–1960) when he opened the first British eye bank in 1948. McIndoe, a New Zealand–born plastic surgeon, before the Second World War, had built up a thriving and fashionable practice in London's Harley Street. During the war, at the Queen Victoria Hospital, a small cottage hospital in East Grinstead in the southeast corner of England, McIndoe had begun the painful and painstaking plastic reconstruction of the face and hands of "Britain's finest," the young aircrew and ground staff who suffered drastic burns in the war against Nazi Germany. Many lost their eyelids and suffered damage to the cornea. In 1947, a corneal transplant unit was attached to the burns unit, and Benjamin Rycroft (1902–1967), an ophthalmic surgeon, who, before the war, had gained some experience in corneal grafting, was appointed. Rycroft began grafting corneas recovered from the eyes of corpses in the hospital mortuary, but they were few and far between: the most he retrieved was four in one week, and, at that rate, it would have taken him at least three years to clear his waiting list. The problem was people who lived in the hospital's vicinity tended to die in their own beds, where no one thought of retrieving their eyes. What McIndoe called an eye bank was mostly a public relations exercise albeit one couched in medical terms.

Giving and taking

The hospital issued pledge cards with a set of instructions which, among other things, advised that the card had to be held separately from a last will and testament, which is read several days after a death, usually following burial or cremation of the body and certainly too late for corneas to be usable. The scheme, in effect, envisaged "donors" as people who would make appropriate arrangements for the redistribution after their death of personal effects such as money, paintings, and jewelry. It exposed a legal vacuum: eyes pledged for the purpose of grafting fell outside the law on bequests because eyes, like every other part of the human body, are not personal effects and no one can determine what shall happen to them after their death.

East Grinstead lies west of Royal Tunbridge Wells, the spiritual epicenter of middle England. Many of its residents opposed the collective egalitarian principles embodied in the postwar welfare state. They rallied round McIndoe, a seasoned fighter against bureaucracy, and supported his campaign for an amendment to the 19th-century Anatomy Acts, which allowed the donation of corpses to medical schools for teaching and research but did not encompass body parts donated for grafting purposes. Their principal opponents were civil servants in the Ministry of Health fearful that publicity encouraging cadaver eye donation would exacerbate people's fear of hospitals as places where few patients left alive, a fear reputed to be widespread in older people. Nonetheless, McIndoe won. In May 1952, the Corneal Grafting Bill was passed by the House of Commons.

The Corneal Grafting Act allowed people to bequeath their eyes during their lifetime either in writing at any time or during their last illness orally in the presence of two or more witnesses. It was a "donation statute." From the mid-1950s onwards, American states began enacting donation statutes that authorized antemortem pledges of cadaver eyes and other body parts – mostly skin and arteries – for medical purposes. American donation statutes explicitly served an additional purpose: they were designed to protect whoever recovers cadaver tissue from an action for damages by distressed relatives. Next of kin in the United States have a common-law right of possession of the dead body, in the same condition as it was at the time of death, for the purposes of burial or other disposition. This right originated in considerations of love, reverence, domestic relations, and blood ties and is sometimes called a quasi-property right [26], although strictly speaking the human body is not property; also, the right is limited to burial: it does not allow, for example, the next of kin to sell the cadaver, but it does permit them to bring an action for damages for intentional, reckless, or negligent removal of cadaver body parts.

The Uniform Anatomical Gift Act (UAGA) 1968, a landmark in the history of tissue banking, is a donation statute. It was drafted during an era concerned with guaranteeing the civil rights of every American adult and celebrates individual autonomy, that is, the right of every citizen to do with his or her body as he or she sees fit. The dead person has the first and deciding voice as long as his or her intentions have been recorded by means of a pledge written and signed in the presence of two witnesses. The pledge in effect disentangles the corpse from inconvenient ties of love and kinship: next of kin cannot abrogate it. The UAGA also, paradoxically, grants the next of kin the right to authorize a donation where no pledge is found. By 1971, the UAGA had been adopted, usually in a modified form, in every state and the District of Columbia.

The UAGA's exceptional popularity was stimulated by enthusiastic media coverage of improving rates of survival in kidney transplants, which had followed the discovery of powerful drugs for immunosuppression in the early 1960s. Before then, with the one exception where donor and recipient were identical twins, the procedure was fatal and almost never performed. The first time a cadaver kidney was transplanted was in 1962 at the Peter Brent Brigham Hospital, Boston. The British Human Tissue Act 1961 was introduced to fill a legal vacuum in relation to the recovery of arteries, skin, and other grafting material from cadavers. The Act allowed people to pledge one or several parts of their body to be used after their death. In other words, it allowed people to "opt in." It also allowed them to "opt out," but in making no provision for how this might happen, it was almost impossible for anyone who wanted to opt out to do so.

The Human Tissue Act 1961 was only partially a donation statute. The section under which most cadaver material was recovered was the one allowing the person in lawful possession of the body to authorize the removal of body parts if, having made such reasonable enquiry as may be practicable, they had no reason to believe that the deceased in his or her lifetime had expressed any objection to it or that his or her surviving spouse or any surviving relatives objected. In including no sanction or punishment of transgressors, the Act effectively insulated the person lawfully in possession of the body, a legal person, usually a hospital manager, from threat of prosecution.

The Human Tissue Act 1961 promoted an ethos within NHS hospital operating theaters and mortuaries of taking without asking, that is, of treating human tissue as waste freely available as salvage. "Taking statutes" in the United States were organized around medical examiners and coroners' cases, that is, around people who die in unexpected or suspicious circumstances. American law allows the withholding of body parts removed during a postmortem examination that might yield forensic clues, but it did not provide for the recovery of cadaver tissue for therapeutic purposes. An action for damages following taking without agreement of the next of kin might succeed.

Baltimore is usually near the lead in the annual competition for murder capital of the United States. Russell Fisher, the Chief Medical Examiner of

Maryland, was a busy man. He was also a transplant enthusiast eager to add to the public good by assisting the Medical Eye Bank of Maryland (MEB) secure more transplant material [27]. In 1975, Fisher and Frederick N. Griffith, Executive Director of the MEB, persuaded Maryland senators to pass what became known as the "Medical Examiner's Law," a statute which allows a medical examiner to agree to the removal of specified body parts from a corpse within his jurisdiction where no objection from the next of kin is known.

The Act introduced what is sometimes called implied or presumed consent, that is, anyone whose death is brought to the attention of a medical examiner is presumed to have agreed to tissue recovery, unless he or she has registered a refusal or his or her next of kin explicitly disagrees. In practice, the circumstances under which a corpse typically falls into the possession of a medical examiner make it unlikely that his or her next of kin will raise an objection. It is more appropriate to call presumed consent a legislative consent because the statutes provide the state embodied in the legal person of the medical examiner with complete authority to agree to, or refuse to, cooperate with a tissue bank.

The law's treatment of the cadaver as a resource is inconsistent. The United States has resisted efforts to move to legislative consent with respect to solid organ donation precisely because it values the right of citizens, or their families as surrogates, to give such a gift and enjoy the associated moral benefit. Nonetheless, legislative consent statutes were introduced in many states in the 1970s and 1980s but most allowed recovery only of corneas and pituitary glands, then being collected in vast numbers for the extraction of growth and other hormones.

Taking without asking is responsible for some of the scandals that periodically have tarnished the reputation of tissue banks, because it abuses the sensitivities surrounding the corpse during its dangerous liminal stage. It takes advantage of public ignorance. The public outrage following the Lions Doheny Eye & Tissue Transplant Bank scandal revealed how few people associate the medical examiner's office with authority to agree to tissue recovery. Few people associate a hospital postmortem examination with withholding of tissue for therapeutic or research purposes. In November 2000, Robert McNeil summed up the responses he had encountered during his 32-year-long career as a mortuary technician in NHS hospitals:

"There are members of the public who had a very clear idea as to what an autopsy was about and they could speak up for themselves, but in the main the majority of people I believe when a doctor asks can they carry out a post-mortem, the main thing that concerned the relatives would be was it going to cause any delay or can they see the body afterwards, and the answer(s) would be no and yes" [28].

McNeil was commenting on the so-called Alder Hey scandal that followed the discovery in 1999 of a large stash of babies' and children's body parts in the basement of the Royal Liverpool Children's Hospital, known locally – and affectionately – as Alder Hey Children's Hospital [29]. This gruesome news was shortly followed by the revelation that throughout the United Kingdom, it was customary for pathologists to withhold, without asking, body parts removed during a postmortem examination, a practice kept hidden from the public. The material was used mostly in teaching and research and to discourage doctors from "burying their mistakes." But some tissue was also taken for a therapeutic purpose. The British government responded to the public's outrage by setting up a review of the law, which resulted in the passage in 2004 of the Human Tissue Act.

Asking

Official policy nowadays emphasizes asking. Consent is described as the golden thread running through the English Human Tissue Act 2004. In the United States, a succession of policies has spawned a host of professionals trained in asking people confronting difficult and tragic circumstances to consider tissue donation. However, the scandals also suggest that public accounts of what giving means have failed to keep pace with developments in the tissue recovery industry. Put another way, cultural work provides an inadequate account of organizational work and has failed to keep pace with the radical changes it has undergone.

Tissue banks have transformed rare and sometimes desperate acts to save life or restore function into routine unremarkable procedures. However, whereas solid organs and corneas are counted both in and out, there are no reliable or published data on tissue banks' activity. Yet far more people provide tissue than provide organs. Of the estimated 1.2 million people who die in American hospitals each year, 11,000–14,000 of them die in circumstances that allow them to be an eligible organ donor. In contrast, at least 100,000 dead Americans meet the criteria of tissue donation [30]. Indeed, tissue was recovered from around 20,000 American corpses in 1999, a cohort far greater than that of 1994, which numbered around 6,000 [31]. How many British corpses "volunteer" is unrecorded.

Fear of cadaver toxins resurfaced in the 1980s in response to the threat of HIV transmission, which was followed by worries about other old and new infectious diseases such as malaria and variant Creutzfeldt–Jakob disease (vCJD). Risk of transmission is being reduced through the imposition of increasingly stringent criteria of donor eligibility organized around where a potential donor lived, his or her lifestyle, and where and how he or she died. Although criteria vary from country to country, tissue from a British corpse is almost universally unwelcome outside Britain because of the belief it might harbor vCJD. What this means is altruism is no longer the only quality sought in a potential donor, a development which cultural work has not yet addressed.

What was once a cottage industry in the United States has become an industrial complex of often interconnected for-profit and not-for-profit organizations with a turnover in billions of dollars. The scope and size of each American bank varies from small local hospital-based programs providing one kind of tissue to regional or national organizations offering several different ones. In the United Kingdom, stashes have mostly been eliminated by the licensing arrangements imposed by the new Human Tissue Act 2004. A few banks provide one type of tissue such as cornea, bone, and heart valves, and the NHS Blood Service, since the early 1990s, has become the major source of bone, skin, and tendons and also provides heart valves.

Processing allows Medawar's laws of transplantation to be circumvented. It can make tissue that might otherwise be rejected into a universally acceptable product. The range of "products" has significantly increased, and diversification in the industry has substantially altered the profile of the typical recipient. The series of articles published in April 2000 in the *Orange County Register* revealed that tissue donated in response to requests emphasizing life-threatening situations, such as a drastic burn, could be diverted into frivolous applications such as puffing up the lips of fashion models or enlarging penises. Each corpse can provide as many as 50–100 "products," which means that hundreds and thousands of people are on the receiving end of them. Yet few are aware that their treatment originated in the mortuary.

People may feel cadavers are defiled when they discover they have been transformed into "off-the-shelf" products, sold at high cost through catalogs and by sales representatives. Processing has widened the gulf separating donor and recipient that characterizes the indirect method. However, advances in processing methods have also increased the usefulness of tissues and the safety of tissue transplantation. Imaginative and responsible cultural work is needed in order to ensure that beneficial developments are facilitated in an open and transparent way without exploitation of donors or donor families. It is crucial to remember that organizational work and cultural work are interdependent and that a tarnished reputation in one has repercussions in terms of public trust in the whole enterprise.

Acknowledgements

I would like to thank The Wellcome Trust for providing research leave award GR066454MA, which allowed me to undertake the extensive research on this project. Grateful thanks to the many people on both sides of the Atlantic who allowed me to look into their filing cabinets and who answered numerous questions.

References

1. Brown JB. Homografting of skin: with report of success in identical twins. Surgery. 1937;1:558–63.
2. Gillies H. Corneal transplantation of an opaque cornea. Proceedings of the Royal Society of Medicine, xxvii, 60 (Sect. Ophthal.). 1933. p. 603.
3. Tudor Thomas JW. Corneal transplantation of an opaque cornea. Proceedings of the Royal Society of Medicine, xxvii, 60 (Sect. Ophthal.). 1933. p. 597–605.
4. Schneider WH. Blood transfusion between the wars. J Hist Med Allied Sci. 2003;58:87–224.
5. Starr D. Blood: An Epic History of Medicine and Commerce. London: Little, Brown and Company; 1990. p. 70–1.
6. Hedges SJ. Tissue imports pose hazards. Chicago Tribune, May 22, 2002. p. 10. The Sklifosovsky Institute came to the attention of the American public in 2000 when the Chicago Tribune revealed that Valery Khvatov, a doctor working in the Institute, was selling bones from Russian cadavers to US tissue banks. The tissue had been taken without permission and proved hazardous.
7. Doughman DJ. Tissue storage. In: Krachmer JH, Mannis MJ, Holland EJ, editors. Cornea: Fundamentals of Cornea and External Disease, Volume 1. St. Louis, MO: Mosby; 1997. p. 509–17.
8. Filatov V. My Path in Science. Moscow: Foreign Languages Publishing House; 1957. p. 27.
9. Hockey J. Changing death rituals. In: Hockey J, Katz J, Small N, editors. Grief, Mourning and Death Ritual. Buckingham: Open University Press; 2001. p. 185–211.
10. I am indebted to the insights in Healy K. Last Best Gifts: Altruism and the Market for Human Blood and Organs. Chicago: The University of Chicago Press; 2006.
11. Brown JB, McDowell F. Massive repairs of burns with thick split-skin grafts. Ann Surg. 1942;155:658–74.
12. Hogle LF. Standardization across non-standard domains: the case of organ procurement. Sci Technol Human Values. 1995;20(4):482–500.
13. Strong MD. The US Navy Tissue Bank: 50 years on the cutting edge. Cell Tissue Bank. 2000;1(1):9–16.
14. Strong WR. The tissue bank, its operation and management. In: Wolstenholme GEW, Cameron MP, editors. Preservation and Transplantation of Normal Tissues. London: J & A Churchill; 1954. p. 220–33.
15. Eldad A. War burns: the blow and the cure. Clin Dermatol. 2002;20:388–95.
16. Scarry E. The Body in Pain: The Making and Unmaking of the World. Oxford: Oxford University Press; 1985.
17. Medawar P. Memoirs of a Thinking Radish. Oxford: Oxford University Press; 1988.
18. Flosdorf EW. Freeze-drying: Drying by Sublimation. New York, NY: Reinhold Publishing Corporation; 1949.
19. Kirn TF. Tissue banking in midst of "revolution of expansion" as more uses are found for various transplants. JAMA. 1987;258(3):302–4.

20. Kearney JN. Yorkshire regional tissue bank – Circa 50 years of tissue banking. Cell and Tissue Banking. 2006;7:259–64. The Yorkshire Regional Tissue Bank is one of the exceptions.
21. Joyce MJ. American Association of Tissue Banks: a historical reflection upon entering the 21st century. Cell Tissue Bank. 2000;1(11):5–8.
22. Starr, D. op cit:5:65–9.
23. Field MG. Soviet medicine. In: Cooter R, Pickstone J, editors. Medicine in the 20th Century. London: Harwood Academic Publishers; 2001. p. 51.
24. Paton D. The founder of the first eye bank: R. Townley Paton, MD. Refract Corneal Surg. 1991;7:190–4.
25. Pfeffer N. Insider Trading. London: Yale University Press; (forthcoming).
26. The concept of "quasi-property" is controversial. Some authorities claim it is a device for avoiding the difficult questions raised by rights in the human body. See for example, Jaffe ES. "She's got Bette Davis['s] eyes": assessing the nonconsensual removal of cadaver organs under the takings and due process clauses. Columbia Law Rev, 1990;90:note 106. Nonetheless, it is widely used to account for the rights of next of kin over a cadaver.
27. Fuller RL. Medical legal issues. In: Krachmer JH, Mannis MJ, Holland EJ, editors. Cornea: Fundamentals of Cornea and External Disease, Volume 2. St. Louis, MO: Mosby; 1997. p. 537–41.
28. McNeil R. Evidence before the review group on the retention of organs at postmortem. 2000. http://www.sehd.scot.nhs.uk/scotorgrev/Documents/final%20auto psy%20technician% (accessed December 20, 2004).
29. Redfern M. The Royal Liverpool Children's Inquiry: Report. London: The Stationery Office; 2001.
30. Anderson MW, Schapiro R. From donor to recipient: the pathway and business of donated tissues. In: Youngner SJ, Anderson MW, Schapiro R, editors. Transplanting Human Tissue: Ethics, Policy, and Practice. Oxford: Oxford University Press; 2004. p. 7.
31. Youngner SJ, Anderson MW, Schapiro R. In: Youngner SJ, Anderson MW, Schapiro R, editors. Transplanting Human Tissue: Ethics, Policy, and Practice. Oxford: Oxford University Press; 2004. p. xi.

2 Recruitment for Tissue Donation

Martha W. Anderson[1] and Esteve Trias[2]

[1] Musculoskeletal Transplant Foundation, Edison, New Jersey, USA
[2] Processing Facilities, Transplant Services Foundation, Barcelona, Spain

Introduction

Tissue donation depends on the development of a strong working relationship between a tissue bank and a hospital or other donor referral agency. There are different operational models that can be explored to achieve the most successful program in a given service area. Two seemingly opposite approaches can both provide positive results, which may point to differences in a society's view of donation for transplantation. When considering implementation of tissue donor recruitment in a region, this chapter should be helpful by offering results and valuable experiences from successful programs.

A particularly successful example of collaboration in the United States between a tissue bank and a hospital is in Michigan, where Gift of Life Michigan (GOLM), the statewide organ and tissue procurement organization, recovers tissue from approximately 900 tissue donors each year. GOLM instituted its tissue donor program in 1987, recovering fewer than 50 donors that year. Programs associated with Gift of Life's donor program include the establishment of organ and tissue donation (OTD) committees in all major hospitals. The OTD committees are composed of physicians, administrators, nurses, chaplains, and social workers; the committees develop hospital protocols for donation and evaluate donor potential and performance of organ procurement organizations (OPOs) and hospital staff involved with donation.

CASE 1

Designated requestor

Gift of Life, like many OPOs and tissue banks in the United States, provides

---

Tissue and Cell Donation: An Essential Guide. Edited by Ruth M. Warwick, Deirdre Fehily, Scott A. Brubaker, Ted Eastlund. © 2009 Blackwell Publishing, ISBN: 978-14051-6322-4.

"designated requestor" training for hospital staff responsible for obtaining informed consent from donor families. However, despite providing in-depth and regular (at least once yearly) education on the donation and consent process, Gift of Life has found (as have many other US OPOs, tissue banks, and eye banks) that hospital staff consent rates fall far below the consent rates obtained by their own personnel. For example, a key hospital with broad support of tissue and organ donation experienced a consent rate of 9% compared with 45% when consent interviews were undertaken by the OPO staff [1].

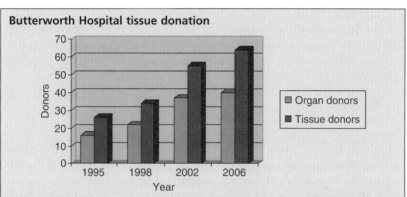

Butterworth Hospital tissue donation

Donation activity increased over time because of several programs including:

1 connecting the need for allograft tissue with the need for donor referrals;
2 federal regulations that require the referral of all hospital deaths to the OPO (Conditions of Participation);
3 implementation of a donation committee and medical record reviews to evaluate the performance of death referrals (98% are referred in a timely fashion);
4 training of designated requestors who obtain consent from the next of kin (NOK);
5 increase in OPO hospital development staff;
6 commitment to the national organ donation goals established by the Breakthrough Collaborative for Organ Donation, which establishes organ donation as a priority for hospital administration and staff [2].

Organized by the U.S. Health Services and Resources Administration (HRSA), the Organ Donation Breakthrough Collaborative brings together donation professionals and hospital leaders to identify and share best practices to integrate organ donation into the hospital's end-of-life continuum of care. Staff from HRSA and the OPOs help participating hospitals identify, adapt, test and implement practices essential to an effective and family-centered donation program. It resulted in an increase of 3,905 more organs being transplanted in 2007 compared to 2003. [© European Communities 1995–2008]

CASE 2

Intrahospital team

The Spanish donation model has resulted in one of the highest organ donation rates per million population across the world. It is based on a transplant coordination unit, or more hospital units, with hospital staff, physicians, and nurses responsible for donor detection, consent, screening, and selection. The hospital-supported team is in charge of OTD, and the specific training they receive results in consent success rates of over 80% for organ donation and between 60% and 70% for tissue donation.

The Spanish model has been applied successfully by other European countries, such as Italy, with improvements in their OTD rates. Professionalism, availability, training, and knowledge of their own hospital have been highlighted as the keys for success in this donation model.

Tissue donation and transplantation occur in most parts of the world, although the recovery of tissues from deceased donors varies. Tissue recovered from living donors ("surgical discard tissue") is a by-product of a medical procedure such as total joint replacement, amputation (e.g. femoral head, distal femur), or childbirth (amnion). While the use of surgical discard tissue is prevalent in many parts of the world, it is limited by the quality and quantity of tissue available. Although skin grafts may be recovered from an unburned portion of a burn patient's body, major burns must be treated with large amounts of donated tissues; skin retrieved from deceased donors is routinely used in these instances. Limb-salvage surgery, tendon replacement, abdominal wall repair, heart defect repair, and corneal transplant require tissue recovered from recently deceased donors. Donated tissues and cells are being increasingly subjected to tissue engineering and prepared in different ways for a wide variety of clinical uses. Both the number and diversity of anatomic parts that can be implanted and the application of processing, preservation, and storage is increasing every year. Tissues donated by a single donor can be grafted into more than 80 different recipients.

Tissue donation from deceased (formerly called cadaveric) donors typically includes the following types of tissues:

1 musculoskeletal: bones, tendons, and ligaments of the upper and lower extremities, pelvis/iliac crest, ribs, meniscus, fascia;
2 cardiovascular: heart valves, blood vessels, pericardium;
3 skin: split thickness (typically, only the epidermis) and full thickness (epidermis and dermis);
4 ocular: corneas, sclera.

Donation for research, either all or part of a body being donated for medical education and research, is a relatively new donation option in many parts of the world, including the United States. This type of donation may occur in conjunction with donation for transplant, or the patient's entire body may be donated. Uses for this type of donation include the following: education of medical and nursing students; development of medical devices and instrumentation; training in surgical techniques; and development of new therapeutic interventions for diseases such as pulmonary fibrosis, diabetes, and Alzheimer's (www.iiam.org). The donation of adult stem cells occurs much less frequently than other types of donation. Adult stem cells may be obtained from the bone marrow (which contains hemopoietic stem cells) from iliac crests and vertebral bodies of deceased donors, as well as from the umbilical cord blood directly following the delivery of a new baby (see Chapter 11).

Keys to a successful tissue program

Tissue donor programs are perhaps most well-organized in the United States and parts of western Europe; the common characteristics of a successful tissue donor program include:

1 governmental regulations or laws that permit and/or encourage donation;
2 public awareness of both organ *and* tissue donation, which results in a willingness to donate and/or to register the intention to donate;
3 systems that facilitate the referral of potential tissue donors – identification, routine medical chart reviews in every case of in-hospital death;
4 adequate training of professionals involved in the identification and referral of potential tissue donors;
5 collaborative relationships among the tissue bank, medical professionals, and people in other disciplines who may be involved with a recently deceased person.

We will present the legislative structures and public policies that guide and govern tissue donation – a worldview of how donation after death is organized, referral processes, the importance of public awareness of tissue donation, opportunities and challenges associated with establishing a tissue donor recruitment program, and the critical role medical professionals play in establishing a well-functioning tissue donation program. In most cases, organizational, legal, and public policy initiatives were developed for organ donation and subsequently applied to tissue donation. In some areas of the world, a common legislative act must be applied in different countries; this is the case for the regulatory framework of human tissue procurement and banking in Europe (Directive 2004/23/EC, Directive 2006/17/EC, and 2006/86/EC). These directives not only focus on quality and safety measures, but also highlight the need to ensure fair and unpaid donation systems and the need to ensure that adequate information is provided to the general public in order to increase their willingness to donate.

Excerpts from Directive 2004/23/EC of the European Parliament and of the Council (March 31, 2004) [3,4,5]

Article 4

Implementation

1 Member States shall designate the competent authority or authorities responsible for implementing the requirements of this Directive.

2 This Directive shall not prevent a Member State from maintaining or introducing more stringent protective measures, provided that they comply with the provisions of the Treaty. In particular, a Member State may introduce requirements for voluntary unpaid donation, which include the prohibition or restriction of imports of human tissues and cells, to ensure a high level of health protection, provided that the conditions of the Treaty are met.

....

(5) It is necessary to promote information and awareness campaigns at national and European level on the donation of tissues, cells and organs based on the theme "we are all potential donors". The aim of these campaigns should be to help European citizens decide to become donors during their lifetime and let their families or legal representatives know their wishes. As there is a need to ensure the availability of tissues and cells for medical treatments, Member States should promote the donation of tissues and cells, including haematopoietic progenitors, of high quality and safety, thereby also increasing self-sufficiency in the Community.

....

(18) As a matter of principle, tissue and cell application programmes should be founded on the philosophy of voluntary and unpaid donation, anonymity of both donor and recipient, altruism of the donor and solidarity between donor and recipient. Member States are urged to take steps to encourage a strong public and non-profit sector involvement in the provision of tissue and cell application services and the related research and development.

....

(19) Voluntary and unpaid tissue and cell donations are a factor which may contribute to high safety standards for tissues and cells and therefore to the protection of human health.

....

(27) Personnel directly involved in the donation, procurement, testing, processing, preservation, storage and distribution of human tissues and cells should be appropriately qualified and provided with timely and relevant training. The provisions laid down in this Directive as regards training should be applicable without prejudice to existing Community legislation on the recognition of professional qualifications.

Finally, we will discuss the interconnection between organ procurement and tissue procurement agencies. Our remarks will be restricted to donation after death; where the term "tissue" is used, it refers to bone, connective tissues, heart valves, corneas and skin.

Public policies

Systems and laws that control and/or facilitate the donation of organs and tissues are widely established throughout the world; they govern the determination of death (including determination of brain death), mechanisms for granting, refusing, or revoking consent for donation, and allocation rules for donated organs and possibly tissues. They may also address financial issues, including whether financial reimbursement or consideration may be exchanged (from a recipient to a donor, from a tissue recovery establishment to a donor hospital, from a recipient to a tissue bank, etc.) (see Table 2.1).

Presumed consent, in either weak or strong versions, exists in much of Europe, including Spain, France, Austria, Belgium, Poland, Slovakia, Portugal, and Italy. The absence of a registered objection (in a will, on a donor registry, or on a donor card) permits donation to occur in these countries. Within the presumed consent model are the opt-in and opt-out systems. In the "opt-out" system (the most common), individuals are required to register their desire *not* to be a donor; otherwise, they are considered to be a donor. In countries with "opt-in" systems, individuals are given the opportunity to register their intent, desire, or consent to donate; and in the absence of an explicit and expressed decision, the default is donation, rather than nondonation. Regardless of laws and policies for presumed consent, it still remains usual practice to consult the family and to allow a family to override an individual's stated preference for or against donation.

Explicit consent (also known as informed consent) requires the explicit authorization of a donor to donate his or her organs and tissues (or the authorization by a legal designee following the donor's death). It is practiced in countries including the United States, the United Kingdom, Canada, Ireland, Germany, and Australia. In countries with explicit consent laws (also known as "first-person consent" and "donor designation"), donor recruitment activities receive significant attention and allocation of resources. Donor registries or donor cards may be used to establish an individual's intent or consent to donate. In some parts of the United States, donor family members are still given the authority to decline donation despite a previously registered intent or consent to donate, although the Uniform Anatomical Gift Act of 2006 removes that capability as does the recently revised legislation in the United Kingdom (http://www.hta.gov.uk/guidance.cfm).

Table 2.1 Regulatory frameworks for donation after death

Country	Legislation	Year	Impact on practice
Argentina	Presumed consent Law 26.066 (modification of the Law 24.193, 1983)	2005	Mandatory referral of brain dead donors.
Australia	Informed consent	Individual state/territorial legislation for donation	No mandatory referrals. Homicide victims not released by coroner for donation; coroner may decline consent in other instances. "Human Tissue Acts" allow for removal of tissues during autopsies without consent, but not typically invoked.
Australia	National Code of Ethical Practice	2002	Outlines need for consent from deceased or next of kin (NOK).
Australia (Western Australia – WA)	Coronial legislation		Allows for referral of all potential donors irrespective of donor registry status.
Bangladesh	Tissue Donation and Transplantation Act	1999	Permits tissue donation from both living and deceased donors. Applied in addition to existing fatwas.
Belgium	Presumed consent	1986	Individuals may register consent or refusal to donate.
Brazil	National Transplantation Law No. 9434/97 incorporating amendments introduced by Law No. 10211 of March 23, 2001	1997	Establishes National Transplant Coordination System to govern transplantation of organs and tissues. Allowed for presumed consent (opt-out). Amended in 1997 to explicit consent.
Brazil	Portarias (ruling on donation)	1998	Establishes retrieval and transplantation teams; requires authorization by the Ministry of Health. Requires the notification of brain dead donors.
Canada	Provincial/Territorial Human Tissue Gift Acts (13)		Precludes exchange of funds for tissue recovery or transplantation. Establishes hierarchy for providing informed consent.

Location	Legislation/Code	Date	Consent/Notes
Canada – British Columbia and New Brunswick	Routine referral		Primarily used for organ donor referrals in British Columbia, as tissue donation is not actively pursued.
Canada – Ontario	Trillium Gift of Life Act	January 2006	Routine notification and request to Gift of Life Trillium Network for organ, tissue, and eye donation evaluation. First-person consent is binding.
Chile	Sanctuary Code referring to good use of tissues or parts of body of a living donor, and the use of cadavers for scientific or therapeutic purposes, which should be provided free of costs		Requires consent from donor NOK.
China	Written consent required	Law July 1, 2006. Human Organ Transplant Regulation on April 6, 2007	Requires consent.
Cuba	Public Health Law	1983	Requires consent from donor. Donors must be over 18. Permission of the family is always required.
England	Code of Practice	July 4, 2006	Establishes specific protocols for consent, donation of organs, tissues, and cells, and recovery and screening requirement. No requirement for referral of potential donors.
England	Explicit consent/first-person consent		Individuals may register consent through the National Health Service Organ Donor Register. First-person consent system precludes family members from overruling the decision.
European Union (EU)	EU Commission Directive 2004-23-EC Commission Directive 2006/17/EC February 8, 2006. Annex IV on donation and procurement procedures, including consent	2004	Establishes requirement to follow national legislation for consent, requires providing "appropriate information" in order to make a decision. Precludes advertising the need for or availability of tissues.

continued p. 26

Table 2.1 *Continued*

Country	Legislation	Year	Impact on practice
France	Presumed consent Loi n° 2004-800 du 6 août 2004 relative à la bioéthique Loi n° 94-654 du 29 juillet 1994	1994	Opt-out – may register an objection, but cannot register as a donor. Presumed consent is not strictly applied, as family members must be interviewed as to potential donor's desires. Strong recommendation for referral of all potential donors. Police/justice administrators may deny recovery.
Germany	Explicit consent	1997	May register consent and objection via donor card.
Hong Kong	Human Transplantation Ordinance Human Organ Transplant Act 1992	1977 1992	An opt-in law requiring consent from the donor or NOK.
India	Transplantation of Human Organs Act	1994	Not yet adopted by many Indian states. Regulates organ donation only; no legal framework for tissue donation as yet.
Indonesia	The Indonesia Health Regulation	1992	Allows tissue procurement from living donors only but not from deceased donors.
	Fatwa for bone, skin, and amnion	June 29, 1997	Passed by the Religious Council permitting tissues to be procured from deceased donors.
Iran	Act of Deceased or Brain Dead Patient Organ Transplantation	2000	Applies to organ donation. The will of the deceased can be approved by written notice of an heir apparent. If the original will is not available, a Ministry of Health consent can be signed by informed heirs.
Italy	Presumed consent	Law No. 91 of April 1, 1999	May register consent and objection. Discussion with family occurs. Families are consulted before extraction.
Japan	Law Concerning Human Organ Transplants Law N° 104	1997	For organs: brain death donation authorized under explicit consent; non-heart-beating donation authorized under presumed consent. For tissues: explicit consent legislated, but consent is always required from the relatives.

Korea	Organ Transplantation Law	2000	Covers organs and tissues. Donor consent required but family has strong veto.
Malaysia	The Human Tissues Act	1974	Act permits the removal of tissues from cadavers for therapeutic, medical education, and research purposes. Requires expressed consent from the donor given at any time in writing or stated verbally during the deceased's last illness in the presence of two witnesses and the consent of the NOK.
	Fatwa on bone, skin, and amnion	September 4, 1995	Passed by the Malaysian Islamic Centre; these were the first fatwas for tissue donation.
Mexico	General Law of Health Reform	2004	Explicit consent for donation in life. Presumed consent for organs and tissues but requires consent from families if donor did not reject donation.
Netherlands	Explicit Consent Law 24	1996	Opting in (explicit consent) – registration is required. At age 18, all citizens are asked to register "yes," "no," "I allow my NOK to decide," "I allow another to decide."
Netherlands	Organ Donor Law ("Wet op de organdonatie – WOD")		Required referral of potential organ or tissue donor to the organ center as determined by treating physician. National donor registry allows four options: yes, no, I leave the decision to NOK, I leave the decision to a specific designated person. In the event of a "yes," NOK cannot officially overturn that decision, although it is the practice to accommodate family wishes. Coroners/medical examiners do not have the formal capacity to deny tissue recovery.
Peru	Law No. 23415 "Transplant of Organs and Tissues of Cadavers and Transplant of Organs and Tissues of a Living Person"	1982	Every tissue and organ of a cadaver can be used for prolongation of human life. It requires consent from donor or NOK.
Philippines	The Republic Act 7170	1991	Organ donation requires explicit consent. No specific law for tissues.

continued p. 28

Table 2.1 *Continued*

Country	Legislation	Year	Impact on practice
Singapore	Medical (Therapy, Education, and Research) Act	1972	Any person of sound mind and 18 years of age or above may give all or any part of his body for education transplantation. The gift takes effect upon death (opting in).
	Human Organ Transplant Act	1987 and amended in 1994	Opting out for organ donation but also covers corneas. Muslims and over-60s are excluded.
Spain	Presumed Consent Law 30/1979	1979	Presumed consent is not strictly applied. In practice, organs are removed only with the consent of families.
	Royal Decree 2070/1999 (organs) Royal Decree 1301/2006 (tissues)		Police/justice administrators may deny recovery.
Sri Lanka	The Human Tissue Transplantation Act No. 48	1987	Consent is required from the donor or the NOK.
United States	Uniform Anatomic Gift Act	1986	Defines who may make an anatomic gift. Includes tissues in definition of organ.
United States	Uniform Anatomic Gift Act	2007	Further defines who may make or revoke an anatomic gift. Establishes "first-person consent," which precludes NOK from refusing authorization for donation.
United States	Conditions of Participation	1997	Routine referral of *all* hospital deaths to OPO or OPO designee. Mandates hospital participation in donation.
United States	National Organ Transplant Act	1986	Precludes OPOs and tissue banks from selling body parts but allows reasonable compensation for activities involved with donation, processing, and distribution.
United States	Medical Examiner Laws – presumed consent	Various	Allows recovery of corneas without family consent if there is no known objection (mostly inactive).
Vietnam	The Human Organ, Tissue Transplantation Act	2006 (effective on July 1, 2007)	Consent needed from the donor or the NOK.

In some states in the United States with first-person consent, a family may not override an individual's registered intent to become a donor, but this does not preclude a family from agreeing to donate organs and tissues when there is no stated preference. In other words, in the United States, a "yes" cannot be overruled, but a family may make the decision in the presence of an "I don't know" or "I don't want to decide," or when there is no documentation found. In these circumstances, family members are informed of the patient's previous declaration that he or she is a donor, and they can be asked to confirm that the patient had not revoked that document of gift. Regardless of which consent model (presumed or explicit) a country follows, mechanisms for referring potential tissue donors must also be established and are likely to be the most important predictor for a successful tissue donation program. (Information on consent is provided in Chapter 4.)

Primary systems of tissue referral and recovery
1 routine recovery;
2 required request;
3 voluntary referral;
4 routine referral.

Routine recovery

Routine recovery "presupposes that the state or society has a right of access to the organs of deceased individuals" [6]. In a limited number of states in the United States, medical examiners are permitted to remove corneas from bodies that come under their authority to determine the cause of death. In Australia, this right was also granted to coroners under the "Human Tissue Acts" and "Transplantation and Anatomy Acts;" coroners could allow the recovery of tissues from individuals undergoing autopsy without the need to consult the NOK. These laws do not require expressed consent, nor do they require opting in or out of donation. Although still allowed in the United States and Australia, these laws are rarely applied in practice because of the need to obtain medical and behavioral information from knowledgeable persons, who are often also the NOK. Prior to the HIV and hepatitis epidemics of the 1980s and 1990s, this practice resulted in huge increases in cornea donation; as reported in the Institute of Medicine report, corneal transplants in Georgia (United States) increased from 25 in 1978 to more than 1,000 in 1984.

Required request

Required request was implemented in the United States in 1986 and is in effect in other countries, including the Netherlands. This process requires that hospitals have a system to: (a) identify potential donors; (b) approach potential donor families regarding OTD; and (c) refer donors for whom consent has been given to the appropriate recovery agent. This system was intended to eliminate the possibility that hospital and/or medical staff would fail to give potential donor families the opportunity to donate. While many hospital staff are supportive of donation and adept at presenting donation options to recently bereaved family members, other hospital staff who are not knowledgeable about, are unsupportive of, or are uncomfortable with donation may still be expected to present the option of donation to a newly bereaved relative. Likewise, the system often provided opportunities for patients with complicated medical histories to be "ruled out" as being unsuitable for donation. It permitted hospital staff to make judgements as to which families are "appropriate" to approach for consent, or to rule out potential donor families whom they identify as being "too upset" to consider donation. It was not uncommon for a family to be told, "By law, I have to ask you if you want your loved one to be an organ and tissue donor. You aren't interested are you?" Not surprisingly, required request did not result in an increase in organ and tissue donors in the United States.

Voluntary referral

Voluntary referral is the most common type of donor referral system, the least standardized, and, in the authors' view, the least fruitful. It is associated with minimal tissue usage, negligible (or nonexistent) financial reimbursement for the costs associated with tissue recovery and processing, and marginally staffed tissue banks. Tissue donors may be referred only from selected hospitals or from the hospital where the tissue bank is located. In general, organ donors are the only patients considered for tissue donation. In a region with minimal tissue needs, this system is adequate. Few activities to increase donation rates (e.g. public awareness or professional educational activities) are undertaken by the tissue bank. This is the most prevalent system in many small hospital-based UK tissue banks where much of the costs of tissue recovery is absorbed into general hospital costs. However, the model of referral varies in the United Kingdom; in the English National Health Service Tissue Services, a routine referral model is used in designated hospitals as described next.

Routine referral

In routine referral, all deaths (typically hospital deaths) are required to be referred to a donation agency, regardless of the age of the patient, the cause of death, whether the patient was registered as a donor, or whether the family is willing to consider donation. Begun in the United States in 1998, it resulted in the annual referral of over 1.2 million hospital deaths. Although the anticipated increase in organ donors was lower than expected (7.5% increase between 1995 and 1999), routine referral resulted in a large increase of tissues and corneas recovered in the United States. The American Association of Tissue Banks (AATB) reported an increase of 65% during that same time frame. The Eye Bank Association of America (EBAA) (www .restoresight.org) reported a 10% increase; however, during that same time period, some eye banks narrowed their age criteria because they had sufficient tissue to meet patient needs, so these data should not be seen as evidence of poor outcome of routine referral.

CASE 3

Routine referral

Routine referral has also been implemented in parts of Canada (British Columbia, Ontario, and New Brunswick). In these provinces, all deaths are reported to a central referral service, with the focus on maximizing potential organ donors. Because tissue recovery programs are not well developed in these provinces, patients with no potential for organ or cornea donation are typically deferred. In Ontario, routine notification and request was instituted in 2006. Its impact on musculoskeletal tissue donation has yet to be realized, but the Trillium Gift of Life Network reported a 153% increase (from 2,554 to 6,453) in referrals and a 93% increase (from 436 to 843) in cornea donations in the first year of its implementation [7].

Routine referral has pros and cons: on the positive side, it provides every potential donor family the opportunity to donate, eliminates the need for hospital staff to determine donor suitability, and standardizes the donor referral system. It dramatically increased tissue availability in the United States and elsewhere. On the negative side, it added huge costs to the organ and tissue procurement field (estimates are upwards of $30 million per year for communication centers, training, and education of hospital staff); it frustrated hospital staff who were required to report all deaths, even those with clearly no potential for donation (e.g. extremely elderly patients, patients with HIV and hepatitis, etc.); and it increased workload for hospital staff who were required to provide extensive medical information on a larger number of potential donors.

Referral sources

Tissue donors may be referred from a variety of sources; hospitals, medical examiners, coroners, and forensic institutes are the most common sources, although funeral homes, emergency medical services, and law enforcement agencies may also provide referrals (see Chapter 9). Potential donor families may initiate the donation conversation, typically at or around the time of a family member's death. In parts of the United States, funeral home recovery programs became more active in the 1990s and into the 2000s, as demand for tissue increased and as funeral home operators identified new ways to increase revenue. This type of program increased the amount of tissue available to some tissue banks, but it is felt by many to have been a system ripe for misuse and abuse. This concern came to fruition in 2005 and 2006, when Biomedical Tissue Services and Donor Recovery Services, two independently run tissue banks, were found to have falsified medical information and/or consents on bodies referred to them by funeral homes. This resulted in some jurisdictions proposing regulations precluding funeral home recoveries (New York State Proposed Guidelines 2007); others increased penalties for falsifying tissue donor information (New Jersey 2007). AATB has responded with numerous changes to its standards to prevent any kind of recurrence of fraudulent acquisition of tissues. Finally the perpetrators of these crimes received lengthy prison sentences.

In the United States, approximately 90% of all recovered-tissue donors are referred through hospitals and approximately 2% by medical examiner's and coroner's offices. The remainder comes from funeral homes or other sources (some data for referral locations were unspecified) [8]. Tissue procurement organizations in the United States focus their greatest efforts on improving hospital donation programs ("hospital development"), although many also have a medical examiner and coroner liaison and/or a funeral home liaison charged with improving communication systems with those individuals and agencies. In European Member States with high donation rates, such as Spain and Italy, it is reported that 99% of tissue donations come from hospital sources, and funeral homes account for very few [9–13]. Funeral homes have a role in donation, without involvement of any revenue, and help the tissue bank solely because of the social benefit that donation implies. It has been suggested that a higher level of safety can be achieved when no economic interest is involved in the detection and selection of potential donors.

Donation stakeholders – Blockers and supporters

There are a variety of stakeholders, and they can function as either active supporters or blockers of a tissue donor program. It is of paramount importance that the tissue bank recognize the role these parties play, be cognizant of the challenges tissue donation presents to them, and develop collaborative and communicative relationships with them. The key stakeholders and their challenges are given in Table 2.2.

Although there are many challenges posed by these parties, there are also many positive opportunities that a relationship with the tissue bank can

Table 2.2 Challenges posed to key tissue donation stakeholders

Person/entity involved	Potential challenges
Public	Unwilling to face death as something that will happen in the future; discomfort or lack of knowledge associated with tissue donation and transplantation
Potential donor family	Grief, lack of understanding about donation, negative attitudes toward medical profession (either preexisting attitude or as a result of problems with hospitalization prior to family member's death)
Hospital staff: RN, MD, ancillary staff	Death of patient; workload from other (living) patients; discomfort or lack of knowledge about the donation system; time required to refer and/or screen potential donor; need for hospital bed for other incoming patients
Organ transplant team	Concern that tissue consent will impact on organ consent (unproven); lack of knowledge about tissue donation
Medical examiner, coroner, or forensic investigator	Potential impact on death investigation (loss of evidence, interruption of chain of custody of body, delay in performing autopsy) (see Chapter 9, Facilitating Donation – The Role of Key Stakeholders: The medical examiner, the coroner, the hospital pathologist, and the funeral director)
Funeral director	Difficulty in preparing body for funeral services, increased time and cost; delay in scheduling funeral services (see Chapter 9)
Law enforcement	Concern over potential (unproven) impact on investigation

present (Table 2.3). Opportunities for collaboration between the tissue bank and related stakeholders abound. The typical collaboration is between a tissue bank and hospital, and generally includes:

- written agreement or memorandum of understanding in which the responsibilities of each party are outlined; hospital responsibilities could include referring potential donors, providing medical screening information, and making operating rooms or mortuaries available for recovery; tissue bank responsibilities include prompt response to referrals, financial reimbursement for supplies, staff, etc., used during tissue recovery, providing education to hospital staff related to donation, and commitments to provide allografts to the hospital; responsibilities for obtaining informed consent would also be outlined (use of hospital staff or the tissue bank staff);
- regular interaction between the tissue bank and the hospital staff, including in-service training of relevant hospital employees on subjects including donor acceptance and rejection criteria and uses of allograft tissue, consent training, and review of medical records used to evaluate the donor during the referral process;
- staff follow-up after each donor or after a particularly challenging case.

Table 2.3 The key stakeholders of a tissue donor program and the potential opportunities

Person/entity involved	Potential opportunities
Public	Learn about tissue donation prior to the death of self or family member; make an informed decision about donation long before one is needed. As a positive message before death, the public can also learn about the success of transplantation and the needs of and benefits to recipients
Potential donor family	Honor loved one's wishes to be a donor; know that a part of the family member "lives on;" gain some control after a sudden death when little is within the family's control
Hospital staff: RN, MD, ancillary staff	Support donor and donor family wishes; extend care to family after knowing there is no hope for the patient; increase availability of tissue for future patients
Organ transplant team	Expand the number of potential donor families reached; maximize donation opportunities for organ donors; collaborate in donor development and public awareness activities
Medical examiner, coroner, or forensic investigator	Obtain tissue and blood samples from the tissue recovery team for investigation; receive cardiac pathology reports on heart valve donors; extend support to families; support local needs for transplantable tissues
Funeral director	Extend support to bereaved families; social recognition of their work
Law enforcement	Extend support to bereaved families

In 2001, the American Nurses Association strongly supported a collaborative relationship between professional nurses and organ/tissue procurement teams. As an example of this type of collaboration, the New York State Nurses Association (NYSNA) formally stated that nurses should:

- acquire necessary knowledge and skills to be able to work cooperatively with the tissue bank;
- serve as a resource to colleagues, patients, and their families by providing information about donation and participating in educational programs and activities, including public awareness;
- be knowledgeable about ethics, cultural, religious, and social issues regarding donation [14].

CASE 4

Highway patrol referral programs

An award-winning example of nontraditional tissue donation collaboration is the Donor Referral Program developed by the Northwest Tissue Center in Seattle,

Washington, and the Washington State Patrol (WSP). The brainchild of WSP Detective Steve Stockwell, it allows WSP officers to contact the tissue center's donation referral line for each fatal motor vehicle accident. The program started in 2003 and, within 12 months, resulted in 22 donors (13 tissue donors and 20 cornea donors). Because traffic fatalities are not normally transported to a hospital, those donors would not have been referred to the tissue bank; approximately 28% of all referrals were registered donors. This program ensures that an individual's desire (or his or her family members') to donate is not dependent on dying in a hospital. The program has since been expanded to other states in the United States, including Oregon, California, Wyoming, Colorado, and New York.

Positive working relationships between tissue bank personnel and funeral professionals are critical – a funeral director can easily impede donation by embalming the body before a family can be contacted regarding donation; he or she can discourage a family from considering donation, or can cause a family to question their decision to donate by disparaging the tissue donation process. Alternatively, a funeral director can offer donation opportunities to bereaved families, allow donation to occur in the funeral home, and actively support a family's decision to donate by including donation information in obituaries and displays during the funeral (see Chapter 9).

CASE 5

"Lasting Legacies"

A particularly effective collaboration between OPO/tissue bank and funeral homes is "Lasting Legacies," a family support program developed by LifeLine of Ohio in Columbus, Ohio. The program includes:

1 a framed remembrance displayed at the funeral home during calling hours;
2 green ribbon lapel pins provided to the donor's immediate family;

3 green ribbons provided to the donor's additional family and friends; the ribbons are attached to a small card, which has a donation message, helping to raise awareness;
4 a brochure display stand filled with general donation educational displays;
5 obituary acknowledgement;
6 remittance envelopes for monetary donations in a loved one's memory.

Newspaper announcements

Increasingly, family members are choosing to publicize their loved one's donation by including information about the donation in newspaper obituaries. This practice has a collateral benefit, in that it provides an additional way to educate the public about organ, eye, and tissue donation. Examples of phrases used in obituaries include:

In keeping with Mr. Smith's loving and generous spirit, it was his decision to donate life so that others may live.

Mr. Smith gave in death as he gave in life; he was an organ/tissue donor.

Mr. Smith gave the gift of life through organ/tissue donation.

Local newspapers may be willing to include an illustration or donation logo in obituaries at no cost to the family. Examples of those illustrations include the "Donate Life" logo and the Circle of Life promoted by the Global Organization for Organ Donation.

It is clear that initiatives such as these will work well only where the culture in the country accepts or expects such public announcements. It is difficult to imagine obituaries explicitly referring to donation in some European countries like Spain or Italy, where a family's decision to donate is considered an intimacy and the society expects anonymity between donors and recipients. In some cases, contact between donor family and recipients is not permitted by law.

Public awareness and support for tissue donation

Public support for OTD varies from country to country, but for the most part is overwhelmingly positive. Concerns about donation are common as well. A 2006 German study found that 90% were in favor of organ donation and that 21% had signed an organ donor card. Concerns raised regarding donation in this study included fears regarding determination of death, removal of organs prior to death, and the fairness of organ allocation [15]. A study commissioned by the Canadian Council for Donation and Transplantation (CCDT) in 2005 found that 96% of Canadians strongly (71%) or somewhat (25%) approved of OTD, that 54% had signed an organ donor card, and that 17% had registered in their provincial registry. Reasons for not donating included the presence of a medical condition that precluded donation, religious beliefs, age, or a desire to keep one's body intact at death [16].

A 2005 poll carried out for the US Department of Health and Human Services found that 95% supported (54.9%) or strongly supported (40.5%) OTD, and that 53% had indicated their desire to donate on an organ donor card or driver's license. Given the diversity of the US population, this study also focused on variables including gender, age, race, and ethnicity. Women are more strongly supportive of donation than men (43.2% versus 36.8%); individuals between the ages of 35 and 54 are more strongly supportive (46.5%) than those in the older (33.1%) or younger (40.8%) groups. Although all racial groups were overall supportive of donation (e.g. strongly support or support), Whites and Asians are more strongly supportive than Blacks or Latinos (42.9% for Whites, 41.0% for Asians, 28.7% for Blacks, and 36.3% for Latinos) [17]. These results point to the need for continued education and outreach to those communities that are less likely to donate.

Promotion of tissue banking to the public

The promotion of tissue banking to the public is increasingly important as agencies attempt to increase donor registrations, to increase public support for tissue donation, and to increase tissue donation. While the public's knowledge of cornea and organ donation is high in most places in the world, awareness of tissue donation and transplantation lags behind. In a survey of 4,500 Americans conducted by the Coalition on Donation (now Donate Life America), 98% had heard of organ donation, while 86% had heard of tissue donation (which included cornea donation) [18]. While 83% would be likely or somewhat likely to donate kidneys, 73% would be willing to donate skin and 12% would be unlikely to do so. Thirty-two percent reported being more comfortable with donating organs than tissue. Presumably, one solution to this situation is education, both of the general public and of healthcare professionals (HCPs) who can be in a position to discuss tissue donation with potential donor families.

Organizations such as Donate Life America, the CCDT in Canada, Australians Donate in Australia and New Zealand, and UK Transplant in the United Kingdom (now part of NHSBT) have developed public awareness campaigns designed to increase the awareness of OTD, and to encourage people to register as donors. Promotional activities include the following: the development of public service announcements and advertising for use on the television, on radio, and in print; brochures, posters, and videos about donation; race/ethnicity-specific advertising; use of celebrities as spokespeople; workplace partnerships; government-sponsored education; fund raisers;

walkathons; and the production of television shows (either fictional or documentary) that present donation in a positive light.

The Internet presents a huge opportunity to educate the public about donation and to allow individuals to register their desire to become an organ and tissue donor. The CCDT survey found that 52% of respondents would go to the Internet for information about donation [18]. An Internet search using the words "organ and tissue donation" resulted in close to one million websites, which were aimed at increasing awareness of OTD. While many are targeted to organ donation, others are equally focused on tissue and cornea donation and transplantation. They include www.organtransplants. org, www.transweb.org, and www.donatelife.net.

Some activities may be nationally organized such as Australia's Organ Donor Awareness Week – this program (www.australiansdonate.org.au) encourages Australians to register to become organ and tissue donors through various activities, including workplace education. In the United States, the month of April is designated as "National Donate Life Month," and donation and transplant organizations participate in activities as varied as walkathons, donor family recognition ceremonies, and health fairs at which donation information is provided. Donate Life America's efforts include general public campaigns as well as those targeted to specific minority communities, most notably the Hispanic and African-American communities.

The International Atomic Energy Agency (IAEA) assisted many countries with the development of tissue banks during the 1990s and into the mid-2000s. One key document developed by the IAEA is "Public Awareness Strategies for Tissue Banks" (June 2002). It includes information about the development of a communications strategy, identifying target audiences and messages for those particular audiences, public awareness activities, dealing with the media, and crisis management. Suggested key messages include the importance of tissue transplants to community health, safety of tissue transplants, focus on compassionate care for the donor family, ethical tissue bank practices, and technical aspects of tissue donation.

One of the major challenges to increasing public awareness of tissue donation is overcoming fears and myths associated with donation and transplant. While some myths are more associated with organ donation (e.g. the kidnapped traveler who wakes up in a hotel room missing a kidney), others are more generally applicable to tissue donation as well.

Fears and myths about tissue donation

1 Registered donors receive poor medical care so that their organs and tissues can be removed (18% agreed with this statement in the Coalition on Donation survey) [20].

2 The transplant system is unfair (e.g. wealthy individuals receive transplants more than poor people) (30% agreed with this statement).

> **3** Donation results in disfigurement.
> **4** Donation is against a particular religion.
> **5** Cancer can be transmitted through tissue transplants.

Education, proactive positive media placements, and the Internet can all be useful in combating these fears and myths, but vigilance and perseverance are required.

Role of HCPs

Hospital staff play an integral role in the donation process; this role is complex and may be the cause of conflict with the tissue procurement agency. From the time of the patient's admission in the hospital, the entire focus is on treatment, patient recovery, and discharge [19]. They may develop relationships with the patient and his or her family during the course of hospitalization – especially in the intensive care unit (ICU), where emotional levels for both family and HCP may run high. When a patient dies, the HCP is asked to change focus away from saving the life of the patient to focusing on the potential treatment of an unknown or unidentified recipient who could benefit from the organs, tissues, and eyes of the deceased.

The connection between a potential donor family's willingness to consider donation of a family member's organs and tissues and their overall hospitalization experience has been noted: families who were more satisfied with the care their loved one received, with the communication they had with medical staff, and who felt the medical staff cared about the family, were more likely to donate. Nondonor family members reported inadequate or insensitive care, as well as concerns with how the request for donation was made [19,20]. Therefore, insuring that hospital staff are aware of their impact on donation potential is important.

Donation-related roles filled by hospital personnel (bedside nurses, attending physicians, and ancillary support staff such as social workers or chaplains) include:

1 providing aftercare for the donor family; providing medical screening information to the tissue bank;
2 obtaining consent from the donor family;
3 preparing the body for donation (placing the body in a refrigerated place, insuring corneas are moist).

Operating room staff may also participate in the recovery process, depending on the hospital and tissue banking protocols.

No matter how positively inclined an HCP may be toward tissue donation, there are issues that may be raised by medical personnel as well as funeral directors and medical examiners that need to be addressed by the tissue bank.

There are opportunities for a tissue bank to build a true collaborative system with HCPs in order to establish, expand, or maintain a highly functioning tissue donor program. Regardless of whether a tissue bank receives donor referrals from a hospital or medical examiner's and coroner's offices, the key components of a successful donor program must include those described in the following box.

Key components of a successful donor program

Champion(s) or influencers. These individuals take tissue donation on as a cause. Although having a champion such as a physician or nurse who serves as the in-house "cheerleader," the tissue bank cannot totally depend on the enthusiasm of one person to build and then sustain a tissue referral program.

Institution-wide support for tissue donation. Support from all levels within a hospital, from administration to physicians, nurses, social workers, chaplaincy, finance, and medical records, is vital. This has been referred to as "top down, bottom up, and sideways buy-in" by the US Organ Donation Breakthrough Collaborative.

Institutional policies and procedures. Policies and procedures that delineate responsibilities and roles of all involved are required. These include referral procedures (who is to be referred as a potential donor, who should make the referral, when the referral should be made), consent policies (who is responsible for discussing donation with the family), notification of the medical examiner, coroner, and funeral home, care of the body, use of the operating room for recovery, etc.

Established performance goals. Goals (e.g. for referral rates, consent rates, conversion rates, etc.) should be set for individual units in a hospital (e.g. emergency department, ICU) or for the whole hospital.

Medical record reviews. The tissue bank should use medical record reviews to (a) determine which hospitals should receive the greatest attention from the tissue bank and (b) monitor ongoing death referral rates. No tissue bank has unlimited resources, either in terms of time, personnel, or funding – each organization must allocate resources in such a way as to maximize potential opportunities. Referral sources with high potential should receive more service, attention, education, etc., than those with little to no potential.

Performance monitoring. The tissue bank and hospital should agree which performance metrics are to be evaluated, and then establish a regular reporting system (monthly, quarterly, annually) process. Donor referral data, regular medical record reviews, etc., can be used.

Feedback. Feedback can take a variety of forms, including debriefing after each tissue donation (especially in a hospital that is new to tissue donation) and providing regular reports of tissue donors from that institution. It can also be helpful to provide reports of local tissue use, reinforcing the need for tissue donors in order to meet the needs of patients. It is vital that the tissue bank ask the hospital for comments, constructive criticism, and advice – how the tissue bank can work more effectively with hospital staff, streamline the process, minimize disruption, etc.

Recognition. Many tissue banks send a thank you letter to staff involved with a tissue donation; others hold annual nursing recognition events, bestow awards for those hospitals that improved the most, provided the largest number of donors, etc. Pens, pins, and other promotional items are cost-effective ways of saying thank you, although they should not be considered as an alternative to education, data, communication, or the development of strong relationships between the tissue bank and referral source.

Education for HCPs

Much has been written about the correlation between the HCPs' knowledge of donation and their comfort level with approaching a family for consent to donate organs. While the great majority of HCPs are positively inclined toward donation (88% in Italy [21], 92% in Spain [22], 89% in Denmark [23], and 99% in Canada [24]), studies indicate that those hospitals with low levels of knowledge about donation have similarly low levels of donation rates [25]. A vast number of studies in countries from the United States to Germany to Italy to India to Hong Kong show that although support for donation is high, actual knowledge about the donation process is low – all of these studies postulate that increasing knowledge will result in higher rates of donation, even more so than improving the public's awareness of OTD.

Educational programs can include special conferences on tissue donation and transplantation, new employee orientation, in-service seminars on topics including donor criteria, tissue transplantation, grief, consent, etc. As hospitals struggle with staffing shortages, the availability of staff for lengthy in-service training days may be limited. Internet-based training (e.g. NYSNA's e-learning program "Think, Care, Act: the Role of the Nurse in Organ and Tissue Donation" is an excellent example) and short, targeted learning tools (e.g. elevator posters) can also be useful. DVDs and CD-ROMs have been developed by many organizations (e.g. Nicholas Green Foundation's "Never Forget, Never Forgotten" video). Continuing education for nurses and physicians is mandatory in some countries or regions, and the tissue bank can often provide approved continuing education credit. Donor family and recipient stories and/or speakers are often the most motivational part of any educational program.

The Australian Medical Association has released its "Doctors and Organ Donation" brochure aimed at general practitioners, raising the issue of organ donation with patients and encouraging two key messages to be passed on to patients: "talk to your family" and "registering is about your decision, not your medical suitability." In addition to the information brochure, Australians Donate has assisted the Royal Australian College of General Practitioners to develop an online module of 25 multiple-choice questions on OTD for transplantation.

In the European Union, the Health and Consumer Protection Directorate General is currently working toward a new project to develop a European Training Program on Organ Donation. In addition, the Information Society Directorate General is supporting the creation of a European online registry on organs, cells, and tissues through the European Registry for Organs, Cells and Tissues (EUROCET) project (https://www.ec.europa.eu/information_society.org/eurocet/).

Donor registries

Donor registries are now common in most countries, regardless of whether the countries have presumed consent or explicit consent systems (see Table 2.4). They are often linked to driver's license bureaus or are managed through governmental agencies such as voter registration or the National Health Service. Organ and tissue donation agencies typically have access to those registries when evaluating a potential donor. Some registries are privately organized, although these are not always linked to OTD agencies. With the spread of the Internet, registries have become more readily accessible. Maintaining confidential information in registries requires the development of secure computer systems.

Table 2.4 Donor registries

Country	Consent system	Registry	Population registered (%)
Australia	Explicit	Yes	26
Austria	Presumed	Only no	0.05
Belgium	Presumed	No and yes	2
Canada*	Explicit	Yes	14
Denmark	Explicit	Yes and no	4.25
France	Presumed	Only no	0.05
Netherlands**	Explicit	Yes, no, other	40
Sweden	Presumed	Yes and no	13
United Kingdom	Explicit	Yes	24
United States	Explicit	Yes	31

Source: Personal correspondence from David Fleming, Donate Life America [26].
*Fourteen percent of citizens from British Columbia are registered.
**The Netherlands registry options are yes, no, I allow my next of kin to decide, and I allow another person (identified) to decide.

In the United States, electronic donor registries have proliferated in the past five years, to a total of 46 in 2008 (up from 14 in 2002). All 50 states (plus the District of Columbia) allow registration as a donor at the driver's license bureau, although access to that information by the OPO, eye, and tissue banks varies. In the United States, it is estimated that approximately 75 million people are registered as donors (31% of citizens between 15 and 80 years old); an initiative to have a total of 100 million people enrolled is being coordinated by Donate Life America.

Donate Life America is a national alliance of geographically organized coalitions dedicated to inspiring all people to save and enhance lives through organ, eye, and tissue donation. Its website functions as a portal for state registries and as a repository of information about organ, tissue, and eye donation in the United States (www.donatelife.net).

In the Netherlands, all citizens are asked on their 18th birthday to register their decision regarding OTD. Unlike most other countries, the Netherlands gives their residents multiple registry options: yes, no, I want my NOK to decide, I want someone else to decide (see Table 2.1). Annually, approximately 38% of those young adults who turn 18 respond to a letter from the Ministry of Health regarding OTD. Of those who have registered (40% of Dutch citizens over age 18), 47.1% have given permission to donate; 9.5% have given permission to donation with some restrictions; 30.8% have refused permission; 10.7% wish to have their NOK decide; 1.8% have asked that a specific person (not the NOK) decide. Most interesting are the restrictions placed on certain organs and tissues, which may point to a lack of understanding or comfort with a particular type of donation (Table 2.5).

Table 2.5 The Netherlands donation restrictions

Skin	61%
Cornea	50%
Bone, tendon, cartilage	32%
Blood vessels	30%
Heart	21%
Heart valves	14%
Kidney	8%

Source: Theo DeBy, BIS Foundation [27].

Collaboration between OPOs and tissue banks

In many parts of the world, tissue banks and OPOs function completely separately, rarely collaborating at all. In these areas, tissue donation often occurs only through the medical examiner's and coroner's offices with very few, if any, donors being identified in hospitals. Reasons for this separation include concerns the organ procurement/transplant teams have (unfounded, in our opinion) that requesting consent for tissue recovery will have a negative impact on organ consent rates, and the OPO staff's discomfort with or lack of knowledge about tissue donation. On the other hand, tissue banks that are not formally affiliated with OPOs often feel that the tissue banks' singular focus on tissue donation allows them to be more effective than an OPO, which is primarily focused on increasing organ donation.

The perception that organ donation and transplant is more important than tissue donation and transplant is rampant, and in many ways is understandable. With the exception of burn patients and pediatric patients with severe congenital heart defects, tissue recipients are not in danger of losing their lives without a transplant, as compared with potential organ recipients who die at alarming rates because of a worldwide shortage of organs. However, this attitude is disrespectful to families who donate tissues and eyes, as well as those who donate for research – their loss is no less painful and their willingness to donate to strangers is no less honorable than that of organ donor families. Even at OPOs that perform both organ and tissue recovery, it is common to hear employees talk about the "organ side" and the "tissue side."

OPO – Tissue Bank Collaboration Options

Collaboration between OPOs and tissue banks may take several forms:

1 consent for tissue donation obtained from the relatives of organ donors;
2 tissue referrals coordinated through the OPO;
3 public awareness activities conducted by or coordinated with the OPO;
4 professional education activities conducted by or coordinated with the OPO;
5 tissue recovery performed by staff of the OPO.

The easiest kind of collaboration between an OPO and tissue bank is for the OPO to obtain consent/authorization for the donation of eye/tissue from the NOK of organ donors. The donor has already been identified and referred; consent has already been obtained, and the donor has been medically screened. The concept of "maximizing donation" (e.g. recovering as many organs and tissues as possible) fits perfectly with recovering tissues (including corneas) from organ donors. In a recent AATB survey of US OPOs with AATB-accredited tissue recovery programs, an average of 36.5% of organ donors were also tissue donors. The range of this reported percentage, collected from 19 OPOs accredited by the AATB, was from 4% to 65%, with a median of 39% [28]. Reasons for this disparity can include strict donor suitability requirements for tissue donation as well as OPO staff perceptions about tissue donation.

Collaborative Public and Professional Education

Working together on public and/or professional education activities is another relatively easy way for OPOs and tissue banks to collaborate:

1 By joining forces and combining resources, more public awareness activities can be conducted.
2 Presenting a unified message about the roles of different procurement organizations can avoid potential confusion.
3 With hospitals limiting time available for HCP education, coordinated professional education efforts are critical and can be an invaluable service.
4 In circumstances where hospital staff are to be educated about donation on a regular basis, presenting one set of protocols, donor criteria, etc., makes it much more likely that the hospital will make its staff available to the procurement organization.

The most complex type of collaboration involves merging the tissue bank and OPO. Such a merger is likely to involve combining governing boards, "rebranding" the organization in order to accurately reflect the activities and mission of the new organization, eliminating redundant jobs (i.e. administrative, financial staff), and developing a new organizational culture that emphasizes the value of all types of donation. Those OPOs that have incorporated tissue recovery into their mission and everyday practice routinely report that the benefits associated with tissue donation have far outstripped their expectations. According to Rob Linderer, Executive Director of the Midwest Transplant Network in Kansas City, Missouri, "Tissue allows us to be in the hospital to talk about any death. When hospitals think about tissue donation, it has a synergistic effect of increasing organ donation" [29]. The number of potential tissue/cornea donors far exceeds that of organ donors (US estimates 15,000 potential organ donors versus 225,000 potential tissue donors per year). Therefore, if an OPO is involved with tissue donation, the OPO is able to interact with hospital personnel more frequently, leading to the development of stronger, deeper relationships.

Benefits of OPO – Tissue Bank Collatoration

1 When an OPO embraces tissue, cornea, and research donation, the philosophy that "donation is donation is donation" becomes pivotal, giving appropriate respect to all donors and their families.
2 Most donors and/or their families state their desire to "be a donor", not to "be an organ donor" – they want to help others and generally make no distinction among tissue, organ, or eye donation.
3 Recovering corneas and tissues from organ donors is one way to expand a tissue recovery program – the donor has already been identified, consent has been obtained, and medical screening has been performed.

4 Collaboration in public and professional awareness activities allows a uniform message and minimizes costly duplicative efforts.

5 Because the public is generally more knowledgeable about organ donation and views the OPO as a "good" entity, affiliations can potentially be positive for the tissue bank – it puts the tissue bank in good company.

6 The OPO is typically seen as the "face of donation," and an affiliation gives the tissue bank increased credibility.

7 Mergers of OPOs, eye, and/or tissue banks can result in vertical integration and financial savings.

8 Recovery of tissues from nonorgan donors is still key, especially in an area with active tissue transplantation practices.

Challenges associated with developing a relationship between an OPO and a tissue bank

1 An OPO's mission requires that it focus primarily on organ donation; a lack of focus on tissue donation can occur, especially when the OPO is short staffed.

2 Adding tissue recovery into an OPO's operations requires a cultural shift that must be driven by senior management throughout the entire organization.

When a single institution manages the process from donation to transplantation: the case of the Clinic Hospital/Transplant Services Foundation in Barcelona (Spain)

At the Clinic Hospital, a university hospital in Barcelona, donation and transplantation are included as priorities in the hospital's strategic plan. A well-trained and experienced donation team works together with a well-designed tissue processing establishment where tissues are processed in state-of-the-art clean rooms. The activity is supported by the central units of the hospital, including testing laboratories, and all types of solid-organ (except lungs) and tissue transplantation are carried out in the hospital. The full process from donation through recovery, processing, and implantation takes place in the same hospital, although the hospital also offers services to other hospitals and institutions. The procurement team works for both organ and tissue donation. More than 90% of organ donors are also multi-tissue donors, although there are also many donors of tissue only. This allows the annual grafting of more than 300 solid organs, the processing of more than 80 different types of tissue from deceased donors, and the distribution of nearly 10,000 units of processed allograft tissues – a reality any region can achieve.

Organ and tissue donors in the Clinic Hospital, Barcelona, Spain

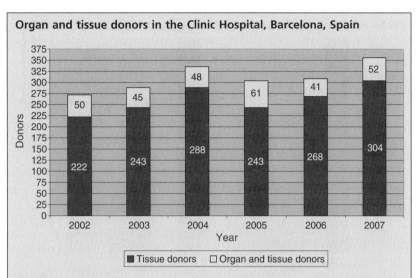

The fact that the full process takes place in the hospital means that there is effective feedback to all units and that the implementation of improvement measures is efficient. Donation teams visit all units where there may be potential donors. When a death is recorded in the Hospital Information System, the donation team is contacted in real time. The clinical chart is reviewed and a preliminary evaluation is performed. Relatives are approached either before leaving the hospital (after their NOK's death) or by telephone in a very short time.

Tissue donation among all deaths in the hospital (excluding organ donors, either encephalic death or donation after cardiac death)

Only 15% of all in-hospital deaths result in a tissue donation. In most cases (70%), a medical contraindication is identified. Between 10% and 12% of all cases are lost as a result of refusal to donate (35% of all interviews). Refusals are more frequent when the donor is over age 65 and when the family is approached by telephone (30–34% versus 42–46%). No differences are noted in relation to the type of tissue (global: 35%; corneas: 35%; bones: 38%; skin: 35%; and cardiovascular: 36%). Main causes for refusal are related to the decision of the deceased while alive and the doubts about body integrity. The model of an integrated hospital team has important advantages in terms of knowledge exchange and smooth interactions among the different units, but most importantly, it gives the possibility of a continuous overview, analysis, and improvement of the processes to support continuous improvement.

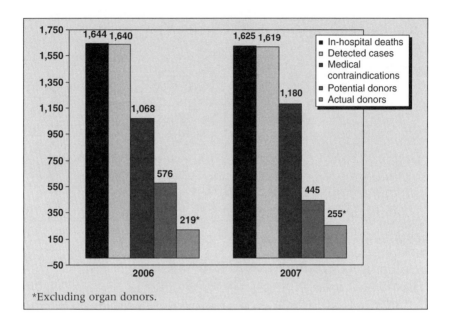

*Excluding organ donors.

Summary

Tissue donation continues to expand in every country of the world. The need for allografts for transplant cannot be met by autografts or surgically discarded tissues. The ability of a tissue bank to meet patient needs requires that multiple efforts be undertaken to increase tissue donation activity. Several classic approaches have proven to have a limited or transient impact on donation rates. A sustained increase requires the implementation of a set of measures, mainly of an organizational nature, such as networks of highly trained and motivated professionals with the main responsibility of developing a proactive donor identification program. The tissue bank, however, does not operate in a vacuum and is dependent on a large number and variety of stakeholders, including the general public, hospital staff, funeral homes, and medical examiners and coroners. Support of donation is significant, which affords each tissue bank the opportunity to build and grow, as long as the needs of those stakeholders are also met. The development of collaborative partnerships and relationships is vital to the success of any tissue donation program, as is insuring that all stakeholders are knowledgeable about the benefits of tissue donation and transplantation.

KEY LEARNING POINTS

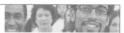

- Tissue donation depends on the development of a strong working relationship between the tissue bank and a hospital or other donor referral entity.

- Common characteristics of a successful tissue donor program include the following: laws that permit and/or encourage donation; public awareness of OTD, which results in a willingness to donate and/or to register the intention to donate; systems that facilitate the referral of potential tissue donors; and collaborative relationships among tissue banks, medical professionals, and people in other disciplines that may be involved with a recently deceased person.

- Primary systems of tissue donor referral and recovery are routine recovery, required request, voluntary referral, and routine referral.

- It is of paramount importance that tissue bank personnel be cognizant of the challenges tissue donation presents to a variety of stakeholders and develop collaborative and communicative relationships with them (e.g. the general public, hospital staff, funeral homes, and medical examiners and coroners).

- The Internet presents a huge opportunity to educate the public about donation and can be useful in combating fears and myths regarding donation in general.

- Insuring that hospital personnel (bedside nurses, attending physicians, and ancillary support staff such as social workers or chaplains) are aware of their impact on donation potential is important.

- Donor families and recipients should be utilized as public speakers because their stories are often the most motivational part of any educational program.

- Donor registries are common and can be used to evaluate public perception about donation and can be used to educate the public and promote recruitment.

- The perception that organ donation and transplantation is more important than tissue donation and transplantation is rampant; however, this attitude is disrespectful to families who donate tissues and eyes, as well as those who donate for research – their loss is no less painful and their willingness to donate to strangers is no less honorable than that of organ donor families.

- Organ transplant organizations and tissue banks should collaborate on public and professional education activities to present a unified message and avoid potential confusion.

- The growing need for tissue grafts for transplant requires that multiple efforts be undertaken to increase tissue donation activity to meet patient needs.

References

1. Personal correspondence from Dennis Rhoda, Gift of Life Michigan, to Martha Anderson, March 12, 2007.
2. Personal correspondence from Joan Bates, Gift of Life Michigan, to Martha Anderson, April 5, 2007.
3. Directive 2004/23/EC of the European Parliament and of the Council of 31 March 2004 on setting standards for quality and safety in the donation, procurement, processing, preservation, storage and distribution of human tissues and cells. Official Journal of the European Union L 102/48 07/04/2004.
4. Commission Directive 2006/17/EC of 8 February 2006 implementing Directive 2004/23/EC of the European Parliament and of the Council as regards certain technical requirements for the donation, procurement and testing of human tissues and cells. Official Journal of the European Union L 38/40 09/02/2006.
5. Commission Directive 2006/86/EC of 24 October 2006 implementing Directive 2004/23/EC of the European Parliament and of the Council as regards traceability requirements, notification of serious adverse reactions and events, and certain technical requirements for the coding, processing, preservation, storage and distribution of human tissues and cells. Official Journal of the European Union L 294/32 25/10/2006.
6. Institute of Medicine (IOM). Childress JF and Liverman CT (Eds), Organ Donation: Opportunities for Action, The National Academies Press, Washington, DC, 2006.
7. Personal correspondence, Lisa MacIsaac, Trillium Gift of Life, and Martha Anderson, March 17, 2007.
8. Personal correspondence from Scott Brubaker, American Association of Tissue Banks, April 15, 2007.
9. Personal communication from Deirdre Fehily Centro Nazionale Trapianti, CNT, Italy http://www.trapianti.ministerosalute.it/cnt/cntDettaglioMenu.jsp?id=58&area= cnt-tessuti&menu=menuPrincipale&sotmenu=istituzioni&label=mti
10. Personal correspondence from Organización Nacional de Trasplantes – ONT, from tissues activity report 2007, and Esteve Trias.
11. Rodríguez-Villar C, Ruiz-Jaramillo, MC, Paredes D, Ruiz A, et al. Telephone consent in tissue donation: Effectiveness and efficiency in post-mortem tissue generation. Transplant Proc. 2007;39:2072–5.
12. Geissler A, Paoli K, Maitrejean C, et al. Rates of potential and actual cornea donation in a general hospital: impact of exhaustive death screening and surrogate phone consent. Transplant Proc. 2004;36:2894.
13. Tandon R, Verma K, Vanathi M, et al. Factors affecting eye donation from post-mortem cases in a tertiary care hospital. Cornea. 2004;23:597.
14. Role of the Registered Professional Nurse in Organ Tissue Donation – Position Statement of the New York State Nurse's Association. www.nysna.org/programs/nai/practice/positions/position10_04.htm (accessed February 1, 2008).
15. Beutel ME. Attitudes towards cadaveric donation – Results from a representative survey of the German population. Z Gastroenterol. 2006 Nov;44(11):1135–40.
16. Canadian Council for Donation and Transplantation. Organ and tissue donation: health professional opinion survey. February 2006.
17. The Gallup Organization, 2005 National Survey of Organ an Tissue Donation Attitudes and Behaviors, www.hrsa.gov

18. Fowler J, Corlett C. Commitment and Compliance as Determinant Factors in Individual Decisions to Donate Organs or Tissues, prepared for the Coalition on Donation, 2004.
19. Study reveals satisfaction with hospital experience major factor in decision to donate. Nephrology News and Issues, June 1998. p. 64–8.
20. DeJong W, Franz HG, Wolfe SM, Nathan H, Payne D, Reitsma W, et al. Requesting organ donation: an interview study of donor and non-donor families. Am J Crit Care. 1998;7(1):13–23.
21. Pugliese MR, Degli Esposti D, Venturoli N, Mayetta Gaito P, Dorian A. Hospital attitude survey on organ donation in the Emilia-Romagna region, Italy. Transplant Int. 2001 Dec;14(6):411–9.
22. Rios A, Consesa C, Ramirez P, Galindo PJ, Rodriguez JM, Rodriguez MM, et al. Attitudes of resident doctors toward different types of organ donation in a Spanish transplant hospital. Transplant Proc. 2006 Apr;38(3):869–74.
23. Bogh L, Madsen M. Attitudes, knowledge and proficiency in relation to organ donation: a questionnaire-based analysis in donor hospitals in northern Denmark. Transplant Proc. 2005;37(8):3256–7.
24. Ibid (see reference 16).
25. Evanisko MJ, Beasley CL, Brigham LE, Capossela C, Cosgrove GR, Light J, et al. Readiness of critical care physicians and nurses to handle requests for organ donation. Am J Crit Care. 1998;7(1):4–12.
26. Personal correspondence from David Fleming, Donate Life America, to Martha Anderson, April 30, 2007.
27. Personal correspondence from Theo DeBy, BIS Foundation, to Martha Anderson, April 3, 2007.
28. Ibid (see reference 6).
29. Anderson M. The History of MTF. Edison: NJ: 2008.

3 The Donor Family Dimension of Tissue and Cell Donation

Robin Cowherd[1] and Jane Pearson[2]
[1] LifeNet Health, Virginia Beach, Virginia, USA
[2] NHS Blood and Transplant, NBS Leeds, Seacroft, Leeds, UK

Introduction

Bereavement and the accompanying mourning are vital coping processes. The painful thoughts and feelings during an acute grief reaction to loss and the subsequent mourning process can, however, be complicated. When approaching a family for consent to donate tissue, transplant professionals must understand the many aspects of an acute grief reaction following a death. By applying their skills and experience, transplant professionals can assist the family's mourning over the subsequent months and years.

This chapter explores the usual and the unusual aftermath of the personal loss felt by family members during and following tissue donation. We attempt to describe how some families have reacted and how tissue procurement organizations can sensitively interact with bereaved families to offer the opportunity to donate, to help the process of grief reconciliation, and, when appropriate, to provide postdonation bereavement support.

The grief process and consent for donation

For most family members, their loss is a life-changing experience, and, in some, it can bring about changes in their religious beliefs, philosophical viewpoints, and the way they look at life. Unusual circumstances surrounding the loss can be so severe that they can lead to intense grief reactions and a prolonged complicated bereavement process (box 1).

Tissue and Cell Donation: An Essential Guide. Edited by Ruth M. Warwick, Deirdre Fehily, Scott A. Brubaker, Ted Eastlund. © 2009 Blackwell Publishing, ISBN: 978-14051-6322-4.

Box 1 Common manifestations of the grief process

1 Shock, numbness, confusion, denial
2 Crying, yelling, screaming, pacing
3 Confusion, bewilderment
4 Bargaining, guilt, remorse, regret
5 Anger, frustration, resentment, blame
6 Depression, despair, disorganization
7 Yearning, searching, philosophical and religious challenge
8 Questioning benevolence of higher being, life's meaning, and religious beliefs
9 Beginnings of acceptance of loss, integration with life, reorganization

---

Donor families have faced the trauma of unexpected deaths as a result of strokes, heart attacks, suicides, homicides, drownings, car accidents, and other accidents. Many deaths are senseless and occur at an early age. Deaths of children are especially difficult because babies are supposed to grow up and outlive their parents, and their deaths are often incomprehensible to their families. In fact, most types of deaths leading to tissue donation are of the types that can lead to complications in the grief process (box 2).

Box 2 Factors complicating the outcome of the grief process

1 Disenfranchised death: difficult to share with others, e.g. homicide, suicide, relationships outside traditional marriage
2 Death of infants and children
3 Violent death: fear, horror when thinking of the final moments of life experienced by loved one
4 Accidental death as a result of carelessness, inattention of family member
5 Death immediately following arguments with the deceased
6 Death of abused or of abusing spouse
7 Preexisting individual or family emotional problems
8 Drug and alcohol dependency of the mourner
9 Lack of available emotional and bereavement support

Donation professionals have to learn to navigate the tense environment of acute grief to obtain a decision about donation that is best for the family. In this environment, the professional must offer support and introduce the offer of tissue donation only if he or she considers that the family member has the capacity to understand the information given.

The act of giving consent and subsequent answering of the long list of questions about the prospective donor's medical and social history may be the first of many times the bereaved gets to review the life of the deceased. Later, memories of the life of the donor will be thought of and reviewed many more times. Although not the subject of many research studies, these initial interactions with the transplant professional and what is triggered about the grief process will have profound effects on some families. Studies have reported that the events surrounding being told of the death of a loved one create some of their most vivid and long-lasting memories. By skillfully facilitating the family's decision to donate or to honor a loved one's previous wish to donate, the transplant professional may be assisting the family with the beginnings of a successful mourning process.

The skilled and sensitive approach to obtain consent

In order to obtain valid and informed consent for donation, professionals must have a conversation with the lawful next of kin. It is a conversation, as opposed to an interview, that must be had because the professional has to skillfully balance the needs of the family for information and support with the needs of the organization, in terms of increasing the donation rate on behalf of waiting recipients. There is an art to conducting successful donation conversations. In the words of Verble and Worth (June 2006) [1], consent is a process, a flow, and not an isolated event. This is true regardless of whether the consent process takes place in a face-to-face setting or over the telephone.

There are reports that both telephone and face-to-face communications are effective in medical care. Advances in information and communication technologies are revolutionizing healthcare delivery by transforming relationships between patients and health professionals [2]. A similar impact might be expected in the relationship between a potential donor family and the tissue procurement organization. Conducting medical care by telephone, or telecare, has been successfully used to deliver psychotherapy to women with postpartum depression, to enable the elderly to remain in their own homes with dignity and independence, and to provide a variety of telephone interventions to mental health patients, preventing situations that may otherwise lead to a hospital admission [3–5]. If the telephone can be used as a method of care delivery in these situations, its use in obtaining consent for tissue donation can also be appropriate. Although there may be some limitations to telecare, it can offer increased, rapid access to specialists and services in a cost-effective manner, with locations of the care provider and the patient no longer limiting the quality of care delivered.

CASE 1

The consent process undertaken by telephone

Kevin Green, in the eyes of his mother Elizabeth, was quite literally "simply the best," and this was the song she had played at his funeral. Kevin's car left the road, hitting a tree, fatally injuring him. There was no one for his mother to blame. It was a tragic twist of fate, which changed her life forever. The same police officer that broke the news of her son's death to Elizabeth also referred her to a team of specialist nurses to discuss the options of tissue donation. Kevin donated his eyes, bone, tendons, heart valves, and skin. This decision was easy for Elizabeth because she knew that Kevin had carried a donor card since he was nine years of age. Still, the conversation about donation was far from easy for her. Elizabeth became a champion for tissue donation and often helped raise public awareness of the need for donors.

Many months after her initial conversation about donation, during which she helped compile a picture of Kevin's medical and social history, Elizabeth explained why the conversation had been difficult for her. She explained that the fact that Kevin was dead became real to her after she had identified him in the mortuary. Kevin died at 2:30 pm on a Sunday afternoon and Elizabeth spoke with the tissue bank the following Monday mid-morning. As she was listening to the information about donation, her mind was still racing. As she tried to listen, she felt an incredible urge to pace, from room to room, from sitting to standing, from house to garden.

When asked how she felt about the conversation and whether it would have been better to have spoken with Sarah (the nurse) face to face, Elizabeth felt that it would have been too traumatic not only for her but also potentially for Sarah. Elizabeth reasoned that with no one looking at her, she could pace, sit, stand, or lie down; she did not feel self-conscious. When she went to the mortuary in the hospital to see Kevin at about 7:00 pm that Sunday evening she was tired and extremely emotional. She subsequently spent about an hour in the chapel of rest and would not have wanted anyone to interrupt at that time. When she had said goodbye to Kevin, she wanted to go home, to the place that would remind her of his life. A face-to-face conversation in her home would have made her feel like she had to be a hostess, and that would have been intolerable for her and embarrassing for Sarah. Elizabeth felt the telephone offered distance as a form of protection for her and yet she still felt cared about and supported throughout.

The experiences of Elizabeth are not unique. Rodrigue et al [6] studied the tissue donation experience, comparing families who became donor families with those families who did not choose donation. Both groups were asked about donation over the telephone and they found that most donor and nondonor families viewed requestors as caring and compassionate. This suggests that the requestors were able to communicate sensitivity and understanding in the absence of a face-to-face interaction. A later study [7] concluded that although the process is inherently stressful and difficult, most families felt the approach was sensitive. They felt they were given adequate time to make the decision to donate, and an approach by telephone was acceptable.

Donation conversations are particularly successful when the family views the conversation as a part of the end-of-life care. Achieving this takes skill, and donation conversations should be undertaken by specially trained professionals who are comfortable with the subject matter and whose practice can be peer reviewed within a competency framework.

As the need for tissue for transplantation increases, donation rates must adequately meet demand, and tissue banks need to invest heavily in donor referral and identification systems. Another need of tissue banks is to improve the consent process as a way of increasing donor rates. Improving the consent process not only can increase donor numbers but also can ensure that families have a positive experience, whether they refuse or give consent to donation.

To improve consent rates, we need to understand why some families give consent and others do not. Table 3.1 includes the observations of the chapter authors on this issue.

Studies have been published about improving the consent process and communicating with the donor family [8–10]. However, the most common reason for giving consent is that it was the known wish of the deceased. Most families want to respect the wishes of the deceased and their willingness to give consent brings them close, one more time. Dodd-McCue et al [11] found that apprehension within tissue procurement organizations surrounding the strict honoring of the deceased's wish (donor designation

Table 3.1 Reasons for giving or refusing consent

Reasons for giving consent	Reasons for refusing consent
He always said he would be a donor.	He has been through enough.
He always carried his donor card.	It is not what he would have wanted.
His sister died of heart failure; he would have given her his heart if he could have.	I do not know what his wish was.
He was always generous in life – help anyone; he would not want to be any different now he is dead.	It might hurt him.
My friend's daughter needs a transplant; we know only too well how much these patients need donors.	His body will not be buried complete.
Our son died 10 years ago and he could not be a donor; that upset my wife very much; she would be pleased that she can be.	Donation does not fit with our religious beliefs.
I want to stop other people from suffering like I have – something positive should come out of this.	I do not want him to have any scars; people will want to see him in the funeral home and I do not want him to look any different.
Why bury or cremate things that will save other people's lives?	He will need his eyes to see where he is going.

or first-person consent) in terms of the potential for ill effects on the donor family were unfounded. In their study, within the state of Virginia, the majority of families found information about the donor's wish helpful, and less than 10% of families studied found the approach stressful or both stressful and helpful. In other countries, donor designation laws are already in place, the difference is in how strictly they are enforced.

Recent legislation in the United Kingdom does not give the family a legal right to interfere with carrying out the deceased's consent to donate that was made in life, but Codes of Practice issued by the competent authority have given professionals an opt-out if it is perceived that to proceed with the deceased's wish, in the face of strong opposition, would cause undue distress to the family. This approach is common across Europe. For instance, Belgium has had presumed consent laws in place for almost 20 years yet families' final wishes are respected, and refusal rates run at about 15% [12].

Other approaches to consent have been widely described and debated, e.g. mandated choice, which requires citizens to decide and record their decision, not merely to opt out. Whether consent is obtained by donor designation, presumed consent, or mandated choice is perhaps less important than the responsibility of the procurement organization to ensure that the public has the opportunity to consider donation. It is clear that from a family perspective, making the decision to donate is easier when the wishes of the deceased are known. Using specially trained and sensitive professionals to make the approach will certainly ease the anxieties of families and allow a sensible risk-based approach to be taken on a case-by-case basis.

Communicating information to donor families about tissue donation: how much is enough?

The amount of information made available to donors in life and donor families after the death of a loved one about the risks, purposes, benefits, and process of tissue donation varies with the type of consent being provided. What constitutes an appropriate amount of information required by a family for consent occupies the thoughts of transplant professionals on a regular basis. And quite rightly, providing information prior to obtaining consent is at the heart of donation and should always be the fundamental principle of the legal and ethical recovery of tissues from the deceased. But what do families think is enough information?

CASE 2

How much information should donor families receive?

Albert felt strongly that when his wife and soul mate Edith died, her wishes should simply be respected and we should just do whatever was necessary for Edith to donate whatever tissue she could. Albert listened intently to the information about the potential uses of the tissue in terms of potential recipient benefit, and he also went through all the options for use in research. Edith was able to donate her eyes. Albert had no problem giving consent for them to be used in research conducted in the health service, universities, or the commercial sector. He also understood that if for any reason the eyes could not be used for any of the purposes for which he had given consent, the tissue bank would not be able to return Edith's eye tissue and instead it would be disposed of consistent with health regulations.

However, Albert did not want to know how they would be recovered, and at this point in the conversation, Albert said he could not continue if he had to listen to anything to do with this aspect. The professional who was talking with Albert felt very uncomfortable about proceeding with the donation of eyes when Albert was not willing to listen to any information about how they would be donated or about the appearance of Edith following the donation. As a compromise, Edith's daughter agreed to listen to the information about the operation and the donation proceeded.

In this case the outcomes were successful for all parties. In terms of the tissue bank, the eyes were recovered and made available to patients. Edith's wishes were fulfilled, and Albert did not have to listen to information he did not want to hear. The outcomes would not have been as good if he had not had his daughter present. This case illustrates that a full description of donation-related information is not appropriate for all families (also see case 3).

CASE 3

How much information should a donor family receive?

After dropping her children off at school and returning home, Stacey opened her front door to find two policemen there. Her husband, Mark, age 45, had been killed in a car crash. During her conversation about donation, Stacey felt she had no choice but to listen to all of the information about which tissue could be donated, the potential uses of those tissues, and how they would be recovered. About six weeks after the death of her husband, Stacey wrote to the tissue bank and accused them of being cruel. Her point was that she should not have had to listen to the details of how the tissue would be donated. The reason she got through the conversation and still said "yes" was that she knew it was what Mark wanted to do and she did not want to let him down. What she had been left with were terrible visions of what he had been subjected to during the surgical recovery of the donated tissue. Stacey further pointed out that as she already knew that she would not want to see Mark again after the donation, he would have a sealed coffin, and there was absolutely no value or benefit in her knowing the details of the donation operation.

In this case, the needs of Stacey and the actions of the donation professional did not match, and harm was done to Stacey. Professional views on these difficult questions are often polarized. One opinion is to only give what information the family actually asks for and the other is that the family must be told absolutely everything: which tissue will be donated, a description of the donation procedure including reconstruction, potential uses of tissue in both clinical practice and research, the method of discard, and the potential need for follow-up in the light of confirmed positive blood tests. These two "extreme" views miss the fact that the family has probably not heard of tissue donation before this event and so does not know what questions to ask. Professionals cannot have the luxury of having "got consent" but in doing so perhaps having caused harm to the donor family and risked converting an interest in donation into a refusal.

Agitation, frustration, and irritability observed in a family member while receiving consent-related information may signal unwanted stressful information and a need for respite and reconsideration as to how much information is needed and wanted. Perhaps the commonsense solution to this dilemma lies somewhere in the middle. Professionals need to decide how much information a reasonable person would want to know, and they need to apply individual judgement as to how much information each family requires.

Deciding what information should be given to a family requires the donation professional to use an evidence-based approach to information giving. Part of the evidence for this conversation should be the concerns that have been expressed by families during donation conversations. The literature is full of these. Verble and Worth [13] described a "ladder of information" that should be used in the donation conversation and offer a sound structure for the conversation that covers opening the conversation, describing the benefits of donation, the right not to donate, the implications of consent, including the funeral arrangements, the disclosure of news about the donation procedure itself, and answering questions. Using this approach, it is possible to standardize the donation conversation in a way that safely allows the professional to provide an individual service and not make any assumptions about what the family needs in terms of information.

General bereavement support

Improved health care and increased life expectancy in developed countries has brought about challenges in bereavement care. Today, many people live into their 50s and 60s without experiencing the death of a close loved one. These changes are positive for the society as a whole; however, when one eventually suffers the death of a loved one, particularly the sudden, unexpected deaths such as those of many prospective tissue donors, there may be few previous grief and loss experiences on which to rely at the time of this most painful life event. Adding to this challenge is the prevalent societal philosophy of denying the inevitability of death and awareness of the need to mourn. Outside of the hospice environment, death education is simply not made available to the public or many healthcare providers.

Tens of thousands of bereaved families every year agree to support the donation of a loved one's tissue and entrust organizations with the recovery of the tissue. Many within the profession believe that the recovery organization should invest in extending this stewardship responsibility to the provision of some level of bereavement support for that family.

Throughout the world where tissue donation programs are more comprehensive, the identification of responsibility for the care and support of individuals grieving the death of a loved one is unclear. Even in cases where there is death without donation, there is no clear delineation of societal responsibility to support bereaved persons. In England, hospitals most often lead the effort of making comprehensive bereavement care available. In Australia, hospital social workers have accepted leadership for donor family advocacy and initial bereavement intervention [14].

In the United States, bereavement care is not coordinated or comprehensive, and healthcare organizations have assumed a limited role in the development of much needed bereavement support programs. Healthcare facilities, hospice programs, the funeral profession, the faith community, and the military community have, to varying degrees, committed resources to some form of follow-up care for grieving family members but rarely in a comprehensive, long-term format. Tissue procurement organizations can have a positive impact by helping to meet the needs for bereavement support.

Research in the field of grief and loss can identify what type of support may be helpful for bereaved persons. Raelynn Maloney and Alan D. Wolfelt [15] wrote of six reconciliation needs of the mourner, which many bereavement specialists find beneficial for organizing support programs. These needs are (a) acknowledging the reality of the death; (b) embracing the pain of the loss; (c) remembering the person who died; (d) developing a new self-identity; (e) searching for meaning; and (f) activating a support system for years after the death. Tissue procurement organizations can consider structuring bereavement support programs for tissue donor families around these needs. Since levels of resources vary among organizations, support efforts can be categorized as basic and comprehensive.

Suggested basic bereavement support services

1 A dedicated staff position to support donor family follow-up is recommended for developing effective donor family care. While the procurement organization's consent coordinators' work with families may be exceptional, the nature of their work might not allow them sufficient time to build a comprehensive system of follow-up support.

2 A basic correspondence program that provides incremental, regular contacts with families. Each correspondence would typically include a letter addressing generic circumstances that may be occurring in the life of the family at various intervals following the death of the loved one. Significant aspects of the follow-up care mailings may include:

- grief literature addressing general information needs such as the uniqueness of grief, how to make birthdays and holidays meaningful, and dealing with sudden, unexpected death;
- written confirmation, upon request of the donor family, of information concerning the distribution and uses of allograft tissue;
- listings of local and regional grief support groups with accurate contact information;
- a survey questionnaire of the donor family's donation experience may be offered; the survey will help identify the donor family's questions and concerns and provide a "risk and quality management tool" for the procurement organization;
- an anniversary card might be sent at the first anniversary of the loss.

3 An annual or periodic donor remembrance event to which the families of donors are invited is considered a standard means of honoring donor families.

4 Programs that encourage tissue transplant recipients to write notes or letters of gratitude to the donor family are gaining popularity across the United States. Donor families report that such letters are helpful in finding meaning and remembering their loved one.

Suggested comprehensive bereavement support services

1 All donor families might receive a quarterly newsletter that chronicles donor family stories, displays letters from transplant recipients, and other items of interest.

2 A telephone call might be made to the donor family in the first few months following the death. The purpose of the call is simply to inquire how the family is getting along and to ask for specific ways in which the procurement organization may be of assistance.

3 Procurement organizations may serve geographically dispersed donor families through an online bereavement support group or through referrals or links to similar online resources available on the Internet. The shared experience helps curb the sense of isolation and promotes healing.

4 Donor family members may benefit from speaking with individuals who have experienced a similar loss. The procurement organization may wish to develop a means of assigning capable and interested donor family members to the newly bereaved.

CASE 4

The transformative effect of donation helps families help others

Maria Diaz at 19 years of age had accomplished much in her short life. As she returned to the University of Virginia for her second year, she and her parents were excited about all the opportunities before her. Less than one hour after leaving home, her car crashed, and Maria's death changed her mother and father forever.

Al and Susie Diaz, Maria's father and mother, followed Maria on the highway that fateful day. Al knew of Maria's wish to be a donor, and, even in the midst of tragic confusion, he asked the police officer on the scene to help contact someone who could make this happen. Within 24 hours, Maria became a donor of bone, related soft tissue, fascia, and pericardium. Al and Susie's only expectation of the donation was that the tissue procurement organization carry out Maria's wish.

Susie Diaz requested information about the distribution of her daughter's gifts about six months following the death. She and Al felt comforted knowing the number of people helped by the donation. At the same time, they were disappointed that they could not learn exactly how the patients were progressing following their surgery.

The Diaz family regularly attended the procurement organization's donor recognition programs. "These programs make me feel comfortable, to be with other families who have gone through a similar loss, to be myself and laugh and cry together," said Susie.

The couple has been trained as grief companions, a special program to help the newly bereaved deal with loss. "Through all the correspondence and calls from the recovery organization, we learned of more resources that were of help to us as we dealt with our loss. The grief companion program allows us to help others who are struggling with a similar situation," describes Al.

Susie is a volunteer educator and visits high schools, technical schools, colleges, and hospitals spreading the word about organ and tissue donation. She describes the reasons for her active volunteerism: "talking about Maria's life and how in death she has been able to help over 50 people allows me to keep her name alive so more people will remember than forget her."

Case 4 describes the beneficial aspects of donor family bereavement support programs. Maria's parents participated in several bereavement programs, have been of help to other donor families struggling with grief, and have educated the public about tissue donation. The activities have helped the parents maintain positive memories of their daughter. Formal recognition ceremonies can strengthen families by adding an element of community and decreasing the sense of isolation.

CASE 5

Healing involving a spiritual journey

Frank Robinson believed in an unspoken contract with his God. "If I followed the rules and lived a good life, devastating events would not happen," Frank thought. In June of 2003, his son Alec was killed in a car accident. Frank's grief journey began with a feeling that God had deceived him.

Frank's life always contained an element of deep spirituality. Following Alec's death, he descended into what he called an analysis of "the deep conflict between his beliefs and his knowledge of the world." He questioned the value of his career, whether his future work or personal efforts had any meaning, and that everything was irrelevant. As he put it, "If the things most valued in your life could be snatched away without any reason, what value was there in anything material or worldly?"

Other perplexing aspects of his journey were numerous incidents and dreams suggesting after-death communications from Alec or the "beyond." Several of these situations are outlined in *Alec's Legacy* [16], a book chronicling Frank's experiences, and many of them occurred immediately following Alec's death. The incidents included experiences such as unexpected fragrances of Alec, the regular appearance of coins in unusual places, the sudden playing of inspirational music on a CD player that was in the "off" position, and an intense dream that conveyed the message that Alec was at peace.

Of more relevance to this writing was Frank's struggle within a culture of reason to try to make sense of, or to even be able to communicate, such experiences. In a rationally based society, he and others more readily accepted that he was mentally unstable than to consider the possibility that these experiences were real.

He was confounded to find the least effective people in dealing with his deep spiritual questions were members of his own clergy. Frank, a Christian, found most help from a Jewish counselor who embraced the spiritual base of these experiences in the Old Testament of the Bible. His prior frustrations with the vague clergy responses turned to an affirmation that he was not crazy. Frank believes that asserting the reality of these experiences and taking an open, public stance was one important step in restructuring his life.

Many donor families find solace and meaning in the donation of a loved one's tissue. Frank did not find this to be the case. Through previous discussions with Alec, he knew he would have been comfortable with the affirmative donation decision. However, the timing of the request and the "horrific," detailed listing of tissues for consent was practically overwhelming. Furthermore, he had no knowledge of the procurement agency and initially believed the call was a "cruel prank." For these and other reasons, his family questions that if they had to remake the decision, or have to make another future decision for donation, they are unsure of the result.

> Despite his obvious and understandably difficult grief journey, Frank believes that all healing requires a spiritual journey. He compares his "shattered soul" to those who speak of a "broken heart." The broken heart relates to the pain and hurt, but it is the shattered soul that seeks answers to the meaning of life, the lost dreams, and the sense of isolation. And these are the lingering challenges of grief.
>
> Today, Frank realizes he has a closer, more intimate relationship with his God. Where in the past he had a passive relationship, this horrendous experience resulted in an active spiritual dialog. As he describes it, "we traveled to hell together and came out on the other side – together."

Grief and loss educators agree that bereaved persons draw upon physical, emotional, social, and spiritual energies as they seek to reconcile the loss in their lives (see case 5). We have discussed previously the seeming lack of attention paid to bereaved persons. However, when attention is paid to those suffering a loss, the emotional component seems to be addressed most. In most moderate-sized communities, there are grief support groups, clinical therapy practices, and some basic community consideration for the emotional well-being of a bereaved family.

The spiritual dimension of grief and loss, however, is vastly misunderstood, regardless of a person's reliance on any formal faith tradition. One may argue that "all losses are spiritual," requiring the bereaved person to go deeply inside oneself to realign the meaning of one's life, investigate a new orientation, and begin to live again without the presence of a loved one.

Here again, however, we encounter a cultural resistance to the needs of mourners. Not only do our communities resist the general needs of mourners, but also many locations resist public displays of spirituality. Literary works from the C.S. Lewis classic, *A Grief Observed* [17], published in 1961, to the more contemporary work of Jerry Sittser, *A Grace Disguised* [18], published in 1995, are examples of the deep spiritual reflection many undertake following the death of a loved one. In these texts, both men write openly about how their faith was challenged following the death of their wives, and in Sittser's case, the deaths of his mother and daughter at the same time. As difficult as it may seem, both grew from the loss, understood their purpose in life far better, and transcended the incredible pain associated with the deaths. In both cases, it was the spiritual aspect of the journey that required attention, reflection, and support.

All bereavement caregivers at some time lend an ear to a bereaved family member expressing the psychospiritual "why" questions: Why did my loved one die? Why this way? Why now? Why am I still here? Why should I go on? Most often, the bereaved family member does not expect an answer. And, of course, as bereavement caregivers, we have no answer. The caregiver who is patient, compassionate, and understanding honors the bereaved person's need to "search" the soul for responses to this tragedy.

Summary

Grief support and bereavement care can be very important to families suffering the loss of a loved one, particularly following the types of deaths resulting in tissue donation. Transplant professionals have a difficult task in offering consent to donate in the face of the acute grief reaction. Tissue procurement organizations can play an important role in bereavement care following donation as the family reconciles the loss into their life.

KEY LEARNING POINTS

- A skilled and sensitive approach to seeking consent for tissue donation may contribute to a family's successful mourning process.

- Donation-related procedures and information communicated sincerely complement the family's early mourning process.

- Transplant professionals' understanding of grief and loss issues, including the impact of spirituality, helps serve the donor family.

- The transformative effect of transplantation can help many donor families begin to reconcile the grief in their lives.

- Donation programs are superbly positioned to provide helpful aids for bereavement, even long after the donation [19].

- The growing need for tissue grafts for transplant requires that multiple efforts be undertaken to increase tissue donation activity to meet patient needs.

References

1. Personal Communication from Margaret Verble of Verble, Worth and Verble Inc, to Jane Pearson.
2. Finch T, Mort M, May C. Mair F. Telecare: perspectives on the changing role of patients and citizens. J Telemed Telecare. 2005;11(S1):51–3.
3. Ugarizza DN, Scmidt L. Telecare for women with post partum depression. J Psychosoc Nurs Ment Health Serv. 2006 Jan;44(1):37–46.
4. Brownsnell S, Blackburn S, Aldred H, Porteu J. Implementing telecare: practical experiences. Housing, Care & Support. 2006 Oct;9(2):6–12.
5. Leach LS, Christensen HA. Systematic review of telephone-based interventions for mental disorders. J Telemed Telecare. 2006;12(3):122–30.
6. Rodrigue JR, Scott MP, Oppenheim AR. The tissue donation experience: a comparison of donor and nondonor families. Prog Transplant. 2003 Dec;13(4):258–64.
7. Wilson P. Family experiences of tissue donation in Australia. Prog Transplant. 2006 Mar;16(1):52–6.

8. Verble M, Worth J. Overcoming families' fears and concerns in the donation discussion. Prog Transplant. 2000 Sep;10(3):155–60.

9. Verble M, Bowen GR, Kay N, Mitoff J, Shaften TJ, Wann J. A multiethnic study of the relationship between fears and concerns and refusal rates. Prog Transplant. 2002 Sep;12(3):185–90.

10. Verble M, Worth J. Fears and concerns expressed by families in the donation discussion. Prog Transplant. 2000 Mar;10(1):48–55.

11. Dodd-McCue D, Cowherd R, Iveson A. Myer K. Family responses to donor designation in donation cases: a longitudinal study. Prog Transplant. 2006 Jun;16(2): 150–4.

12. Van Gelder F, Van Hees D, de Roey J, Monbaliu D, Aerts R, Coosemans W, et al. Implementation of an intervention plan designed to optimize donor referral in a donor hospital network. Prog Transplant. 2006 Mar;16(1):46–51.

13. Verble M, Worth J. Adequate consent: its content in the donation discussion. Prog Transplant. 1998 Jun;8(2):99–103.

14. Forbe-Smith L, Haire M, Doneley M. Social work practice in the donation of human tissue for transplantation: utilising social work values and competencies to achieve effective outcomes for transplant patients and donor families. Soc Work Health Care. 2002;35(1/2):377–89.

15. Maloney R, Wolfelt A. Caring for Donor Families Before, During and After. Fort Collins, CO: Companion Press; 2001. p. 97–101.

16. Robinson F. Alec's Legacy. Richmond, VA: ALR LLC; 2006.

17. Lewis CS. A Grief Observed. New York, NY: Harper Collins; 1961.

18. Sittser J. A Grace Disguised. Grand Rapids, MI: Zondervan; 1995.

19. American Association of Tissue Banks, Guidance Document, No 4; Providing Service to Tissue Donor Families. March 10, 2007. http://aatb.timberlakepublishing.com/ files/2007bottetron3Gattachment.pdf

4 Consent[1]

Annette Rid[1] and Lisa Dinhofer[2]

[1] Institute of Biomedical Ethics, Centre for Ethics, University of Zurich, Zurich, Switzerland
[2] Hood College, Frederick, Maryland, USA

Introduction

To lead an autonomous life is important for us as persons. We do not want others to decide for us what to do or what to desire, nor do we want merely to submit to our own uninformed or unreflected desires. We want to decide freely about matters that are essentially our own.

Views about the concept of autonomy, its implications and importance, differ as much as views about the body's relation to the self. Yet most people agree about the body's important contribution to our sense of selves. Our body falls in the realm of matters that are essentially our own. Autonomy, at the least, implies bodily control and makes informed consent a general ethical requirement for medical interventions.

Obtaining informed consent is relatively straightforward in most interactions with patients prior to a therapeutic intervention or with research subjects, among them possible living cell and tissue donors. However, it is less clear how respect for autonomy applies to decisions or action after death. Views about the existence of posthumous interests and their scope and weight differ as much as views about the weight of the next-of-kin's interests – in particular, burial arrangements or society's interests in obtaining tissues. Yet most people agree that bodies of the deceased should not be conscripted for further clinical, research, or educational use. What makes postmortem tissue procurement ethically defensible is consent to donation.

---

[1] For consent issues in the reproductive setting, in particular in relation to embryo donation for embryonic stem cell lines, please turn to Chapter 12.

Tissue and Cell Donation: An Essential Guide. Edited by Ruth M. Warwick, Deirdre Fehily, Scott A. Brubaker, Ted Eastlund. © 2009 Blackwell Publishing, ISBN: 978-14051-6322-4.

Even though it is a matter of debate whether consent should be informed or presumed, obtained from the individual or the next of kin, and so forth, consent is a general ethical requirement for procuring tissue from the deceased [1].

This chapter explores the central issues relating to consent for post-mortem cell and tissue removal in three parts: The section on "The concept of informed consent in clinical practice" provides a brief outline of informed consent prior to therapeutic intervention in clinical medicine. This is adapted to consent for cell and tissue donation by living persons in the section "Consent for cell and tissue donation from living donors". The section on the "Consent for tissue removal from a deceased person" discusses the particularities of deceased-tissue donation that limit a simple adaptation of the informed consent model and offers practical guidance for obtaining consent in this context.

The concept of informed consent in clinical practice

Conceptual analysis of informed consent in clinical medicine and biomedical research customarily distinguishes two different meanings of informed consent. The first meaning implies the autonomous authorization of a medical intervention. A person gives informed consent if he or she, with substantial understanding and in absence of control by others, intentionally authorizes a health professional to proceed with the proposed medical intervention.

The second meaning of informed consent implies that a patient approves of a medical intervention in a way that conforms to the rules governing a specific institution. The two meanings of consent are not always equivalent. Informed consent can be legally or institutionally effective even if it does not meet all criteria for an autonomous authorization [2: 274–87]. *The present chapter focuses on consent as autonomous authorization*, not on consent processes conforming to institutionally required procedures. However, an overview of different existing legal or regulatory frameworks for consent to deceased-tissue donation is provided in Table 4.1 [3].

There are three elements of informed consent in clinical medical care contexts. *Threshold elements* mark the preconditions of informed consent: competence to understand and decide and voluntariness in deciding. *Information elements* comprise disclosure of material information, recommendation of a plan, and understanding of both the information and the recommendation. Decision in favor of a plan and authorization to proceed with the chosen plan are the *consent elements* of consenting [2: 287–336]. Giving and obtaining informed consent thus goes far beyond signing a consent form. It is an interactive process.

Table 4.1 Selected legal frameworks and international or professional guidelines for consent to deceased-tissue and/or organ donation

Existing frameworks and guidelines (year)	Consent model
1 *Legal frameworks*	
EC Directive 2004/23/EC (2004)	Unspecific: "mandatory" consent or authorization in line with individual Member State laws
Austrian Law on Medical Institutions (1982)	Presumed consent ("opt-out") • No NOK veto and no requirement to inform the family in the absence of an individual premortem veto
Spanish Act No. 30/1979 and Royal Decree No. 2070/1999 (1979/1999)	Presumed consent ("opt-out") • NOK veto (according to the hypothetical will of the deceased) in the absence of an individual premortem veto
Belgian Law on the Removal and Transplantation of Organs (1986)	Presumed consent ("opt-out") • NOK veto in the absence of an individual veto • No NOK veto and no requirement to inform the NOK in the presence of premortem designated donation
UK Human Tissue Act (2004) US Uniform Anatomical Gift Act (2006)	Legal authorization (United States) or "appropriate" consent (United Kingdom) ("opt-in") • NOK consent in the absence of premortem designated donation • No NOK veto in the presence of premortem designated donation
Dutch Organ Donation Act (1998)	Informed consent ("opt-in") • NOK consent (at full discretion) in the absence of premortem designated donation • No NOK veto in the presence of premortem designated donation
2 *International guidelines*	
IAEA "International Standards on Tissue Banks" (2005)	Unspecific: no open or presumed objection on the part of the deceased
WHO "Guiding Principles on Human Organ Transplantation" (1991)	Unspecific: consent required by law
3 *Professional guidelines*	
AATB/AOPO/EBAA "Model Elements of Informed Consent for Organ and Tissue Donation" (2000)	Informed consent by a family member or other legally authorized person. Additionally, AATB Standard D2.100 authorization requirements describes that "a consenting person is (a) the potential donor; (b) a person legally empowered to grant consent in accordance with federal, state, and/or local laws and/or regulations; or (c) the deceased donor's *next of kin* in order of legal precedence."

continued p. 70

Table 4.1 *Continued*

Existing frameworks and guidelines (year)	Consent model
EATB Ethical Code (2000)	Appropriate consent from the next of kin according to national regulations
National Donor Family Council under the National Kidney Foundation "Informed Consent Policy for Tissue Donation" (2001)	Informed consent of the family

Regulatory frameworks may not be fully implemented in practice [3]. Where applicable, separate regulations on research with tissues from deceased donors or use of such tissues for educational purposes may have to be considered.

The World Health Organization's (WHO) Global Knowledge Base on Transplantation contains further country-specific information about legal frameworks regarding cell, tissue, and organ transplantation (available online: http://www.who.int/transplantation/knowledgebase/en/ [accessed April 25, 2008]).

NOK, next of kin; IAEA, International Atomic Energy Agency; AATB, American Association of Tissue Banks; AOPO, Association of Organ Procurement Organizations; EBAA, Eye Bank Association of America; EATB, European Association of Tissue Banks.

Consent for cell and tissue donation from living donors

Applying the clinical model of informed consent to living cell and tissue donation is relatively straightforward as living autonomous persons donate in most of these cases. Nonetheless, the particularities of living cell and tissue donation require some elaboration and adaptation of the model. The following paragraphs cover consent issues in the most frequent forms of living cell and tissue donation, notably the donation of hematopoietic stem cells, reproductive cells, amniotic membrane, and surgical residues such as femoral head bone tissue discarded as a consequence of hip replacement surgery.[2]

The substantial difference between clinical and donation interventions

The donation of cells and tissues is an altruistic act. Because donors assume risks and inconveniences for the benefit of others, making a tissue or cell donation is substantially different from being treated as a patient who undergoes an intervention for his or her own benefit. A tissue or cell donation – for example, hematopoietic stem cell donation – is performed to enable the treatment of other patients, not to promote the individual donor's best

---

[2] Consent issues in unrelated bone marrow donation are covered in Chapter 11.

interests. Donation therefore implies, to some extent, a trade-off between individual welfare and social utility. It has an inherent potential for the abuse and exploitation of individual donors. As a consequence, obtaining individual consent becomes crucial to assure that donation conforms to the individual's goals and values.

Competence and voluntariness: general preconditions of the decision to donate

Competence, the ability to understand, to weigh the alternatives, and to decide, is a general precondition of consent [2: 287–97]. If donation entails no health risks, such as the donation of amniotic membrane or placental cord blood after the placenta has been delivered or donation of surgical residues such as femoral head bone tissue that has been removed and is ordinarily discarded after hip replacement surgery, the donor may not necessarily be competent, and surrogate consent for donation can be appropriate. However, when donation entails significant health risks, such as the donation of hematopoietic stem cells, the competence of the donor becomes a stronger or even necessary requirement. Blood should generally not be collected from incompetent donors because the intervention entails no medical benefits, but more than minimal risks and inconveniences for the individual, and usually no compelling medical reasons exist to turn to blood from incompetent persons as the pool of blood donors is large.

When a competent person donates cells or tissues, the potential for abuse and exploitation makes *voluntariness* in deciding particularly important. *A donor should will donation without being under undue control or influence of others, above all coercion or manipulation.* Professionals dealing with potential donors should assure that the individual's motivation for donation is authentic. They must rule out that a person is coerced to donate through any credible and severe threat of harm or force [2: 338–46].

Professionals should obviously not coerce or manipulate donors themselves. Overenthusiastic dedication to collecting cells or tissues can compromise the objective and adequate transmission of information. Informational manipulation, for example, through withholding of information, misleading exaggeration, or excessive emotional appeal about the need for donation, can undermine the donor's voluntary decision to donate. Professionals should be conscious that encouraging donation can be suggestive [4]. They should also be aware of the potentially manipulative effects of inducements for donation, such as financial or material incentives. Whereas the reimbursement of donation-related expenses are appropriate, larger payments can become monetary inducements to donate. Excessive payments can lead to acceptance of risks the donor otherwise would not have assumed, and they can lead to giving mistruths during the donor's risk assessment interview and an increased risk of disease transmission to patients receiving the tissue or cell donation.

Providing *material* information to prospective cell and tissue donors

Potential donors must be informed about the individual risks and inconveniences of donation just as information is given to patients prior to undergoing a medical intervention. In addition, information regarding the purpose of cell or tissue donation and associated purposes has to be disclosed to justify a medical intervention that is not being performed in the donor's best interest. The list of relevant information for consent (Table 4.2 [5]) can be even longer than in the clinical setting.

Theoretically, all relevant information should be provided because *consent is not transitive*. One may consent to A which entails B; however, if one is blind to the logical implication, consent to A does not imply consent to B. If consent for skin donation means consent for use in patients undergoing nontherapeutic cosmetic surgery rather than for burn treatment and reconstructive or other therapeutic applications, one cannot assume that the donor or donor family intend for their donation to be used in that context. The information provision needs to ensure that these potential purposes are understood before consent is given. As a propositional attitude, consent does not reflect logical implications or causal connections [6].

Intransitivity of consent, permitting use of a donation for some but not all possible purposes, is not a primary concern when the purposes of donation are rather uncontroversial. For example, in blood donation, living autonomous persons incur minimal risk for usually life-enhancing or life-saving effects. General consent to the clinical use of donated cells or tissues is usually sufficient in similar cases. However, *if practices are more controversial, it is important to be aware of the intransitivity of consent*. In tissue donation by deceased donors, for example, consent to the processing of skin as acellular dermis for reconstructive surgery on burn victims does not necessarily imply consent to using acellular dermis for penile enlargement or lip plumping. If two purposes are not structurally similar – as is the case in using the same processed tissue for lifesaving or for cosmetic purposes – it cannot be assumed that both of them conform with the donor's goals and values. Similarly, some donors may feel differently in making tissue or cell donations to a not-for-profit organization compared with a for-profit one [1].

At the same time, it is both unreasonable and practically impossible to obtain specific consent to all potential future uses of cells or tissues and to comprehensively inform about associated methods of processing and distribution. Not all relevant features that contribute in any way to understanding donation are equally important. The goal is therefore to *disclose material information that allows substantial understanding by the consenting party*. It must be assured that a person understands those propositions about donation that are germane to his or her evaluation of whether donation is an act or intervention he or she wants to authorize [2: 302].

Table 4.2 Potentially relevant information for informed consent to cell or tissue donation by *living* donors

Information relating to . . .	Elements of information
Donation interview	Right to be assisted by an independent donor advocate in hematopoietic stem cell donation
Intended purposes of donation	Often lifesaving purposes of hematopoietic stem cell donation in malignant disorders (e.g. leukemia, lymphoma, myeloma) and nonmalignant disorders (e.g. autoimmune disorders, thalassemia major, Fanconi anemia)
	Usually life-enhancing purposes of surgical residues and amniotic membrane donation (e.g. bone grafting in hip replacement revision, amniotic membrane transplantation in various conjunctival and corneal diseases)
	Occasional lifesaving purposes of skin (e.g. burn applications) donated by living donors and amniotic membrane donation, which can also be used for burn applications
	Primary or secondary uses of donated cells or tissues for ethically reviewed research
	• Where research is offered as the primary purpose of the donation, the research and all associated protocols must have been reviewed by an independent research ethics committee.
	Educational or training uses of donated cells or tissues
Recovery or collection	Hematopoietic stem cell donation may not be immediate after registration in a registry for volunteer hematopoietic stem cell donors
	Donation process with regard to the:
	1 risks, burdens, potential benefits, and alternatives;
	2 alternative donation procedures and the right to elect the donation method;
	3 individual risks and inconveniences of each donation procedure, including their likelihood, magnitude, duration, and reversibility;
	4 time commitment involved in the donation procedures and the subsequent recovery period;
	5 continued contact to monitor postdonation recovery in hematopoietic stem cell donation;
	6 voluntary decision about multiple donations in hematopoietic stem cell donation (a donor may be approached for a further donation for the same patient and the rationale for such requests should be disclosed).
Donor-eligibility evaluation	Necessary steps to determine medical suitability of the donor through:
	1 completion of the medical history and behavioral risk assessment;
	2 physical examination;
	3 laboratory tests (list specific tests for infectious disease markers, HLA and blood typing);
	4 sample material may be stored for an indeterminate period for future testing.
	Medically unsuitable cells or tissues will be disposed of in a safe and lawful way.

continued p. 74

Table 4.2 *Continued*

Information relating to . . .	Elements of information
Donor data	Recording and protection of donor data (includes confidentiality measures) Regular updating of contact details and changes in medical status that preclude donation temporarily or permanently is necessary for a functioning registry for hematopoietic stem cell donation (registries may try to trace volunteers who fail to provide updated contact details) Institutional policies regarding disclosure of test results that indicate a high risk of serious and preventable harm to third parties, either to the next of kin (with the offer of appropriate advice) or to necessary affiliated agencies in case of an imminent public health threat
Processing and storage	Processing and modification of donated cells or tissues Storage of cells or tissues for extended time periods and use on the basis of need Involvement of multiple organizations in the processing, storage, and distribution process
Costs and profits	Donation-related costs to the donor (if applicable, refunding of out-of-pocket expenses and compensation for loss of earnings) Affiliations with both for-profit and not-for-profit establishments in the transportation, testing, processing, distribution, transplantation, or research use of donated cells or tissues No donor payment as a result of products or devices derived from donated cells or tissue(s)
Distribution	Institutional allocation criteria National or international circulation of donated cells or tissues and transplantation abroad
Withdrawal of consent	Right to withdraw from registries for hematopoietic stem cell donation at any time Right to withdraw consent for hematopoietic stem cell donation while understanding the consequences for the recipient if consent is withdrawn after the transplant protocol has commenced Criteria for withdrawal of consent
Access to further information	Ways to reach the procurement organization or registry following donation (contact name, address, and phone number) Recipient anonymity in hematopoietic stem cell donation will only be abolished if the recipient himself or herself elects this

Material information for potential donors must be determined with regard to institutional, legal, and cultural contexts.

The table was primarily compiled from the guidance document on informed consent of the Ethics Working Group of the World Marrow Donor Association [5].

HLA – Human leucocyte antigen ABO – Blood group testing.

What counts as material information for the donor largely depends on the specific informational needs of the individual person. These needs differ and should be explored by professionals during the consent discussion. Yet, exclusive reliance on a subjective standard for information disclosure is insufficient because donors often do not know what information would be relevant for their deliberations (in particular regarding activities with limited public awareness such as tissue transplantation). Thus, a reasonable range of information must be communicated in donation discussions. While immutable and precisely knowable priorities for information disclosure are impossible to delineate, a reasonable person would probably agree with the following priority scheme for information disclosure to complement the assessment of individual informational needs.

First, because cell or tissue donation is an altruistic act, providing information about its purposes is primary. This type of information should be detailed in relation to public controversy about the prevailing practices. The more controversy, the more information should be given to assure that the purposes of donation as well as the means to achieve them conform to the individual's goals and values.

Second, there should be a general priority for information directly concerning the donor's health or self-determination. Individual risks and inconveniences of donation, confidentiality of test results and other donor data, as well as the possibility or impossibility to rescind consent later on are paramount items to communicate.

Third, considering that not all potentially relevant information can be provided in the donation discussion, the person seeking consent should not only seek to answer all questions at the time of the consent discussion, but also inform the potential donor about ways to access further information at a later date. A good way to achieve this is to provide written material that covers content beyond the consent discussion and indicates how to follow up with the tissue or cell procurement establishment in case of further questions.

Omitting the recommendation to donate

In contrast to the clinical context of obtaining consent from a patient, *an explicit recommendation for or against cell or tissue donation should not be given*. Clinicians are in a fiduciary relationship with patients and thus are obliged to act, within the constraints of the patient's autonomy, in the patient's best interest. Donation and transplantation professionals, however, offer an opportunity to donate, to be generous, and to help patients in need. They should provide balanced information about donation and assure it is understood. The decision to donate rests with the individual donor himself or herself.

Consent for tissue removal from a deceased person

In contrast to living cell and tissue donation, there are added particularities of tissue donation by deceased individuals – processing, distribution, and use – that limit a simple adaptation of the clinical informed consent model. Most importantly, the prospective donor is no longer a living, autonomous person. Obtaining "real-time" informed consent from him or her is thus impossible. However, death does not abolish all interests about donation that existed when alive. Deciding about one's own demise can be an integral element of leading an autonomous life.

Simultaneously, other interests and needs emerge with the death of a person, which may align, but also contrast, with the premortem wishes of the deceased. The bereaved want to bid farewell to a beloved person now lost in ways that are not only, or not, in concert with the decedent's wishes but also meaningful to them. Patients and doctors need organs and tissues from the deceased to save or enhance lives. Individuals from organ and tissue procurement establishments need to earn a living while serving to meet the needs of patients and doctors. The death of one demonstrates the interdependency of the individual with the community at large.

Most people reject the removal of deceased-donor tissues without consent [7: 143–66] because they believe there are interests that can survive and be fulfilled or defeated after we die (Joel Feinberg and Ronald Dworkin have provided philosophical justifications for this view). For example, if someone is convinced about the importance of bodily integrity after death and wishes that his or her body remain intact postmortem, others should not interfere with the realization of his or her 'life' plan. Respect for autonomy in some way extends beyond death. Existing models of consent for tissue removal from a deceased person capture this belief in different ways.

Who should decide, and according to what?[3]

The informed consent or "opt-in" model
The informed consent or "opt-in" model rests on the assumption that people do not want to donate tissues unless explicit consent is available, either during lifetime by the individual himself or herself or, in the absence of designated donation, after death by the consenting party or next of kin who are considered as surrogates for the deceased. Donor cards, indication of the donor status on the driver's license, enrollment in donor registries, or inclusion of a donor clause in advance care directives are the primary instruments

---

[3] Much of the following discussion applies to deceased donation not only of tissues but also of organs.

to consent to postmortem organ and tissue donation during lifetime. Through these methods, an individual is said to become a "designated donor."

However, today's designated donation practices pose a number of problems with regard to tissue donation. Designated donation is usually centered on organ – not tissue – donation, and the transitivity of consent between the two is questionable. In addition, most designated donations do not fulfill the requirements for informed consent and serve more as a vehicle for expressing the premortem intent to exercise a postmortem donation if circumstances allow. For example, the information provided during Internet enrollment for organ donation is primarily promotional and may not comprehensively reflect the donation process adequately. Also, the given information may not be applicable to other procurement programs outside a specific region. Primary examples are those few programs that currently recover facial, ovarian, and uterine tissues or entire limbs. These activities are not commonly featured on organ and tissue bank websites or in promotional materials [8]. In addition, as the number of potentially recoverable tissues outnumbers recoverable organs and the modalities of tissue recovery, processing, and use remain largely unfamiliar to the general public, transmitting comprehensive information about tissue donation can be difficult to achieve. Designated donation of tissues is thus far from straightforward.

Moreover, voluntary designated donation is unlikely to become comprehensive. As an example, 53% of 2,000 surveyed Americans had granted permission for organ and tissue donation on their driver's license in 2005 [9]; similar data exist from other countries. To make everyone's donor or nondonor status explicit during lifetime, a comprehensive system of required response would have to be installed [7: 175–81]. However, its implementation remains controversial and perhaps unfeasible for postmortem tissue donation considering the practical constraints discussed earlier. Finally, recognition of the "designated donor" status may vary from state to state. When a person perishes while traveling abroad, realizing his or her wish to donate (or not) can be complicated.

But even if all the practical obstacles of designated donation were overcome, the issues related to consent for postmortem tissue recovery would not be entirely resolved. There is considerable controversy whether realizing "posthumous autonomy" should always trump the wishes and needs of families, next of kin, or groups. The next of kin have rights, obligations, and often strong beliefs about the disposition of their loved one's body after death. It is through others that the dead are woven into a web of meaning and respect. Cultural, spiritual, and religious acts have an important role to play in this. How the corpse is treated may be of great importance not only for the life of the person who was, but also for the life of the family or group of which the deceased was a member. If tissue donation proceeds without agreement by the next of kin, it can have adverse psychological consequences for them and impair the grieving process. The role of the next of kin in deciding about donation therefore lies in an area of potentially great dispute [10].

In fact, today's practices are often ambivalent in this respect. Consent from a next of kin[4] or a legal nominated representative with durable power of healthcare attorney is the most frequent form of consent in "opt-in" systems, given the limits of designated donation. Because the informed consent or "opt-in" model is based on the principle of respect for "posthumous autonomy," it requires the next of kin to act as surrogates when the deceased has not indicated his or her wishes or given explicit consent to donation during their lifetime. In "opt-in" systems, the next of kin are expected to give *surrogate consent* by providing their substituted judgment for the deceased. Theoretically, they are asked to appraise whether tissue donation is compatible with the decedent's goals and values, ideally based on previous discussions about the issue. In reality, however, it is often difficult to unravel whether the next of kin act as surrogates or whether they are, to some extent, acting on their own behalf as empirical studies suggest [11] – particularly when a discussion about donation did not occur before death. This becomes especially evident when the next of kin resist honoring an unbeknownst designated donation of the deceased and refuse to cooperate in the provision of necessary medical and behavioral information in an effort to impede recovery. In such cases, it is likely that they are reacting negatively to the idea of donation or to the perception of having the last vestige of control over the deceased removed from them.

The presumed consent or "opt-out" model

In contrast to the informed consent or "opt-in" model, the presumed consent or "opt-out" model for deceased-tissue donation rests on the assumption that people are willing to donate tissues after death even if they did not explicitly consent to donation or share their respective intention during lifetime. Because polls show a general willingness to donate organs after death [9], presuming consent is held to be a better way to respect "posthumous autonomy," provided the opportunity for an *individual veto* is provided during lifetime in an "opt-out" system and, possibly, the next of kin can exercise a veto on behalf of the individual after death [12]. However, caution is warranted when transferring this argument in favor of the presumed consent model from the organ to the tissue context.

---

[4] We generally use the term "next of kin" instead of "family" and in doing so to refer to the deceased's closest living blood relative(s) or relative(s). Depending on the relevant regulations, the first next of kin to address would usually be the spouse, live-in partner, or same-sex partner in a civil union and domestic partnership. If the deceased did not have a spouse, the closest relative of the age of majority is usually contacted (a parent or a sibling, an adult child, a first cousin, aunt, uncle, or grandparent). Some states also provide a hierarchy for who should be contacted first.

First, polling is always subject to a potential social desirability bias. Individuals may wish to be perceived as altruistic without actually being altruistic, or without being prepared to act according to their general attitude.

Second, existing data conflate attitudes toward organ donation with attitudes toward tissue donation. The public is generally unaware of the extent that tissues are used today. Because the circumstances of tissue transplantation are, in many cases, less dramatic than those in organ transplantation – they are used relatively less for lifesaving interventions and scarcity is less marked – there has been comparatively little debate about tissue transplantation.

Third, the existing debates have often been extremely controversial. The controversy about certain practices in the tissue sector, most importantly commercialization and use of tissues for cosmetic purposes,[5] questions the assumption of a general willingness to donate tissues in some countries.

Yet, where clinical use of tissues is generally uncontroversial and the necessary preconditions of a presumed consent scheme are met, notably strong community ties and the existence of a well-publicized opportunity for opting out of donation, it can be ethically acceptable to presume consent.

There are two versions of presumed consent systems. If donation is effected without involving the next of kin, the allegation of a procurement system that resembles conscription more than presumed consent is, to some extent, plausible [7: 167–74]. However, if tissues are recovered after involving the next of kin in the donation process to guarantee that tissues are not removed on false assumptions, presumed consent can be ethically sound within the listed constraints. By being able to object to tissue recovery, a next of kin ensures that a person who failed to opt out during lifetime did not oppose to having his or her tissues removed for transplantation, research, or education. The presumed consent model, if it is based on respect for "posthumous autonomy," should include the opportunity for the next of kin to *veto* donation – not to *consent* to it, which would amount to the informed consent model.[6] The next of kin are asked for their *surrogate veto*. But again, it is difficult to evaluate in practice to what extent the next of kin object on their own behalf rather than on behalf of the deceased.

---

[6] It is also possible to justify a presumed consent or opt-out model on utilitarian grounds as presuming consent is often held to increase procurement of useful tissues. However, it is controversial whether presumed consent actually increases donation rates. The strength of the utilitarian argument is limited as tissues are not as scarce as organs – some are not scarce at all – and are most often used for life-enhancing, not for lifesaving, purposes.

Conflicting preferences between the deceased and the next of kin

The contradiction that occurs when the wish of the deceased opposes that of the next of kin creates some inconsistency. Both the informed consent or "opt-in" model and the surrogate veto version of the presumed consent or "opt-out" model are based on respect for "posthumous autonomy." The role of the next of kin is thus to provide surrogate consent or veto, which is by definition "patient" centered. Allowing the next of kin to decide according to their goals and values instead of those of the deceased (as may be factually true in many cases [11]), therefore, contradicts the fundamental premise of autonomy in both consent systems. Shifting to literal next-of-kin consent or veto would conflict with the common belief that respect for autonomy in some way extends beyond death. Giving priority to the next-of-kin's goals and values would also sharpen the question why the next of kin, and not society, should have priority in deciding. An appeal to "family autonomy," or autonomy of some other group of next of kin, would justify why the family or next of kin should have the power to overrule the deceased's wishes, rather than the state [13].[7] Indeed, even though to some extent existent in practice, legal or institutional systems do not endorse a next-of-kin consent model in European countries, and in the United States, the Uniform Anatomical Gift Act (UAGA) does not define the standard according to which surrogates should decide about donation.

However, in cases where the deceased's preferences about tissue donation conflict with those of the next of kin, the question about giving priority to one of them recurs in both informed and presumed consent systems. As both systems are based on respect for "posthumous autonomy," *priority should be given to the individual deceased person's veto if the next of kin desire donation although the deceased objected during lifetime.* For example, the US UAGA expressly forbids the recovery of tissues (and organs) for any purpose with a known objection to donation from the decedent (but instructs that an objection to donating one part does not imply an objection to donate another and that the next of kin should be queried about any ambiguity).

How to deal with conflicting preferences is less straightforward if the deceased is a designated donor but the next of kin object to donation. Taking the US UAGA again as an example, designated donation is not legally contingent on family consensus and expressly takes precedence over any objection. However, the next of kin are not required to cooperate, and procurement organizations are mandated to comply with designated donation to the best of their ability. Indeed, there is ample evidence that legal and regulatory frameworks are not fully implemented, in particular regarding the role of the

---

[7] However, even if the – yet unelaborated – concept of "family autonomy" was fully developed, it is difficult to see how the justifiable sphere of family decision making can be derived from it (the very issue at stake).

next of kin in decision making [3]. Historically, those within the donation community have usually acquiesced to the discontent of the next of kin for fear of negative publicity. However, the trend to include the next-of-kin's wishes is changing with the recent change in the UK Human Tissue Act and the 2006 US Uniform Anatomical Gift Act. Likewise, individual procurement organizations in the United States are adopting policies to proceed without secondary approval of the next of kin. Nonetheless, some authors make the argument that respect for "posthumous autonomy" requires an organization to proceed with donation, despite the next-of-kin's objection [14]. But it should be kept in mind that being offered the opportunity to receive a gift does not oblige one to act on it unconditionally, or to obey at all. Similarly, potential recipients of tissues as well as procurement establishments have the right to refuse a gift. If recipients were to accept donated tissue only on the condition that the next of kin also consented, based on a concern for their wishes and needs, the deceased's right to offer tissues for donation would not be infringed [13]. Respecting "posthumous autonomy" can thus be limited by the autonomous decisions of others. However, the fact that conflicting preferences are dealt with in extremely divergent ways [15] shows again that these issues lie in an area of potentially great dispute.

Conflicting preferences among the next of kin

Giving weight to the next-of-kin's preferences raises the controversial question how autonomy in the context of tissue donation can be conceptualized for a group of closely related people outside the political setting, such as a group of next of kin. Up to now, there has been no convincing account of "family autonomy" that justifies its value and clarifies the relation of family autonomy and the decedent's "posthumous autonomy." But even if an account of "family autonomy" was elaborated, its scope would probably be limited. Some families are too split or disengaged to be capable of making collective decisions or to realize family values. Indeed, family values may themselves be a matter of dispute when a mix or change of cultures and values occurs within the family. Family disintegration is frequent in Western societies. Among those families who have common values and mechanisms for making decisions, some of these mechanisms will be unjust [16].

From a theoretical standpoint, any donation decision that involves two or more next of kin therefore deserves scrutiny regarding "family dynamics," as both agreement and disagreement can rest upon unfair procedures within the group. Practically, however, it seems reasonable for procurement professionals to act on the assumption that next of kin are in accord unless there is clear evidence for disagreement or unfair decision-making procedures. In some countries, however, procurement professionals are legally required to inquire and ensure that no disagreement or objection exists among the next of kin (for example in the United States). When disagreement is intractable and conflicting parties stand in roughly the same degree of closeness to the deceased, *professionals can attempt to resolve disputes through nondirective mediation*. They should recognize, however, that the means, time, and parameters for dispute resolution are limited and that it may be legally required to forego donation if the next of kin remain divided. The role of the family in tissue (and organ) donation is, and will continue to be, controversial in most societies. Binding dispute resolution rules, which would be necessary for procedurally fair dispute resolutions, are thus unlikely to be established.

Enabling an informed decision of the bereaved next of kin

Approaching the bereaved

Despite the ongoing disputes about who should decide about tissue donation and according to which standard, most informed and presumed consent systems require involving the next of kin in the decision (see Table 1). How to sensitively approach the recently bereaved therefore becomes a central issue in all deceased-donation systems. How does one work with persons experiencing the trauma of often sudden and unexpected death in order to sensitively integrate the option of tissue donation and obtain a valid informed surrogate consent or veto? How does one perform this task without manipulation while knowing of severe shortages of organs or tissues and being aware that the evaluation of one's job performance may be largely predicated on successfully obtaining consent?

Professionals pursue a dual goal when discussing donation with the next of kin. *The discussion should enable next of kin to make an informed, voluntary decision about donation on behalf of the decedent. Simultaneously, the donation discussion should convey respect for the mourners' situation and consideration of their emotional and funereal needs.* Among the potential benefits of deciding to donate, being asked to donate tissues makes the irreversibility of the loss concrete for the family.

Fear of mutilation and spiritual consequences

The primary difficulty in presenting the option for tissue donation to the next of kin is discussing the realities of a graphically invasive procedure upon the body of the decedent at a highly sensitive juncture. The majority of tissue donation emanates from sudden, unexpected and often, traumatic death. Mourners often continue to view the deceased as in an antemortem state, susceptible to injury and embarrassment. In almost every culture traditions, rituals, and obligations for the disposition of remains exist that encompass protection and respect for the deceased individual. Those most immediate in relation to the decedent are tasked and often legally mandated to ensure that the body is cosseted and honored according to custom, which frequently includes eschatological concepts of wholeness. Indeed, the realization of these customs was often part of the decedent's wishes during lifetime. Bodily integrity after death is seen by many as a qualification for the survival and successful entrance or progress of the decedent's spiritual essence to a subsequent destination, as prescribed within a myriad of spiritual belief systems.

The majority of literature on how spiritual beliefs affect donation decisions of individuals or, in the absence of designated donation, their next of kin focuses primarily on the perspective of the next of kin and the organ donation context. The literature reports that some next of kin experience donation as giving a piece of the deceased's soul, rather than just an anatomic gift, and reveals sensitivities about specific organs and tissues, particularly the heart and eyes [17–22]. Taken as symbols for sentiment and person-hood, the next of kin can experience conflict and anxiety about "giving away" the essence of the decedent rather than just his or her physical remains. Conversely, some next of kin will only consent to specific anatomic gifts, like the heart and eyes, hoping to transfer the spirit of their loved one to another person and thereby providing a sense of immortality for the decedent.

Donation can be interpreted as representing either a threat or a benefit to the decedent in the afterlife: beliefs about negative consequences for the soul emanating from a "mutilated body" coexist with beliefs about positive consequences, for example, that donating the cornea would enhance the deceased's ability to see God through their beneficence [17,21]. Conversely, donation has also been questioned as an act against nature, which blurs the lines between what belongs in the afterlife and what should remain in the world of the living [18].

While tissue donation possesses high moral value in its potential to save or enhance lives, the perceived threat of harm or mutilation to the dece-dent can create conflict for the next of kin who become responsible as the agent of the deceased. Requestors should provide adequate information about tissue and organ recovery procedures, but avoid provoking unneces-sarily graphic images of the recovery. The delicacy of the conversation must be facilitated through direct and cogent but sensitive language with the sense of how much information is actually desired. It is also incumbent upon the requestor to continually monitor the consenting party for fatigue and emotional capacity, and to carefully assess how quickly to proceed and the level at which the donor family member is digesting the information. Donor families have voiced vigorous discontent about the terminology and nomenclature often lacking sensitivity, as testified by clinically accurate but impassible phrases such as "cadaveric donation" and "harvesting." Simi-larly, referring to donated tissue as a "product" after processing has been heavily criticized, resulting in the request that packaging for processed tissues should include a statement indicating that it was donated with the intention to save or enhance life [23]. Requestors should realize that *the bereaved can perceive 'objective' professional language as insensitive or even offensive.*[8]

---

[8] As a consequence, the corresponding terminology in this chapter oscillates between more objective "professional" terms and more empathic terms (deceased and loved one, next of kin and family, etc.).

Understanding the next-of-kin's motives for consent

Grief is universal among humans. It is an emotional rather than an intellectual response to loss and not easily relieved by thought or information. As such, grief rarely responds to logic or educational intervention. Success in increasing both satisfaction levels of the bereaved next of kin and consent rates for deceased donation requires understanding of the motives that drive decision making. The needs the bereaved have at the time we ask them to deliberate about donation must be considered.

Consenting to donation is an altruistic act. Simultaneously, it is an immediate opportunity for the next of kin to mitigate their grief by realizing one of the decedent's final wishes and by focusing on his or her likely accomplishing the relief of suffering [11]. Donation can provide potential meaning through the next of kin's personal existential or spiritual beliefs for the reasons and circumstances of the death. It can instill hopefulness and empowerment by making one of the final decisions on behalf of the deceased and by altering, at least to some degree, the perception of senselessness about the death. The bereaved often reconstruct and transform the narrative of the death story by creating a living legacy to the deceased and softening the finality of the physical separation, knowing that "he or she still lives on in others." The altruistic drive that inspires donation can be part of the next-of-kin's immediate coping. In fact, the improved fate of tissue recipients may motivate donation to a lesser extent than previously assumed. Recipients are sometimes regarded as the lucky beneficiaries while a central motivation to authorize tissue removal can rest with the meaning created for the bereaved [11].

Overall, the double task of beneficently working with the bereaved to enable an informed decision or refusal to donate, and to serve the collective good in increasing consent rates is challenging and requires *specific education and training that extends beyond discussing donation*. Knowledge about the physical, cognitive, behavioral, and social responses to sudden or traumatic loss, effective communication, and short-term grief counseling skills are necessary to discuss donation sensitively and effectively. Choosing the appropriate timing and circumstances for the discussion; meeting the challenge of locating and contacting the next of kin as a stranger on the phone; being equipped to handle overt grief reactions and responses of offense or anger subsequent to a request for donation or previous treatment by hospital or other agency personnel; compassionately terminating an interview subsequent to discovering the decedent is an unsuitable candidate for medical or behavioral reasons; and so forth – these are practical skills that must be acquired on the basis of sound knowledge through specific training programs. Those with academic and professional backgrounds within a mental healthcare or counseling discipline seem to be some of the best candidates for this function, as their comfort level when working with the bereaved is often high. It is unproven, but possible, that tissue (and organ) procurement organizations that embrace hiring policies favoring such academics and professionals may see an increase in their consent rates and employee retention.

Voluntariness: a necessary precondition of the decision to donate

To obtain consent for tissue removal and at the same time attend to the emotional, cultural, communal, spiritual, and psychological issues of the mourner is a difficult task, in particular when the overall performance of requestors is evaluated more through the number of consents obtained than through donor family or public satisfaction with the ways in which tissue donation is requested. While many requestors may not consciously acknowledge the feeling of anxiety, the pressure to "make the numbers" is an invariable aspect of their professional lives. Subliminal conflicts of interest can lead to subtle informational manipulation in the donation discussion and thereby undermine voluntariness of the consenting party [4].

Similarly, empathy for the bereaved can easily be transformed into emotional manipulation. Sentences such as "I understand your situation and offer you a nonrecurring opportunity to make something good out of the bad" may be well intentioned, but can unduly influence the decision maker. Expressing empathy is appropriate; however, *it is up to the next of kin to assign positive meaning and value to the act of consenting to donation on behalf of the decedent, not the requestor. A sensitive approach should thus be clearly distinguished from suggestive or directive communication.* Suggestive communication is particularly evident when requestors ask family members if they want to manifest a "miracle" for someone else to save a life, as if consent to donation guaranteed that outcome, or characterize the decedent as a "hero" provided that he or she donates. Such language not only risks undermining voluntariness, it can also suggest that the decedent was a failure if the donation is not successful or if the next of kin choose to forgo the option. Similar statements can border on emotional blackmail and can have long-term psychological consequences for the bereaved.

Requestors should also refrain from other forms of manipulation, above all informational manipulation. Taking a neutral stance in donation discussions is essential to allow for an informed and voluntary decision about donation. In contrast, some consent models openly criticize neutrality and advise the use of strong emotional appeal on behalf of recipients. They recommend the presentation of compelling data about those in need, in particular pediatric transplant candidates, without also offering some of the unfortunate, but realistic, statistics on negative outcomes when donation or transplant is not successful. Unbalanced emotional material can unfairly compel a person to give consent. Such measures suggest that donation is so counterintuitive to what next of kin would voluntarily elect that partial and emotional provision of information is the only way to ensure consent.

Requestor neutrality is not equivalent to apathy or indifference. It is a precondition of informed and voluntary decision making.

Providing material information about deceased-tissue donation

The list of relevant information about the purposes of tissue donation and associated processes is too long to be entirely covered in the donation conversation (see Table 4.3 [24–27]). The practical difficulties therefore consist in determining the *material* information that needs to be shared with decision makers and how this information should be shared, without overburdening the bereaved and potentially exacerbating their emotional distress. This again emphasizes the need for requestors to be proficient in working with the bereaved.

The consent discussion must include all material information associated with the decision to donate *for the decision maker, not the beneficiary of the donation*. It is important that professionals consider the intransitivity of consent and expand the list of material information accordingly. As public controversy about current practices in tissue procurement, processing, distribution, and use prevails in some countries, the consent process must be strengthened. By acknowledging current controversies, the consent process can foster accountability and good stewardship for donated tissues within the sector [28,29]. It is therefore incumbent upon requestors to *openly and comfortably address controversial issues* during the donation discussion.

As long as deceased-donation systems are based on respect for "posthumous autonomy," it must be assured that the various and structurally dissimilar purposes of tissue transplantation conform with the decedent's goals and values and take a general precedence over avoiding the burden of an extended discussion for the next of kin. *Careful assessment of individual informational needs is important. At the same time, a reasonable range of information must be communicated in the donation discussion.* As suggested earlier (in the section "Providing *material* information to prospective cell and tissue donors"), this implies that the purposes of donation should be detailed in relation to public controversy about prevailing practices. The use of tissues for cosmetic purposes, management of surpluses, or profits that stem from tissue processing, as well as the possibility of the international distribution of cells and tissues, can be material information in some contexts. For example, in the United States, there is considerable controversy about these issues,[9] and empirical data show that significant minorities of 2,033 American tissue donors and actual majorities of nondonors surveyed in the year 2000 rejected the notion that the next of kin should not be informed about controversial practices, even if they may be perceived as upsetting [29]. In addition, a general priority should be given to information that directly

---

[9] See Chapter 1.

Table 4.3 Potentially *relevant* information for consent to, or authorization for, tissue donation by *deceased* donors

Information relating to . . .	Elements of information
Donation interview	Recording of telephonic consent (preferably the entire conversation, not just the authorization): **1** coverage of recordings by data protection legislation; **2** secured storage of recordings on tape, CD, or a central server; **3** uses of recordings (e.g. case documentation, auditing/sampling, research, staff training); **4** use of electronic methods such as facsimile or encrypted electronic mail to obtain signatures on the authorization form(s)
Intended purposes of donation	Lifesaving and life-enhancing purposes of tissue transplantation for clinical applications in up to 50–100 recipients Primary or secondary uses of donated tissue for ethically reviewed research Educational or training uses of donated tissue
Recovery	Tissue removal process with regard to the: **1** risks, burdens, potential benefits, and alternatives; **2** nature and amount (whole or in part) of tissue(s) that can potentially be recovered, including those necessary to procure as part of the donor eligibility assessment (e.g. spleen, lymph nodes, blood); **3** location and extent of incisions, postrecovery reconstruction measures and their ramifications for the deceased's appearance (e.g. appearance of the deceased for viewing, clothing considerations for funeral viewing); • It is important that the requestor remains conversant with the local tissue establishment recovery process to ensure that the information given is accurate and the consent is consistent with local practices. **4** estimated duration of recovery and time-related consequences for funeral arrangements; **5** location of the procurement procedure and any necessary relocation of the deceased; **6** transportation of the body to forensic agency or mortuary. Reasons for the potential inability to recover tissues (e.g. unknown medical unsuitability) Offer to see the deceased after the procurement procedures, if allowed by medical facility and feasible to facilitate
Donor eligibility evaluation	Necessary steps to determine medical suitability of the donor through: **1** completion of the medical history and behavioral risk assessment, including access to the deceased's medical records and contact with the general practitioner or any other relevant health professional; **2** physical examination and assessment of the deceased; **3** laboratory tests (list specific tests for infectious disease markers); **4** sample material may be stored for an indeterminate period for future testing If the deceased is under 18 months of age and/or has been breast-fed in the last 12 months, an additional medical history and behavioral risk assessment from the birth mother is usually required (check regional requirements).

continued p. 88

Table 4.3 *Continued*

Information relating to . . .	Elements of information
	If the deceased is less than one month of age (28 days), a blood sample from the birth mother is usually required (check regional requirements). Potential medical unsuitability of donated tissues (e.g. unacceptable test results, clinical incompatibility with transplantation or research) Medically unsuitable tissues will be disposed of in a safe and lawful way.
Donor data	Recording and protection of donor data and guaranteed confidentiality Institutional policies regarding disclosure of confirmed test results that indicate a high risk of serious and preventable harm to third parties, either to the next of kin (with the offer of appropriate advice) or to necessary affiliated agencies in case of an imminent public health threat
Processing and storage	Modification of donated tissues that can allow for greater clinical applications Storage of tissues and tissue products for up to five years or more Involvement of multiple organizations in the processing, storage, and distribution process
Costs and profits	No donation-related costs applicable to the deceased's next of kin Affiliations with both for-profit and not-for-profit establishments in the transportation, testing, processing, distribution, transplantation, or research use of donated tissues No payment or personal gain as a result of products or devices derived from donated tissue(s)
Distribution	Institutional allocation criteria (e.g. medical urgency, expected medical outcome, regional balance) National or international circulation of donated tissue(s) and transplantation abroad
Future use	Future uses of donated tissues and their products 1 clinical use: <ul><li>transplantation for lifesaving purposes (e.g. burn care, cardiac valve repair or replacement)</li><li>transplantation for life-enhancing purposes and reconstructive and esthetic surgery (e.g. restoration of sight, limb salvage, cardiac and venous repair surgery, spinal fusion and soft tissue repair, cosmetic interventions)</li></ul> 2 nonclinical use: <ul><li>primary use for ethically reviewed research – where research is offered as the primary purpose of the donation, the research and all associated protocols must have been reviewed by an independent research ethics committee</li><li>secondary use of nonutilizable tissue for ethically reviewed research</li><li>primary use for educational or training purposes</li><li>remaining tissues will be disposed of in a safe and lawful way following the completion of research, education or training projects</li></ul> Right to limit or restrict the future use(s) of tissue, if feasible
Property rights	No property rights are inferred with donated tissues or their products

Table 4.3 *Continued*

Information relating to . . .	Elements of information
Withdrawal of consent	Criteria for withdrawal of consent
Aftercare and access to further information	Time frame for mailing a copy of the consent form and additional information Ways to reach the procurement organization following donation (contact name, address, and phone number) Agency services for donor families postdonation Ways to obtain information about the outcome of donation and information about the time frames involved

Material information for potential donors or their surrogates must be determined with regard to institutional, legal, and cultural contexts.

The table was primarily compiled from one of the authors' experience in requesting deceased-tissue donation in the United States (L.D.) and from various guidance documents and organization's internal documents describing how requesting deceased tissue donation is undertaken [24–27].

concerns respect for the deceased and his or her "posthumous autonomy." Confidentiality of donor data must be assured and justified exceptions, such as the communication of confirmed positive test results posing a high risk of serious and preventable harm to the next of kin or others, should be disclosed. Unfortunately, some state confidentiality laws within the United States regarding disclosure of such information to individuals other than the decedent have not taken into consideration the unique circumstances of postmortem donation. Conditions and criteria for withdrawing consent before recovery commences should also be mentioned; this is a requirement under the US UAGA. Finally, information must be provided about ways to access extendable information after the discussion, in particular regarding ways to reach the procurement organization following donation.

Obtaining the authorization

Once the material information has been disclosed in comprehensible language and time to ask questions has been granted, the next of kin will be asked to make a decision and, if they choose to donate, to authorize tissue recovery. Authorization is obtained through the affirmation of a legal document, provided the next of kin has demonstrated decision-making capacity. Requestors must ensure, based on the donation discussion, that the next of kin meets the following four requirements: the ability to understand the information provided; the ability to evaluate the information according to his or her personal situation and values; the ability to conclude with a reasonably defensible decision; and the ability to communicate a decision (which can include verbal and nonverbal communication through physical affirmations). If requestors determine during their discussions that the next of kin does not meet these criteria, they must seek another legal representative for consent as outlined in relevant regulations. Decision-making capacity should not be confused with legal capacity, which can only be ascertained by a legal authority.

It is strongly advised and usually legally mandatory that the authorization process be recorded. Recording can be accomplished in different ways, depending on the setting and relevant regulations. A signature is required in face-to-face discussions; it is often a legal requirement to also have a third-party witness present during the discussion who cosigns the authorization documents. Tape or digital recordings are standard in telephone consent. If recorded, the recording device is considered a witness by many legal statutes. If not recorded, a second individual must confirm with the decision maker the elections indicated on the form. In both instances, the consent document should be read to the next of kin verbatim (not paraphrased) with periodic inquiries for questions and indication of comprehension. Requestors are advised not to assume literacy by handing the document to a decision maker for private review. If the decision maker is skilled in concealing his or her illiteracy, consent will not only be invalid, but the concerned person can also be embarrassed. It is an essential part of completing the authorization to donate to make a copy of the signed consent form as well as to retain copies or evidence of providing further written information about tissue donation and transplantation proactively made available after the donation discussion.

The practical steps of obtaining consent or authorization are summarized in Table 4.4 [27].

Realizing donor intent and the future uses of tissue

Donor designation and surrogate consent or veto by the next of kin are not only instruments to safeguard respect for autonomy. They also serve to gather information about the deceased's medical history and behavioral risk,[10] to explore the expectations associated with donation, and to specify, to some extent, which future uses of donated tissues conform with the individual's or the decedent's intention to donate. A central motive for donation is usually to help patients in need and, by doing so, to also create meaning for one's own death or the death of a relative. For example, the National Donor Family Council states that families expect donated tissues to be used in a way that promotes healing for people with the greatest need [23].

However, some practices, in particular transplantation of tissues for cosmetic purposes or tissue use in research, may conflict with this customary donor intent. It cannot be assumed that all existing practices in tissue banking and transplantation correspond to the donor's goals and values. *Donors or next of kin should therefore be able to veto uses of donated tissues for*

---

[10] See Chapter 5.

Table 4.4 Steps of obtaining consent or authorization for deceased-tissue donation

Steps of obtaining consent	Elements of action
Step 1. Clarify designated donor status	Ascertain if the deceased is registered as a designated donor or has expressed his or her intent to donate tissues during lifetime (e.g. donor card, advance directive, enrolment in a donor registry). Check for accuracy of the decedent's name and factual information about the death.
Step 2. Exclude forensic or legal objection	Explore any forensic or legal restrictions to donation and obtain release for donation. Some offices may require procurement organizations to contact them only after consent is obtained.
Step 3. Initiate contact	Introduce yourself and identify your organizational affiliation. If conducting the interview in person, choose a quiet and private place with no background noise or distractions from the donation conversation. If conducting the interview by phone, ensure privacy for the individual and eliminate background noise for the requestor. If the requestor works out of a private residence, a separate phone line should be used. Seek approval for voice recording during telephone interview, for those recording the entire conversation and not only the authorization, or for the presence of a witness in face-to-face interviews. Serve as a source of information and support.
Step 4. Establish nominated representative or appropriate next of kin	Identify the appropriate legal party or next of kin according to state or regional law, usually in the highest qualifying relationship to the deceased. Document the rationale for taking consent from someone not in the highest qualifying relationship. If the next of kin as stipulated within the hierarchy cannot be located, is unable or unwilling to make decisions, ascertain whether the deceased had a legally nominated representative other than the next of kin (i.e. healthcare power of attorney) to act on his or her behalf for the purpose of executing healthcare decisions or obtaining consent for organ or tissue donation in the event of incompetence. In some countries, a legally nominated representative may have legal precedence over the next of kin listed within the hierarchy.
Step 5. Explain purpose of contact	If the deceased is a *designated donor*, explain that the following conversation serves to inform about the deceased's designated donor status and the tissues and/or organs included in the designation and their intended procurement and to complete the medical history and behavioral risk assessment. Do not seek consent for procuring the tissues and/or organs designated for donation, but provide information about the recovery procedure and its impact on clothing choices for viewing, the estimated duration of the procedure to allow for funeral planning, and the location and possible transport of the body.

continued p. 92

Table 4.4 *Continued*

Steps of obtaining consent	Elements of action
	If the decedent is medically suitable, seek consent for those recoverable tissues that are not included in the designation and/ or for research in the event that donation for the purpose of transplantation is not possible.
	Review a disclosure document rather than an authorization form and close the conversation. *Steps 6–9 do not, or only partially, apply in designated donation.*
	If the deceased is *not a designated donor*, explain that the following conversation serves to explore the opportunity for potentially donating tissues for transplantation, research, education, or training or, in the case of evidence of previous donor designation, that this conversation can facilitate donation but there may be no expectation to authorize it.
Step 6. Provide disclosure of material information	Neutrally discuss all material information necessary for informed decision making (see Table 3 for potentially relevant information).
	Explain the voluntariness of donation.
	Explain that donation is a possibility and that the final determination will be made during or after recovery once medical suitability and other criteria have been assessed.
	Use language that is sensitive and unlikely to provoke unnecessarily disturbing graphic images.
	Frequently assess for understanding and invite questions.
	Pace the discussion according to the needs of the individual.
Step 7. Ascertain competency	Assess the decision-making capacity (not "legal" capacity) of the consenting party.
Step 8. Request donation	Make the request for donation.
Step 9. Obtain the authorization	Conduct the authorization or witnessed procedures according to state or regional laws.
	Ascertain which tissues are being donated for which purposes, notably transplantation, research, education, or training. Be explicit regarding the nature, whole or part, of all tissue(s) to be retrieved.
	Read the entire consent form *verbatim*, i.e. without paraphrasing, and frequently assess for understanding and comfort with what is read.
	Notate any restrictions requested by the consenting party. Discontinue the authorization procedure if a discriminatory or unlawful restriction is required.
Step 10. Close conversation	Ask again for understanding and any further questions.
	Explain the procedures ensuing the donation discussion (e.g. transmission of the consent form, letter confirming the details of donation).
	Discuss available aftercare services, organizations, and support services provided to donor families.

Table 4.4 *Continued*

Steps of obtaining consent	Elements of action
	Provide contact information for the immediate period following the conversation (contact name, address, and phone number).
	Explain clearly the organization's policy regarding the provision of recipient information to donor families.
	Express reassurance, sympathy, and thanks.
	When deferring donation, explain the rationale for the deferral and thank them for considering donation.
	Investigate further informational or support needs.

Some of the listed steps may not apply to certain institutional or legal contexts.
The table was primarily compiled from one of the authors' experience in requesting donation in the United States (L.D.) and relevant material from the UK National Health Services Blood and Transplant [27].

research, cosmetic, or educational purposes that are contrary to their personal reasons for donating. If uses of donated tissue for purposes other than transplantation are anticipated, providing specific information and obtaining consent are necessary. Providing specific information about and obtaining explicit consent for corresponding uses is a precondition for being able to veto these uses of tissue. For example, some tissue establishments have donation schemes that include secondary use for research if tissues do not meet the criteria for therapeutic use. If applicable, this possibility must be made explicit in the donation discussion and endorsed by the consenting party for an effective authorization. Where research is offered as the primary purpose of the donation, the research and all associated protocols should have been reviewed by an independent research ethics committee. Consent and review by an ethics committee is particularly important if there are data links that might compromise donor confidentiality or if the research use might lead to financial gain by third parties, for example, by the creation and selling of continuous cell cultures.

Similarly, decision makers should be able to restrict future uses of donated tissues for controversial applications, such as lip plumping, penile enlargement, or other elective cosmetic procedures. Cosmetic applications are less frequent than reported in the media; their form in application is similar to that of generally approved uses, and the capability of tissue establishments to prevent off-label use may be limited, if not impossible. However, if donors understand that there is no absolute control over every use of tissue as well as the consequences of vetoing certain application or processing options, such as creating potential tissue shortages for patients in need, then *procurement organizations should promote donor autonomy by respecting restrictions regarding controversial future uses of tissues (provided this is realistically feasible).*

Similar policies also seem to conform to donor attitudes. For example, the majority of American tissue donors and nondonors disagreed or strongly disagreed with the statement that the next of kin should not have a say in how tissues are distributed [29]. The largest organized group of donor families worldwide, the US National Donor Family Council, also claims a right to limit or restrict the use of donated tissues [25]. Allowing the restriction of specific future uses of donated tissues is particularly difficult to achieve in premortem designated donation for reasons previously discussed (in the section "The presumed consent or 'opt-out' model").

There are, however, also limits to realizing donor intent. Facilitating family requests for discriminative choices regarding future uses of donated material, such as exclusive use in patients of a particular race or religion, is already highly controversial in organ donation – and illegal in most countries. Because the scarcity of material is less marked in tissue than in organ transplantation and because tissue recipients are less likely to suffer from life-threatening conditions (heart valves and skin being possible exceptions), *realizing discriminatory choices is ethically unacceptable in tissue donation*. Again, being offered a gift does not oblige its unconditional acceptance or its acceptance at all. Fairness, justice, and rejecting racism are powerful reasons against accepting discriminatory gifts.

Safeguarding confidentiality of the tissue donor and recipient

Safeguards for confidentiality and respect for privacy are a precondition of controlling personal information and thus a precondition for protecting donor autonomy. Consequently, the confidentiality of donor data is a central element of any deceased (organ and) tissue donation system that is based on respect for "posthumous autonomy" and endeavors to realize, to the extent justifiable and feasible, the decedent's wishes, goals, and values regarding donation.

There are, however, limitations on safeguarding donor confidentiality. In particular, when donor testing reveals a positive test for infectious disease, indicating a previously undiagnosed infection and a high risk of serious and preventable harm to either the next of kin who were close contacts or to the wider public, it is well recognized that disclosing this information overrides confidentiality.[11] Notification of the next of kin as a duty to warn them and of the public health authorities because of public health laws and regulations is required. Potential donors or their next of kin should be informed about this in the donation discussion and consent process.

At the same time, confidentiality pertains not only to the tissue donor, but also to the recipient of tissues. There is an increasing demand to provide recipient information to donors or, in the case of deceased donation, their

---

[11] See Chapter 7.

next of kin. According to the National Donor Family Council, for example, the next of kin have a right to receive upon request timely information about which tissues were or were not removed and why, and how any donated tissues were used [30]. Indeed, many anecdotal examples exist of donor families who have been comforted by learning the specific benefits that resulted from their relative's donation. The expectation of the next of kin to be provided with specific recipient information is probably transferred from the organ donation context, where it is common practice in many countries to inform families about the age, sex, diagnosis, and geographic area of the organ recipient. The increasing emphasis on the "heroic" outcomes of tissue donation in the donation discussion may also create the wish for the next of kin to witness these outcomes face to face.

However, providing tissue recipient information poses specific problems beyond safeguarding the right to anonymity between donor and recipient. As tissues can be transplanted to up to 50–100 recipients, providing reliable and accurate information about the ultimate recipient of every tissue graft requires a high investment into tracing and extracting this information. It is also questionable whether the next of kin would be comforted to hear about the frequent discarding of medically unsuitable donated tissues, owing to their insufficient physical quality, accidents during processing, and falsely positive infectious disease markers. For both reasons, *the provision of specific recipient outcome information should not be routine, but on individual request only* [31,32]. Any given information should be provided with *respect for the right to anonymity between donor and recipient*. To avoid the identification of the recipient, information should probably be limited to whether the tissue was issued, the type of transplantation use, and the probable number of patients. Information about the current health status of recipients should be excluded. It is also advisable to inform donor families that there may be considerable delay before any information is available and that the information provided may not necessarily be what they expect to hear.

KEY LEARNING POINTS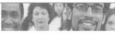

- Respect for autonomy requires that informed consent be obtained for cell or tissue donation from living donors.
- Respect for "posthumous autonomy" of a deceased donor requires obtaining the consent either from the donor during his or her lifetime or, in the absence of antemortem designated donation, surrogate consent or authorization on behalf of the donor from the next of kin after death.
- Consent for cell or tissue donation should be voluntary. This requires requestors to refrain from coercion and informational or emotional manipulation.

- Potential donors or their consenting next of kin should be provided with *material* information about tissue donation, processing, distribution, and use.

- Material information must be determined with regard to institutional, legal, and cultural contexts: the purposes of donation should be detailed in relation to public controversy about prevailing practices, such as profit making or use of tissues for cosmetic purposes; a general priority should be given to information that directly concerns respect for the deceased and his or her "posthumous autonomy," and information should be provided about ways to access additional information after the donation discussion.

- To promote donor autonomy, procurement organizations should respect nondiscriminatory restrictions regarding future uses of donated tissues for research, educational, or cosmetic purposes.

- The double task of beneficently working with the bereaved to enable an informed decision to donate and to serve the collective good in increasing consent rates is challenging and requires specific education and training that extends beyond discussing donation.

References

1. Schulz-Baldes A, Biller-Andorno N, Capron AM. International perspectives on the ethics and regulation of human cell and tissue transplantation. WHO Bull. 2007;85(12):941–8.
2. Faden RR, Beauchamp TL, King NMP. A History and Theory of Informed Consent. New York, NY: Oxford University Press; 1986.
3. Gevers S, Janssen A, Friele R. Consent systems for post mortem organ donation in Europe. Eur J Health Law. 2004 Jun;11(2):175–86.
4. Truog RD. Consent for organ donation – Balancing conflicting ethical obligations. N Engl J Med. 2008;358(12):1297–8.
5. Rosenmayr A, Hartwell L, Egeland T. Informed consent – Suggested procedures for informed consent for unrelated haematopoietic stem cell donors at various stages of recruitment, donor evaluation, and donor workup. Bone Marrow Transplant. 2003 Apr;31(7):539–45.
6. O'Neill O. Some limits of informed consent. J Med Ethics. 2003 Feb;29(1):4–7.
7. Veatch RM. Transplantation Ethics. Washington, DC: Georgetown University Press; 2002.
8. Woien S, Rady MY, Verheijde JL, McGregor J. Organ procurement organizations Internet enrollment for organ donation: abandoning informed consent. BMC Med Ethics. 2006 Dec 22;7(1):E14.
9. Gallup Survey. National Survey on Organ and Tissue Donation Attitudes and Behaviors. Washington, DC: Gallup Inc.; 2005.
10. Boddington P. Organ donation after death – Should I decide, or should my family? J Appl Philos. 1998;15(1):69–81.

11. Sque M, Long T, Payne S. Organ donation: key factors influencing families' decision-making. Transplant Proc. 2005 Mar;37(2):543–6.
12. Gill MB. Presumed consent, autonomy, and organ donation. J Med Philos. 2004 Feb;29(1):37–59.
13. Wilkinson TM. Individual and family decisions about organ donation. J Appl Philos. 2007;24(1):26–40.
14. May T, Aulisio MP, DeVita MA. Patients, families, and organ donation: who should decide? Milbank Q. 2000;78(2):152, 323–36.
15. Wendler D, Dickert N. The consent process for cadaveric organ procurement: how does it work? How can it be improved? JAMA. 2001 Jan 17;285(3):329–33.
16. Wilkinson TM. Racist organ donors and saving lives. Bioethics. 2007;21(2):63–74.
17. Klein HK. Parental bereavement in organ and tissue donation. Presentation held at the Association for Death Education and Counselling Annual Conference in Chicago on March 22, 1998.
18. La Spina F, Sedda L, Pizzi C, Verlato R, Boselli L, Candiani A, et al. Donor families' attitude toward organ donation. The North Italy Transplant Program. Transplant Proc. 1993 Feb;25(1 Pt 2):1699–701.
19. Pittman SJ. Alpha and omega: the grief of the heart donor family. Med J Aust. 1985 Dec 9–23;143(12–13):568–70.
20. Sque M, Payne SA. Dissonant loss: the experiences of donor relatives. Soc Sci Med. 1996 Nov;43(9):1359–70.
21. Soukup M. Organ donation from the family of a totally brain-dead donor: professional responsiveness. Crit Care Nurs Q. 1991 Feb;13(4):8–18.
22. Snell J. Life from death. Nurs Times. 1997;93(27):30–2.
23. National Donor Family Council Executive Committee. Position Statement on Tissue Donation. New York, NY: National Kidney Foundation; 2000.
24. European Association of Tissue Banks, Ethical and Legal Committee. Ethical Code. Berlin: EATB; 2000.
25. National Donor Family Council Executive Committee. Informed Consent Policy for Tissue Donation. New York, NY: National Kidney Foundation; 2000.
26. American Association of Tissue Banks, Association of Organ Procurement Organizations, Eye Bank Association of America. Model Elements of Informed Consent for Organ and Tissue Donation. McLean, VA: AATB; 2000.
27. UK National Health Services Blood and Transplant. Management Process Description MPD/MED/CM/051/03. Management of the Deceased Donor Family Donation Conversation. London: NHSBT; 2003.
28. Department of Health and Human Services, Office of the Inspector General. Informed Consent in Tissue Donation. Expectations and Realities. Washington, DC: DHSS; 2001.
29. Youngner SJ. Informed consent. In: Youngner SJ, Anderson MW, Shapiro R, editors. Transplanting Human Tissue Ethics, Policy and Practice. New York, NY: Oxford University Press; 2004. p. 168–85.
30. National Donor Family Council Executive Committee. Bill of Rights for Donor Families. New York, NY: National Kidney Foundation; 1994/2002.
31. UK National Health Services Blood and Transplant. DATASHEET DAT/PTI/TB/044/01. Rationale behind the Policy on the Provision of Recipient Information to Tissue Donor Families. London: NHS; 2005.
32. UK National Health Services Blood and Transplant. POLICY POL/PTI/TB/004/01. Provision of Recipient Information to Tissue Donor Families. London: NHS; 2004.

5 Gathering Donor History: Ensuring Safe Tissues for Transplant

Blanca Miranda,[1] Alessandro Nanni Costa,[2] Jacinto Sánchez-Ibáñez,[3] and Eliana Porta[4]

[1] Transplant Services Foundation and the Transplant Coordination Unit Hospital Clinic, Barcelona, Spain
[2] Italian National Transplant Centre, Rome, Italy
[3] Coordination Autonomica de Transplantes de Galicia, Galicia, Spain
[4] Italian National Transplant Centre, Rome, Italy

Introduction

Tissue donor selection is a risk reduction process, which ideally precedes testing of the donor and which may highlight risks of transmissible disease that cannot be identified by testing alone. This chapter examines a number of cases that demonstrates the principles behind this process. The transplantation of human tissues and cells always carries risks; one of the most significant of these is the transmission of a donor-derived disease. The objective of the donor selection process is to reduce that risk, minimizing factors that could, potentially, harm the recipient. Blood testing methodologies have greatly improved, and many risks are significantly reduced by testing for infective agents in donor blood samples or in the tissue or cells to be transplanted. However, it is not possible to test for all transmissible agents, or for malignant disease, in every donor, and even negative test results cannot guarantee total absence of risk of infection or other transmissible disease from the donor to the recipient. The selection of the donor on the basis of medical and behavioral history, therefore, continues to be a crucial safeguard for the protection of the tissue or cell transplant recipient.

Tissue and Cell Donation: An Essential Guide. Edited by Ruth M. Warwick, Deirdre Fehily, Scott A. Brubaker, Ted Eastlund. © 2009 Blackwell Publishing, ISBN: 978-14051-6322-4.

CASE 1

Importance of donor medical and behavioral history

In 1997, a woman died in a Scottish hospital. She was 53 years of age and she had been diagnosed as suffering from inoperable lung cancer. For some time before her death, there had been medical concerns about her abnormal gait and her behavior. Because uncertainty over the cause of her undiagnosed neurological problems persisted at the time of her death, a postmortem examination was requested and readily agreed to by her relatives. She had wanted to donate after her death and the hospice staff contacted the ophthalmology staff at the hospital where the postmortem examination was carried out.

The family members gave consent to donation but were not interviewed about the donor's medical and behavioral history. The doctor who removed the corneas was unaware that the patient, while dying of cancer, also suffered from an unexplained neurological condition, and that a postmortem examination had been requested. Only a primary cause of death was entered on the Cornea Donor Information form filled in by the ophthalmologist to accompany the eyes when these were subsequently transferred to an eye bank in England. The corneas and a piece of sclera were transplanted to three patients. Some eight months later, a diagnosis of Creutzfeldt–Jakob disease was confirmed following the tests on the donor's brain tissue, and it came to light that ophthalmic tissue, which should never have been retrieved, had been transplanted into healthy patients [1,2].

In this case, a transmission risk for prion disease was not appreciated because a donor medical history was not fully explored and a postmortem report was not routinely reviewed as part of the assessment of the medical history. In the more than 10 years since this incident occurred, the systems and procedures for eye donor selection in the United Kingdom have radically changed. Donor selection on the basis of medical and behavioral history gathered by trained professionals is now recognized as an essential step in the donation process. Unexplained neurological disease is a universally accepted contraindication to donation.

Facts do not cease to exist because they are ignored.

Aldous Huxley

The risks of disease transmission by tissue and cell transplantation

The literature demonstrates that the risks of disease transmission by tissue and cell transplantation are similar to those associated with blood transfusion. Viruses, bacteria, fungi, and prions have all been reported to be transmissible [3,4]. Despite testing for HIV and hepatitis, these viruses have been transmitted because of inadequate testing (see cases 2, 3, and 4) and/or during the serological window period of infection (see cases 3 and 4). These documented transmissions underline the importance of thorough screening for behavioral risk.

Other viruses that have been transmitted by human allografts in recent years include the West Nile virus and lymphocytic choriomeningitis virus (LCMV) and rabies. The transmission of West Nile virus, initially in the east and subsequently in the west of the United States, has been documented in blood transfusion and then in organ transplantation, so that many agencies now take a medical history of donors to ensure that they were not in an acute phase of a flu-like illness, or that they have not been exposed while in an endemic area for a variety of infectious diseases. LCMV is found in rodents, and because these animals are occasionally kept as pets, animal bites to the donor may have occurred; exposure to pet rodents resulted in two transmissions of meningoencephalitis. In the first case, the donor died of head trauma and donated organs; in the second case, the donor had a cerebral infarct diagnosed by imaging. A number of organ recipients died as a consequence of LCMV transmitted disease. While this virus has not been shown to infect tissue recipients, but only organ recipients who received immunosuppressive drugs to prevent organ rejection, some agencies include questions about animal bites in their medical history taking. However, recent transmission of rabies by an organ donor in 2005 has occurred and transmission by corneas has been recognized since 1979. Again, recent animal bites and travel to rabies endemic areas need consideration on a case-by-case basis [5].

However, identifying transmissions and improving not only testing regimes, but also the evidence to justify guidance on how a medical history should be obtained to reduce risk are all important learning points. All the cases in this chapter were published and provided clear evidence for a considerable need to assess the medical and behavioral risk of the donor to avoid the risk of disease transmission, either because of a disease for which a test was not available or to exclude a donor with a window period infection (undetectable by testing). The knowledge gained strengthened the professional appreciation of the importance of identifying donor-related risks (including hemodilution and prion disease), of not relying on testing alone, and of the usefulness of behavioral or other risk factors, which, either singly or together with other information, may help exclude a donor who poses a risk to potential recipients.

When tissue transplantation began, the potential benefits were considered greater than the perceived risk (principally because the professionals did not recognize all the associated risks), but, gradually, cases of disease transmission were described and practitioners began to identify them with donor origin more than 50 years ago [4]. It is now well accepted that a careful evaluation of the donor's history is a key step to reducing the risk of disease transmission [4].

There are some significant differences between the risk:benefit ratios in organ and tissue transplantation. While organ transplantation usually represents the only chance of survival for the recipient, there are normally other therapeutic alternatives to tissue transplantation; for example, a mechanical heart valve can be used in place of a human valve, and an artificial material can be used instead of a bone graft. Organs must be retrieved as soon as possible after cardiac arrest (warm ischemia time), but tissues can be removed 15 hours after death if the body was at ambient temperature or up to 24 hours after death if the body was refrigerated soon after death; in some organizations, this time limit to tissue procurement can be extended to 48 hours. Organs must also be transplanted in a very short period of time after perfusion of the organ commences (cold ischemia time), but some tissues can be maintained for years after donation because they can be preserved by freezing or freeze-drying. This means that there is considerably more time available to research the medical and behavioral history of the tissue donor and to assess the risk of disease transmission from that donor. For these reasons, a lower level of risk is acceptable for tissue donors compared with organ donors and very strict selection criteria must be applied, which are reflected in ever more complex donor and donor family questionnaires.

As in every field of health care, professionals learn from mistakes and incidents and apply this knowledge to improve quality and safety of human substances for transplantation and transfusion. Scientific and professional associations play an important role in implementing guidelines for donor selection, and regulators build minimum requirements for donor selection into binding laws for the protection of public health.

Donor information requirements

The recently published European Union (EU) Directives on tissues and cells [6–8] provide a list of conditions that should exclude donation – unless there is a documented risk assessment that justifies an exception. The list of exclusions is shown in Table 5.1. Similar regulatory criteria exist in the United States [9], Canada (from Health Canada), and Australia (from Therapeutic Goods Association) and are in development elsewhere.

There are also specific requirements for child donors. Any children born from mothers with HIV infection or that meet any of the exclusion criteria described in Table 5.1 must be excluded as donors until the risk of transmission of infection can be definitely ruled out. Generally, children aged less than 18 months born from mothers with HIV, hepatitis B, hepatitis C, or Human T-lymphotropic virus (HTLV) infection, or at risk of such infection, and/or who have been breast-fed by their mothers during the previous 12 months (any age), cannot be considered as donors regardless of the results of the analytical tests. Children over 18 months of age born from mothers with HIV, hepatitis B, hepatitis C, or HTLV infection, or at risk of such infection, but who

Table 5.1 European Union criteria for exclusion of tissue or cell donation [© European Communities 1995–2008]

Commission Directive 2006/17/EC – General Criteria for Exclusion [7]

For deceased donors, cause of death unknown, unless autopsy provides information on the cause of death after procurement and none of the general criteria for exclusion set out in the present section applies.

History of a disease of unknown aetiology.

Presence, or previous history, of malignant disease, except for primary basal cell carcinoma, carcinoma *in situ* of the uterine cervix, and some primary tumours of the central nervous system that have to be evaluated according to scientific evidence. Donors with malignant diseases can be evaluated and considered for cornea donation, except for those with retinoblastoma, haematological neoplasm, and malignant tumours of the anterior segment of the eye.

Risk of transmission of diseases caused by prions. This risk applies, for example, to:
(a) people diagnosed with Creutzfeldt–Jakob disease, or variant Creutzfeldt–Jakob disease, or having a family history of non-iatrogenic Creutzfeldt–Jakob disease;
(b) people with a history of rapid progressive dementia or degenerative neurological disease, including those of unknown origin;
(c) recipients of hormones derived from the human pituitary gland (such as growth hormones) and recipients of grafts of cornea, sclera and dura mater, and persons that have undergone undocumented neurosurgery (where dura mater may have been used).
For variant Creutzfeldt–Jakob disease, further precautionary measures may be recommended.

Systemic infection which is not controlled at the time of donation, including bacterial diseases, systemic viral, fungal or parasitic infections, or significant local infection in the tissues and cells to be donated. Donors with bacterial septicaemia may be evaluated and considered for eye donation but only where the corneas are to be stored by organ culture to allow detection of any bacterial contamination of the tissue.

History, clinical evidence, or laboratory evidence of HIV, acute or chronic hepatitis B (except in the case of persons with a proven immune status), hepatitis C and HTLV I/II, transmission risk or evidence of risk factors for these infections.

History of chronic, systemic autoimmune disease that could have a detrimental effect on the quality of the tissue to be retrieved.

Indications that test results of donor blood samples will be invalid due to:
(a) the occurrence of haemodilution, according to the specifications in Annex II, section 2, where a pre-transfusion sample is not available; or
(b) treatment with immunosuppressive agents.

Evidence of any other risk factors for transmissible diseases on the basis of a risk assessment, taking into consideration donor travel and exposure history and local infectious disease prevalence.

Presence on the donor's body of physical signs implying a risk of transmissible disease(s) as described in Annex IV, point 1.2.3.

Ingestion of, or exposure to, a substance (such as cyanide, lead, mercury, gold) that may be transmitted to recipients in a dose that could endanger their health.

Recent history of vaccination with a live attenuated virus where a risk of transmission is considered to exist.

Transplantation with xenografts.

have not been breast-fed by their mothers during the previous 12 months and for whom analytical tests, physical examinations, and reviews of medical records do not provide evidence of HIV, hepatitis B, hepatitis C, or HTLV infection may be accepted as donors. This was, in part, a recommendation made in the Centers for Disease Control and Prevention's (CDC) original guidance on the prevention of HIV transmission by tissue transplantation [10].

Very few studies have been published that critically review the medical history and behavioral risk assessment questionnaires being used in organ, tissue, and eye donation. It is not fully understood whether the formats being used provide expected results and add sufficient value to donor screening. There is a project currently being undertaken by the American Association of Tissue Banks with others to develop a uniform donor history questionnaire for organ, tissue, and eye donation by using a format developed by the AABB and recommended by the United States Food and Drug Administration for blood donation. By using survey design experts in conjunction with the evaluation of carefully constructed cognitive interviewing methods and focus group interview studies, the blood bank profession in the United States has qualified a new donor history questionnaire. To be effective, this questionnaire is used in conjunction with accompanying flow-charts for the interviewer to follow for each question, a user brochure, a medication deferral list, and an education form for the donor. These studies support the use of short, direct questions as well as the use of capture questions that are more general and broad but become more detailed if an initial yes answer is provided. Another finding was that medical personnel tend to use medical terms that the general public may not understand; so word selection has changed. To obviate memory and recollection of events, questions should be arranged in sequential time so the historian mentally travels from now to pertinent history during periods of time in their past that could be relevant to disease risk as we know or perceive it. These proven concepts should be used when screening all donors of blood, cells, organs, tissues, or eyes and is a goal to be pursued.

Emerging diseases and the need for horizon scanning to detect new risks

With the introduction of formal adverse event and reaction reporting in Europe [8] and similar initiatives in the United States [11,12] and Canada [13], the reporting of these events has become mandatory. In the EU, they must be reported nationally to competent authorities and, hence, to the European Commission, allowing the identification of trends and the implementation of corrective and preventative action. Such action may result in evidence-based improvements in donor screening and questions being asked when obtaining a donor's history to assess risk. Identifying emerging risks and rare events will become easier when large numbers of institutions report together so that learning will be faster than if it relied on individuals identifying trends from smaller numbers of donors and use of fewer allografts. This will be particularly relevant to preventing transmission of emerging diseases and the need for horizon scanning to detect new risks. It may also contribute to the detection of reemergence of old diseases, such as tuberculosis, which is particularly relevant. Improving proper recognition of tissue-related adverse outcomes, including educating end users to report them, is a key to the success that this surveillance can offer. Lack of recognition of disease transmission and subsequent communication was evident in cases 2 and 4 described in the following discussion. Vigilance is an attitude that can drive such success.

Obtaining history for different types of donors

While the evaluation of some donor risks should be the same independent of the type of donor, the challenges posed and the methods applied are different depending on the donor type – particularly whether the donor is alive or deceased. Also, some risks will only be pertinent to some types of donation.

In the case of living donors, the situation is very similar to blood donation. The donor is a willing participant in the process, can provide a detailed medical history during a face-to-face interview, and can exclude himself or herself from donation when he or she becomes aware that some aspect of his or her lifestyle or medical history poses a risk, however small. Questions about recent travel, risk behavior involving drugs, previous medical treatment, recent travel history, and sexual behavior all need to be discussed. These donor interviews should be conducted following a predefined structured questionnaire to ensure that every known risk is addressed. The wording of questions needs to be carefully considered to ensure optimal understanding. The potential donor's confidentiality should be protected during this process, both to ensure good ethical practice and to encourage truthful and complete disclosure of relevant information.

In the case of hematopoietic stem cell donors, the risks that are shared with other types of donor, such as risk for hepatitis and HIV, will also exist. However, there may be other risks associated with this type of donation that only pertain to hematopoietic stem cell transplantation. In these cases, for example, a recipient receiving a bone marrow donation in order to treat his or her own sickle-cell disease or thalassemia might obtain a better transplant result if the donor did not carry a trait for the same condition. For this reason, the medical history of a hematopoietic stem cell donor should include a history of familial hematologic abnormalities. The same applies to bone marrow transplantation used to treat metabolic disorders or immune deficiencies. In cases of related donation of hematopoietic stem cells, either through bone marrow, cord blood, or peripheral blood stem cells, there is a one in four chance that any two individuals with the same parents will have a tissue type match, but if the patient to be treated has a recessive hemato-logic or immunologic condition, then there is also a risk that the donor may share the same genetic risk for that disorder and needs to be excluded as a carrier or as a sufferer of the same condition. Not all genetic diseases will have the same severity in all individuals in the same family, e.g. a patient with sickle-cell disease may have a sibling with a matching bone marrow but an unrecognized form of the same genetic disorder. A careful donor assessment may elicit these findings.

In the case of cord blood donation, the assessment of the donor at birth may not identify diseases that present after birth and there should always be the opportunity for the family to provide information back to the cord blood bank, in the case of unrelated donations and also in the case where a related cord blood donation is made. In these instances, the donor of the cord blood may not prove suitable for use for another individual, but might be appropriately stored in case, at some time in the future, gene therapy (for example, if the donor has an immunologic condition) becomes a reality and may be pertinent to the donor of the cord blood. Donor selection in such instances requires there to be an opportunity for the donor family to provide late donor information back to the banking institution so that cord blood can be removed from the general inventory for use by others, but may be maintained in an autologous bank for potential future use.

Late donor information may be relevant to stored material, not only in the context of cord blood, but also in any tissue inventory that has a long shelf life. Tissue banks and hematopoietic stem cell banks and bone marrow donor registries need to be able to review their inventories and take appro-priate action in light of late donor information becoming available as part of the management of donor selection information. There are other circum-stances where particular information may be relevant as highlighted by the special requirements for donor selection in donors of gametes. Very exten-sive genetic information is sought in these circumstances and the process is subject to some of the challenges that are described in Chapter 12, "Ethical and Consent Issues in the Reproductive Setting: The Case of Egg, Sperm, and Embryo Donation."

Obtaining an accurate donor history for a deceased donor is a considerably more complicated and challenging task. The range of circumstances is very broad: brain death in the intensive care unit of a hospital followed by organ and tissue donation, death on a hospital ward or in the accident and emer-gency department, death on the road with the body moved immediately to a forensic department or a mortuary, or death in the home or in a long-term care facility. In these various circumstances, someone must identify and contact the most relevant individual(s) who can quickly provide a history that will be equivalent, in terms of accuracy, to that provided by a living donor on their own behalf.

In general, best practice in these circumstances is to use a number of sources of information until a picture can be formed of the risk posed by the potential donor.

CASE 2

The importance of documenting the volume of blood and fluids given

In August of 1986, in Winston-Salem, North Carolina [14], a patient with brain trauma was admitted following a severe traffic accident and became an organ donor. Because of hemodynamic instability and blood loss, he received a total of 56 units of blood components (whole blood, packed red blood cells, plasma, and platelets), and possibly some colloids and crystalloids, all within 11 hours of admission. After surgery, prognosis was poor, brain death was declared, and he became a candidate for organ donation. During screening procedures applied at that time for organ donation, no identified risk factors for infectious or malignant disease were provided by the donor's parents.

Blood was collected and tested and the HIV antibody test (HTLV-III), along with tests for hepatitis and syphilis, were negative. Within 48 hours, three organs were being recovered and before the second kidney was implanted, the organization involved with the transplantation of the liver received results of infectious disease tests they had rerun. This blood sample was collected during the recovery of the liver and it tested highly reactive for HTLV-III Ab (three times higher than the cut-off value for a negative test). This was immediately communicated to all transplant centers and the organ procurement agency, and halted the transplantation of the remaining kidney. (The HTLV-III Ab test was used as the HIV test of that time.)

Within 10–12 weeks, two organ recipients (liver and one kidney) developed HIV infection (the recipient of the transplanted heart did not survive the operation). An investigation by the CDC uncovered that the original testing that was performed was flawed because the blood sample used was collected soon after massive amounts of blood transfusions had been administered, rendering the blood sample too dilute for accurate testing to be performed. This original sample that tested negative was retested by two laboratories and again tested negative for HIV Ab as well as negative using the Western blot assay.

A different blood sample was found that had been collected from the donor upon admission, prior to massive blood transfusions, and it tested highly reactive for HIV Ab and was confirmed by Western blot testing. This was the first documented discovery that transfusions had diluted the patient's plasma and thus masked the presence of HIV antibodies in the donor's blood.

Of further interest in this case, although not reported in the literature, was that the donor sustained massive head injuries after wrecking his car when being pursued during a high-speed police chase. Dealing illicit drugs was known to be a reason for the pursuit and possibly a link to the positive infectious disease test results that the two blood samples, drawn days apart, had shown. This case not only demonstrated that an infectious donor can receive transfusion and infusion therapy to the point of diluting circulating antibody to nondetection by testing, but also showed that this antibody level may return to a detectable level in a few days.

This three-sample blood collection/testing example of "positive, negative, positive," occurring over a specific time period of two days, drives current plasma dilution evaluation algorithms used by tissue banks worldwide. To date, a plasma dilution calculation is not generally mandated for organ donor evaluation.

From this case, the lessons of plasma dilution were learned. Since the incident was published, the assessment of hemodilution has become a routine step in the evaluation of tissue donor suitability. Details of blood, blood products, and other infusions given in the 48 hours prior to death or blood sampling (whichever is earlier) are recorded, and algorithms are used to evaluate the risk that the degree of plasma dilution might be sufficient to hide a marker of a transmissible viral infection. The requirement to include this in the donor medical history assessment is now incorporated into professional guidelines, and it has been mandated in regulations in the United States, Canada, Australia, and the EU.

Who should ask for the donor history?

It is essential that those who collect and collate donor history be appropriately trained for the task and have the communication and interpersonal skills to carry out this work effectively. This is particularly true in the case of deceased donor evaluation when families must often be interviewed in very painful circumstances.

Transplant coordinators who speak to potential organ donor families may have the opportunity to spend some time with the family in the intensive care unit and to develop a relationship that can help facilitate the donor history interview. Those that interview the family or partner of someone who died suddenly, perhaps in a road accident, will not have that opportunity and will have to communicate with people who may be in deep shock and who are often physically separated from the potential donor – indeed, the interview may have to be conducted by telephone. These challenging circumstances should not be used as an excuse to shorten, simplify, or avoid the interview. The coordinator's task is to conduct the interview thoroughly, ensuring that the family has understood what is required in terms of information and how important the accuracy of their responses is. Interviewers need to keep in mind that, although families may be very distressed, they are participating because they (or their deceased relative) want to help others, so the interests of the potential recipients are also their interests.

Given the challenging nature of this kind of donor information gathering, it is not generally appropriate to ask hospital staff to obtain donor information from the families of potential donors. They may play an essential role in the initial identification of potential donors and in establishing that the family wishes to speak to a professional about donation, but the detailed deceased donor family interview should be carried out by dedicated professionals trained for this role.

Who represents the best source of deceased donor history?

An interview with the next of kin or partner of the donor is a key step in the process. Even if the next of kin is not familiar with intimate details of the potential donor's behaviors in life, or in recent years, he or she can often provide details of a person who could provide more accurate information – perhaps a friend or a flatmate. The first question to be asked of a family member who has given consent may be "Will you be able to give me detailed information about his or her life or is there someone else that I should also speak to?" This is particularly important where the next of kin is a parent and the donor is an adult. The important message to convey is that the information required is detailed, and sometimes intimate, but crucially important for ensuring the safety of potential recipients. Donors and their families are participating in the process through a simple motivation to help others. In this context, it would be irrational for them to provide false information or withhold information as long as they understand that the information, as much as the donation itself, is for the benefit of potential recipient patients. Here also, a predefined questionnaire should be used to ensure completeness and consistency. A predefined questionnaire also offers the opportunity for the donor family member participating in the discussion to appreciate that all the questions are asked universally of all donor families and that the request for information is not designed to be different in their individual circumstances. The interview should be frank, and confidentiality should be protected.

Another important source of donor history is the family doctor, who can provide complementary information or confirmation of details already recorded. For "tissue-only" donors, there is adequate time for the family doctor to be contacted; indeed, this could be done even after tissue retrieval, if it is a secondary source of information. If the donor died in a hospital, the medical history notes must be checked for relevant information.

Physical examination of the donor prior to tissue retrieval is a further important source of donor history. The donor's body may provide evidence of behavior that poses an infection risk, e.g. drug injection, tattooing, or anal intercourse. Scars may point to previous surgery that can be significant and skin lesions may represent symptoms of transmissible illness. Physical examination should be carried out systematically by trained individuals and should be recorded on standardized documents. The findings of a physical examination might, in some circumstances, indicate the need to recontact the donor family or partner for further information. In those circumstances where a postmortem examination is to be undertaken, the physical assessment will be more comprehensive and will also include information about the internal organs of the donors. Where a postmortem examination is undertaken, the findings of that examination are an essential part of the donor medical history and selection but this does not preclude the need for tissue recovery personnel to document a thorough assessment of the donor.

In general, where no next of kin or partner of a deceased potential donor is available for interview, the donation should not proceed, unless there are special circumstances that mean that another individual can be identified as having the required very intimate knowledge of the potential donor.

CASE 3

The Donor Questionnaire and the importance of tissue traceability

In October of 1985 in Virginia, an innocent man was shot during a petrol station robbery. He became a donor of organs and tissues, which were transplanted to 50 recipients. In the weeks following the transplant, two organ recipients experienced complications related to "immune deficiency," but since they were being treated, as usual, with immunosuppressive therapy, a link to the donor was not evident. When three organ recipients showed seroconversion for HIV, risk in two patients was attributed to receipt of blood transfusions before 1985 from untested blood donors. Only one recipient met the established criteria and was reported to the state health department as an AIDS case, but no formal system was in place to link these events to the common donor. No report to the regional tissue or eye bank was made from the organ transplant system or from the health department.

A few years later, in 1991, a report to the tissue bank revealed a physician's concern that his asymptomatic, elderly patient had been found to have seroconverted, testing positive for the antibodies to HIV. She had no known medical or behavioral risk factors for HIV with the exception of receiving a tissue graft during hip replacement surgery in December of 1985. The graft was a minimally processed, fresh-frozen femoral head, and as the tissue bank investigated the report, it became apparent that the bone graft was recovered from the same donor who had also provided organs in 1985. The tissue bank requested information regarding the organ recipients from the transplant center programs. The aforementioned descriptions of the recipients were relayed and the donor became identified as the common source. The donor had tested negative for HIV antibodies (anti-HTLV-III) twice using two blood samples collected at different times during his hospital course and testing was performed at two different laboratories. (The HTLV-III Ab test was used as the HIV test of that time and is not to be confused with the HIV Antibody tests used today.) The investigation revealed that plasma dilution was not a factor when testing blood samples as the donor had received only two units of plasma protein fraction (albumin), some crystalloids, and no blood or blood products during the hospital admission.

No serum or plasma samples had been archived by the organ procurement agency or the tissue bank, but, using a section of frozen donor spleen that was located in the freezer at the tissue typing laboratory, donor lymphocytes cultured positive for HIV-1 and also tested positive by polymerase chain reaction (PCR) methods. Neither of these tests was available at the time of donation six years earlier. Another new test, the p24 antigen for HIV, was performed using donor cells but these results were indeterminate. Bone marrow from the donor's lumbar vertebrae was also donated, and these frozen cells were located and used for some disease testing during this investigation.

Of the 48 recipients identified, 41 were tested, and 7 were positive for HIV. These included the four organ recipients plus two who received fresh-frozen femoral head allografts and one who received a fresh-frozen patellar ligament. After an extremely thorough investigation, which included interviewing friends and relatives, and testing friends and some sexual partners, the donor was not identified as having any risk factors for HIV. He was reported to be a patron of men's clubs (striptease bars), which is a history that, today, is still not recognized as a behavioral risk associated with HIV. This 22-year-old donor's parents were the historians when initially interviewed for the risk assessment.

In this case, an early generation HIV test missed an HIV infection in a donor who may have had risk factors in his lifestyle, but which were not available or apparently not obvious enough to be appreciated at the time of donation. Since this incident was published [15], organ and tissue donor medical history and behavioral risk assessment questionnaires developed into formats using long, detailed questions, which are read in entirety. Although this format was not qualified or verified as being effective, it became the method widely used at the present time.

Another outcome was a rejuvenated focus on training needed for organ and tissue donation specialists who administer risk assessment interviews to donor historians. Such professional educational programs heighten awareness about the potential for disease transmission and improve knowledge regarding the safeguard expectations of this critical step during donor screening.

A further lesson learned from this incident was the value of routine archiving of serum and plasma if any remain after all testing has been completed. There was a renewed recognition of the importance of the association of disease in an allograft recipient with the tissue transplant as well as the identification of subsequent reporting and communication gaps.

How much investigation (police work) must be done?

Part of the training of a health professional who is gathering potential donor information is to know how to decide whether the information gathered is adequate and reliable and when more investigation should be carried out. Coordinators can find themselves asking "Should I speak to the surgeon who carried out this procedure five years ago to confirm that there was no malignancy?" or "Should I interview the neighbors of this man who lived alone to know who called regularly to his home – were there young men among the callers?" In some cases, the coordinator can begin to feel like a private investigator! This is a question of judgement and experience, but there are some useful indicators. A reassuring sign is when the same information is repeated from different sources. A warning sign is when there are unanswered questions or inconsistent details emerging. Professionals working in donor selection should always have access to support from a peer group and expert advice to help with decisions of this nature. Such peer groups not only provide expert advice to deal with individual cases, but also provide a means of supporting a professional working in difficult circumstances (see Chapter 9 "Facilitating Donation – The Role of Key Stakeholders: The medical examiner, the coroner, the hospital pathologist, and the funeral director").

CASE 4

The importance of understanding risk behaviors

A more recent case, also in the United States, demonstrated that a donor with undetected hepatitis C viremia may infect several recipients [16]. The donor was a man in his 40s with a history of hypertension and heavy alcohol use who had died of an intracranial hemorrhage in October 2000. In this case, 91 tissues and organs had been recovered from the donor and 40 patients received transplants in 22 months. The donor was anti-hepatitis C virus (anti-HCV) negative but was HCV RNA positive (genotype 1a) (test performed after the transmissions were reported using PCR [or nucleic acid technology]). HCV transmission occurred in eight recipients: three of three organ recipients, one of two saphenous vein recipients, one of three tendon recipients, and three of three tendon with bone recipients. These eight recipients had viral isolates genetically related to those of the donor. This case also demonstrates that there are inherent limitations to obtaining an accurate history for organ or tissue donor as it is from someone other than the donor. It is also understood in a general sense that many people do not understand which behaviors can pose a risk for infectious diseases such as HIV and viral hepatitis.

Who decides donor suitability?

In general, the final decision regarding donor suitability should be made by a medical doctor or, in certain circumstances with the appropriate audit mechanisms and control measures, by a clinician or nurse specifically trained to undertake the task and to seek help from a supervising medical officer. In the latter case, both must be specialized in the field of donation and trained in the professional and regulatory requirements for donor selection. There should be no conflict of interest in deciding whether a potential donor is suitable and with meeting donor recruitment targets. There should be a clear distinction between history gathering and decision making, although the history gatherer should be competent to know when to put a stop to the process to avoid wasting time and resources. The final evaluation of all the donor information collected, not just history but also test results and possibly autopsy findings, should be a clearly defined step carried out by individuals with professional responsibility for that task. They should carry it out following a defined procedure and should record the process in a standard way. This defined donor evaluation procedure should be regularly audited against standards and peer reviewed to ensure consistency and high standards are followed. There will always be individual cases that fall outside of standards because every donor case is different, and important learning opportunities arise from such cases, which may influence policies and procedures at the facility, national, and international levels.

Risk management in donor selection

Donor selection is essentially an exercise in risk management. When the potential donor had traveled to an area with an endemic disease, or received a treatment indicating a possible underlying disease, or has a positive marker for past infection with syphilis, someone must identify and assess the risk, consider if there are risk mitigating steps that can be applied (e.g. conduct additional blood tests, contact a treating physician for more information), and consider whether the residual risk is acceptable, given the potential benefit.

The first question that must always be asked is "What could go wrong and what is the hazard?" The severity or impact of the hazard needs to be assessed (*Could it cause death or serious injury? How many people might be harmed?*) along with the probability, or likelihood, that it might happen (*What are the chances that tissue processed in this way might transmit this agent? Has it ever happened before?*). The total risk is the severity times the probability. Quantitative scores can be allocated to these judgements to allow comparison. Scores can be reduced by introducing mitigating steps (e.g. additional tests, tissue sterilization steps).

In general, only very low risk is acceptable for tissue or cell transplantation. An elevated risk is acceptable in circumstances where the transplant might be lifesaving and there are no safer alternatives, e.g. where bone marrow cells from a donor who has had malaria are the only tissue type match for a recipient in urgent need of transplant and facing death if no matching donor is found. When elevated risks are to be taken, the potential recipient and the recipient's physician should participate in the risk assessment.

Risk assessment is a useful tool to help ensure that decisions about donor suitability are taken in a consistent and rational way and to provide the kind of documentation that regulators want to see. However sophisticated the procedure for deciding on donor suitability may be, it should never be forgotten that donor selection criteria are only as good as the donor medical and behavioral history information on which they are based.

KEY LEARNING POINTS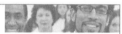

- Tissue donor selection is a risk reduction process, which ideally precedes testing of the donor and which may highlight the risks of transmissible disease that cannot be realized by testing alone.

- Donor selection on the basis of medical and behavioral history gathered by trained professionals is recognized as an essential step in the donation process.

- Donor and donor family interviews should be conducted following a predefined structured questionnaire to ensure that every known risk is addressed.

- Gathering medical and behavioral history in the context of deceased donation poses particular challenges. The family doctor, hospital notes, physical examination, and autopsy findings are important sources of complementary or confirmatory information.

- Where no individual who knew the potential donor well is available for interview, the donation should not generally proceed.

- Final evaluation of all the donor information collected should be a clearly defined step carried out by an individual with professional responsibility for that task. There should be no conflict of interest in the decision to accept or reject a potential donation.

- There should be systems in place for the management of donation inventories in the case where a donor risk is identified "late," i.e. after the donation has been procured or released.

- Professional education programs for those interviewing donors or their families are essential to heighten awareness about the potential for disease transmission.

- Professionals working in donor selection should have access to support from a peer group and expert advice.
- Scientific and professional associations play an important role in implementing guidelines for donor selection, and regulators build minimum requirements for donor selection into binding laws for the protection of public health.
- Vigilance and surveillance are a crucial aspect in identifying risk and preventing potential disease transmission.
- Risk assessment is a useful tool to help ensure that decisions about donor suitability are taken in a consistent and rational way and to provide the kind of documentation that regulators want to see.
- Professionals learn from mistakes and incidents, and application of this knowledge will improve quality and safety of human substances for transplantation.

References

1. Tullo AB, Buckely RJ, Kelly T, Head MW, Bennett P, Armitage WJ, et al. Transplantation of ocular tissue from a donor with sporadic Creutzfeldt-Jacob disease. Clin Experiment Ophthalmol. 2006;34(7):645–9.
2. Moffatt SL, Pollock GA. Creutzfeldt-Jacob disease: perceptions and realities of risk. Clin Experiment Ophthalmol. 2006;34(7):635–6.
3. Eastlund T, Strong DM. Infectious disease transmissions through tissue transplantation. In: Phillips GO, Kearney JN, Strong DM, vonVersen R, Nather A. Advances in Tissue Banking. Volume 7. Singapore: World Scientific. 2003;51–131.
4. Eastlund T. Bacterial infection transmitted by human tissue allograft transplantation. Cell and Tissue Banking 2006;7(3):116–47.
5. Griffiths PD. Transmission of viruses with human allografts. Rev Med Virol. 2007;17(2):147–9.
6. Directive 2004/23/EC of the European Parliament and of the Council of 31 March 2004 on setting standards for quality and safety in the donation, procurement, processing, preservation, storage and distribution of human tissues and cells. Official Journal of the European Union L. 2004 Apr 7;102/48.
7. Commission Directive 2006/17/EC of 8 February 2006 implementing Directive 2004/23/EC of the European Parliament and of the Council as regards certain technical requirements for the donation, procurement and testing of human tissues and cells. Official Journal of the European Union L. 2006 Feb 9;38/40–38/52.
8. Commission Directive 2006/86/EC of 24 October 2006 implementing Directive 2004/23/EC of the European Parliament and of the Council as regards traceability requirements, notification of serious adverse reactions and events, and certain technical requirements for the coding, processing, preservation, storage and distribution of human tissues and cells. Official Journal of the European Union L. 2006 Oct 25;294/32.

9. US Department of Health and Human Services, Food and Drug Administration. Final guidance for industry: eligibility determination for donors of human cells, tissues, and cellular and tissue-based products (HCT/Ps). August 2007. http://www.fda.gov/cber/gdlns/tissdonor.pdf (accessed June 2, 2007).

10. Centers for Disease Control and Prevention. Guidelines for preventing transmission of human immunodeficiency virus through transplantation of human tissue and organs. MMWR 1994;43(RR-8):1–17.

11. FDA. Guidance for industry. http://www.fda.gov/cber/gdlns/advhctp.htm (accessed June 2, 2007).

12. The Transplantation Transmission Sentinel Network. http://www.unos.org/news/newsDetail.asp?id = 754 (accessed June 2, 2007).

13. Health Canada. Regulations and guidance for cells, tissues, and organs. 2007. http://www.hc-sc.gc.ca/dhp-mps/compli-conform/info-prod/cell/index_e.html (accessed June 2, 2007).

14. Centers for Disease Control and Prevention. Human immunodeficiency virus infection transmitted from an organ donor screened for HIV antibody – North Carolina. MMWR. 1987;36(20);306–8.

15. Simonds RJ, Holmberg SD, Hurwitz RL, Coleman TR, Bottenfield S, Conley LJ, et al. Transmission of human immunodeficiency virus type 1 from a seronegative organ and tissue donor. N Engl J Med. 1992;326(5):726–32.

16. Tugwell BD, Patel PR, Williams IT, Hedberg K, Chai F, Nainan OV, et al. Transmission of hepatitis C virus to several organ and tissue recipients from an antibody-negative donor. Ann Intern Med. 2005;143(9):648–54.

6 The Role of Testing in Determining Suitability of Donors and Tissues

Paolo Grossi[1] and Michael Strong[2]

[1] University of Insubria, Varese, Italy; Italian National Transplant Centre, Rome, Italy
[2] Northwest Tissue Center/Puget Sound Blood Center, Seattle, Washington, USA

Introduction

Viral, bacterial, prion, and fungal infections have been transmitted via tissue allografts such as bone, tendon, skin, cornea, dura mater, pericardium, blood vessels, and heart valves [1]. Over the past several years, improvements in tissue donor suitability requirements and donor blood testing have greatly reduced this risk. For example, improved tissue banking standards and practices currently in place would have prevented previously reported cases of disease transmission that resulted from the use of hemodiluted blood samples for infectious disease testing (there have been human immunodeficiency virus [HIV] transmissions by organs because of hemodilution), accepting donors with behavioral risks for HIV infection, and using early generation, less sensitive tests for HIV and hepatitis C virus (HCV) antibodies. The recent availability of viral nucleic acid testing (NAT) has further reduced the risk of disease transmission by detecting the early stages of HIV and HCV infection before antibody tests are positive.

In addition to donor testing, there are several other tissue bank processes responsible for the low risk of disease transmission that exists today. A review of the donor medical and behavioral history is undertaken to exclude donors with risky behaviors for HIV and hepatitis, and other diseases for which donors are not tested such as Creutzfeldt–Jakob disease, malignancies, and other recent infections that are potentially transmissible. During tissue processing, many, but not all, allografts are exposed to antibiotics, disinfectants,

Tissue and Cell Donation: An Essential Guide. Edited by Ruth M. Warwick, Deirdre Fehily, Scott A. Brubaker, Ted Eastlund. © 2009 Blackwell Publishing, ISBN: 978-14051-6322-4.

and sterilization steps such as gamma irradiation, which further reduce or remove the risk for disease transmission. It is critically important to minimise bacterial and fungal contamination, by using aseptic surgical technique in conjunction with maintaining a controlled environment during critical steps. This is important when removing tissue from the donor, during processing and storage, as well as during implantation.

In this chapter, donor blood testing, its rationale, the challenges associated with testing in general, bacterial and fungal testing of tissues and new technologies for viral and bacterial testing are discussed.

What is tested for and what is not? – what is the rationale?

Tissue transplantation therapy is a rapidly developing field improving the health and saving the lives of many. Voluntary donations by screened and tested individuals have made tissue transplantation quite safe. One drawback, however, is the potential for transmission of infectious diseases. Cases of tissue-transplant-transmitted HIV and HCV infections of donor origin have occurred, illustrating the limitations of donor testing. During the past two decades, the disease transmission risk associated with tissue transplantation has been greatly reduced by the implementation of testing requirements set by professional organizations, such as the American Association of Tissue Banks (AATB), the European Association of Tissue Banks (EATB), the Eye Bank Associations of America and of Europe (EBAA and EEBA), and governmental regulations and statutes of the United States Food and Drug Administration (US FDA), United Kingdom Code of Practice for Tissue Banking, Canadian National Standards for Cells, Tissues and Organs, European Commission Directives, and Australia's Therapeutic Goods Administration (TGA). In addition, new tests with improved sensitivity have also played an important role in reducing the risk.

The donor tests listed in Table 6.1 are requirements of the AATB [2], EBAA [3], and EATB [4] and are used by tissue banks in the United States, Canada, Australia, Europe, and countries worldwide to reduce the risk of transmitting communicable diseases. Donor testing requirements and safety requirements to reduce microbial contamination of tissues are fairly uniform, but there are variations in the national regulations and statutes set by the US FDA [5,6], Canada [7], European Union [8–10], and the Australian TGA [11]. Testing must be carried out by a qualified laboratory, e.g. certified under Clinical Laboratory Improvement Amendments (CLIA) in the United States or local regulatory agencies, using US FDA-approved or European Community (EC)-marked testing kits, where appropriate. The type of test used must be validated for the purpose in accordance with the requirements.

Table 6.1 Tissue donor blood testing

---

1 HIV, type 1; HIV, type 2: antibody screening test or combination test for anti-HIV-1 and anti-HIV-2 is required.* In some countries, screening nucleic acid testing (NAT) for HIV-1 RNA, or combination NAT for HIV and hepatitis C virus (HCV), is performed.**
2 Hepatitis B virus (HBV): screening test for hepatitis B surface antigen and for total antibody detecting IgG and IgM to hepatitis B core antigen.
3 HCV: screening test for anti-HCV is required. In some countries, screening NAT for HCV RNA, or combination NAT for HCV and HIV is performed.**
4 *Treponema pallidum* (screening test)
5 Anti-HTLV-I/II***

---

*US tissue establishments not utilizing a United States Food and Drug Administration (US FDA)-licensed screening test that detects group O must defer donors at risk for HIV group O infection [5]. Donors at risk are persons – or their sexual partners – who were born or lived in certain countries in Africa (Cameroon, Central African Republic, Chad, Congo, Equatorial Guinea, Gabon, Niger, or Nigeria) after 1977, or persons who have received a blood transfusion or any medical treatment that involved blood in the listed countries. For tissue establishments outside of the United States, requirements vary.
**US tissue establishments are required to perform a US FDA-licensed NAT for HIV RNA and HCV RNA. For tissue establishments outside of the United States, requirements vary.
***Requirements varies among countries, but a common requirement is that tissue donors are required to be tested for HTLV-I and HTLV-II Human T Lymphotrophic virus antibodies. Being a leukocyte-associated virus, testing is especially relevant for viable, leukocyte-rich cell donations, including reproductive cells or tissues if they are considered to be viable and leukocyte rich. Testing requirements vary in some countries, e.g. Australian Therapeutic Goods Association requires testing for tissue donors but not for cornea donations. In the EU, testing is required for donors from high incidence areas or with partners or parents from those areas.

Viral testing

The earliest methods that were widely used for diagnosing viral infections detected antibodies or antigens. Blood testing for viral antibodies is still widely employed for donor testing. It is important to use sensitive assays for this purpose because antibody levels are low during the early phase of an infection and levels may also decline to low levels later, years after the infection. The assay used should also have good specificity so that false-positive rates are low. This is important to prevent loss of potentially lifesaving tissue grafts in scarce supply. When available, only assays licensed by regulatory authorities for donor screening should be used, to assure optimal sensitivity and specificity and predictive value.

Rapid viral screening became a practical reality during the 1980s as laboratories implemented monoclonal-antibody-based assays to detect a wide variety of viral antigens and antibodies. The sensitivity of viral testing of tissue donors has greatly advanced in the past few years by the application of NAT. These techniques detect specific nucleic acid sequences and can be applied to the detection of virtually any virus or groups of viruses. The latter characteristic is particularly advantageous because it allows NAT to be applied to groups, such as the enteroviruses, for which antigenic diversity has precluded successful application of antigen detection techniques. Nucleic acid amplification technology, including polymerase chain reaction (PCR) and transcription-mediated amplification (TMA), is increasingly used to detect numerous viruses and to assess prognosis, monitor response to treatment, and assess progression of infection. In the United States, NAT assays have been recently licensed for screening deceased donors for HIV RNA, HCV RNA, West Nile virus (WNV) RNA, and hepatitis B virus (HBV) DNA. As a consequence, testing for HIV and HCV RNA in the United States is routine and is also applied in some European countries or in individual establishments in those countries. Testing for WNV RNA and HBV DNA varies but is not routine in the United States, Canada, Europe, and other countries.

Seronegative infectious window period and the importance of NAT

Viral infections can be transmitted if the donor has a viral infection and the viral antibody or antigen levels are too low for detection. In asymptomatic donors who have been recently infected, a transient viremic phase can exist prior to the development of a positive donor screening test for antibodies (the infectious window period). Preventing donor-to-recipient infectious disease transmission relies heavily on ensuring safe donors not only through testing, but also by medical and behavioral screening to select donors without behaviors placing them at risk for recent infection and thus less likely to be in the infectious window period.

The incidence–window period model

The incidence–window period model for estimating residual risk was developed in the mid-1990s and in recent years has been widely used internationally to estimate the residual risk of transfusion-transmission of agents for which donor antibody testing is in place (e.g. HIV, HCV, and HBV). The prevalence rates of HBV, HCV, HIV, and HTLV infections are lower among tissue donors than in the general population. However, the estimated probability of undetected viremia at the time of tissue donation is significantly higher among tissue donors than among first-time blood donors. The addition of NAT to the screening of tissue donors can reduce the risk of these infections among recipients of donated tissues [12]. Table 6.2 summarizes the window periods for HIV, HBV, HCV, and HTLV infections.

Table 6.2 Window period for HIV, HBV, HCV, and HTLV infections by testing individual donations. Adapted from *New Engl J Med* [12]

Agent	Infectious window period (days)	
	Serology	Nucleic acid testing (NAT)
HIV	22	7
HBV	59	20
HCV	70	7
HTLV	51	?

Despite the improvement in detection of window period donors using nucleic acid testing (NAT), it is expected that infections may still be missed because of early infections and low viral copy numbers resulting in false-negative test results. A few cases of transfusion-transmitted HIV from donors tested negative by NAT have been reported, but this is a very rare event. Transmission of HIV or HCV through tissue transplantation from a NAT-negative donor is expected to occur even less frequently as so many tissues are processed, leukocyte free, disinfected, and often sterilized.

Stored blood samples for future viral testing

Testing of donor blood samples after storage for years can be important. There have been examples of HCV transmission by tissues from a donor tested and found negative for HCV antibodies using the first generation, relatively insensitive test with a long window period. Two years later, when a new generation, more sensitive test with a shorter window period was available, the tissue bank tested stored samples from donors with tissue remaining in the inventory. They found positive results, confirmed by NAT, and this led to discovering infected patients who had previously been transplanted with tissue from these donors [13].

The implementation of NAT for the detection of HCV and HIV-1 has undoubtedly contributed to the viral safety of blood transfusion and tissue transplantation. This screening increases the safety margin for allograft use by decreasing the "window period" not detectable by traditional antibody testing. As of March 9, 2005, the AATB required NAT for HIV-1 RNA and HCV RNA in tissue donors. NAT uses a highly sensitive PCR or TMA test for HIV and HCV. This requirement does not apply to tissues prepared before March 9, 2005 and currently stored in inventory by AATB-accredited banks. However, because of the testing stability of frozen blood samples, the testing of inventory could be performed. NAT for deceased donors is not required by the EU directives though it is often applied.

There are other advantages of saving stored samples from tissue donors. The recognition of emerging communicable disease agents or diseases, for which a donor screening test becomes available at a later date, requires the availability of a stored sample for donor testing. It is advisable to archive donor blood samples, with attention to validated storage conditions, to allow for further testing of tissues in inventory when new tests are required. New generation tests with improved sensitivity and new specificities for testing become available over time. This means tissue or cell inventories may need to be reviewed for future testing requirements; thus banking facilities need to develop policies for storing archive samples based on validated studies. This is particularly important for tissue or cells with long inventory lives, such as cord blood, where the donations may be kept for decades. Tissue and cell facilities also need policies for review of inventories when a significant change in donor selection or a new generation test is introduced or when new microbiological specificity is required to be tested.

Generally, frozen storage of donor blood samples does not adversely affect viral antibody testing, but multiple freeze–thaw cycles may affect HCV RNA testing [14,15]. One important matter related to the reliability of NAT is the effect of the storage conditions on the stability of viral RNA and DNA in the blood sample. Many authors have reported that the storage conditions of samples may affect the stability and, hence, the detectability of nucleic acid of viruses, although apparently discrepant conclusions have been drawn. Various factors may have an effect on nucleic acid stability, including shipping conditions and handling of samples. Furthermore, long-term storage conditions (samples stored at −70°C versus samples stored at −20°C) are of great importance to minimize logistics problems, especially at reference testing laboratories [16].

HTLV-I/II

Approximately 10–20 million individuals are estimated to be infected with HTLV-I worldwide. The virus is endemic in southwest Japan, the Caribbean islands, countries surrounding the Caribbean basin, parts of Central Africa, and South America. In Japan, about 1.2 million individuals are estimated to be infected by HTLV-I, and more than 800 cases of adult T-cell leukemia are diagnosed each year. It is thought that the virus is cell associated, being present in CD4+ lymphocytes, and is transmitted in these cells parenterally via blood or semen, or from mother to infant via breast milk. There have been reports of HTLV transmission through blood transfusion and one case reported of transmission through the use of a frozen bone allograft. Asymptomatic HTLV-I infection (antibody seroconversion) was transmitted by transplantation of a fresh-frozen unprocessed femoral head bone allograft donated by a person previously infected by blood transfusion [1,17].

In the United Kingdom, all tissue donors are tested for anti-HTLV-I/II. The EU Directive 2006/17/EC requires that HTLV-I antibody testing must be performed for donors living in, or originating from, high-incidence areas or with sexual partners originating from those areas or where the donor's parents originate from those areas [9]. In Australia, the TGA requires tissue donor testing for anti-HTLV except for cornea donations [11].

In the United States, the US FDA recommends that donors of viable, leukocyte-rich cells and tissues, including reproductive cells or tissues if they are considered to be viable and leukocyte rich, should be screened for antibodies to HTLV-I/II by a US FDA-licensed test labeled specifically for use in donor screening [6]. The AATB requires testing of tissue donors for anti-HTLV-I/II. In general, because confirmation tests and HTLV NAT have not been fully developed, donor acceptability has been based on results of antibody screening tests.

Treponema pallidum (syphilis)

Syphilis, caused by the spirochete *T. pallidum*, is a sexually transmitted infection with a worldwide distribution. There were a few cases of syphilis infection transmitted by transfusion of fresh blood decades ago, but there have been none transmitted by tissue transplantation. Although *T. pallidum* does not survive cold storage, but regulatory authorities continue to require it to be included in donor testing.

Donor screening tests for syphilis may be either nontreponemal or treponemal-based assays. These tests for syphilis are acceptable for use in donor screening. Because of the potential for false-positive results using nontreponemal assays in noninfected persons and persistently positive tests using treponemal-based assays after successful treatment for syphilis, US FDA-approved or cleared confirmatory testing may be used to determine the syphilis status of a potential tissue donor.

Nontreponemal assays, such as the venereal disease research laboratory test, the rapid plasma reagin test, and the automated reagin test, detect nonspecific antibodies (reagins) to an antigen called cardiolipin present in human tissues as well as in treponemes. Reactive tests may be a result of diseases other than syphilis (i.e. biological false positives). Nontreponemal test results usually become nonreactive within a year or two after successful treatment of syphilis. Samples that give positive or reactive results using nontreponemal assays may be retested using a treponemal-based assay as a confirmatory test.

Treponemal assays incorporate specific treponemal antigens into the testing system and detect specific antibodies to these antigens. With a few exceptions, unlike nontreponemal assays, the results of tests for treponemal antigens remain positive or reactive for specific antibodies throughout an individual's life, even after successful treatment for syphilis. Treponemal assays include the fluorescent treponemal antibody with absorption test (FTA-ABS), the *T. pallidum* immobilization test, and the *T. pallidum* hemagglutination assay. In general, treponemal assays have a higher sensitivity in detecting primary and late syphilis than do nontreponemal assays.

Because of the lack of specificity of nontreponemal donor screening tests, both the US FDA and the European Commission consider a donor to be eligible whose blood tests reactive (or positive) on a nontreponemal screening test for syphilis but negative or nonreactive on a confirmatory test, e.g. FTA-ABS, as long as all other required testing and screening results are negative or nonreactive. A donor whose specimen tests positive or reactive on a confirmatory test is not eligible per US FDA guidance, while the European Commission is more flexible and requires a thorough risk assessment to determine eligibility for clinical use. Syphilis testing is required for tissue donor testing in Australia but not for cornea donors.

Prion diseases

Transmissible spongiform encephalopathies (TSEs) are a group of animal and human brain diseases, including Creutzfeldt–Jakob disease (CJD) and variant CJD (vCJD), caused by prions. They are uniformly fatal and are often characterized by a long incubation period, multifocal neuronal loss, spongiform changes, and astrogliosis in the brain. Creutzfeldt–Jakob disease has been transmitted through transplantation of corneas and dura mater (Table 6.3). Because of the lack of reliable blood tests for TSE, preventing donor-to-recipient disease transmission relies heavily on selecting safe donors by evaluating medical history (i.e. screening for neurological symptoms and residency or travel history screening) and preventative measures relating to equipment, procurement, and processing. Regulatory authorities and professional standards have defined donor selection criteria [2–5]. For vCJD consideration, alternative analytes other than blood may be useful such as tissue from the reticuloendothelial system, e.g. tonsil and spleen. These may carry markers of abnormal prions [18].

Testing for bacteria and fungi

Although contaminated bone, tendon, cartilage, cornea, heart valve, skin, and pericardium allografts have all caused bacterial infections in recipients (Table 6.3), very few cases have been reported. Until recently, the threat to patients has been thought to be minimal. However, the prevalence of bacterial and fungal infectious disease transmission by various allografts has not yet been studied. The risk of bacterial and fungal transmission is greatest using heart valves, vessels, tendons, fresh cartilage, and cornea as they are not exposed to strong disinfectants or sterilization steps. Transmission of bacterial disease can occur from infected donors [19]. Exclusion of donors infected by bacteria, fungi, or mycobacteria is accomplished by excluding infected persons with signs or symptoms of infection. Specific tests for bacteremia in asymptomatic prospective tissue donors, such as blood cultures for bacteria and fungi, antemortem or postmortem, are not required but are used by some tissue banks even though their predictive value is unknown.

Bacterial contamination can also be acquired during surgical recovery of tissues from the donor or during tissue processing by the tissue bank, and it has been missed at the time of final sterility testing [20]. Microbiological

Table 6.3 Microbial diseases transmitted by tissue allografts [1]

Allograft	Infectious disease
Bone	Bacteria
	Mycobacteria
	Viruses
Tendon	Bacteria
	Viruses
Cartilage	Bacteria
Cornea	Bacteria
	Fungus
	Prions
	Viruses
Dura	Prions
Heart valve	Bacteria
	Mycobacteria
	Fungus
	Viruses
Skin	Bacteria
	Viruses
Pericardium	Bacteria

monitoring of each step of the tissue banking process should be performed. Monitoring for contamination of tissue during recovery or in the processing environment, along with using adequate and validated tissue sampling techniques and validation of final sterility testing methods, is essential. Bacterial testing has given false-negative tests at the time of recovery as a result of insensitive sampling methods, and at the time of final sterility testing as a result of the carryover of residues of antibiotics used during processing.

Aseptic surgical technique preferably in an environment in which the air quality is specified and controlled, when removing the tissue from the donor, when processing and storing the tissue, and during implantation, is critically important to prevent bacterial and fungal contamination. Procedures are in place at most tissue banks to control bacterial contamination, including environmental monitoring, disinfection, sterilization, and sterility testing. Despite much attention to these issues, no standard approach is used by all tissue banks, and there is great variability in the use of disinfection and sterilization steps and final sterility testing.

Most transplantable tissues such as corneas, bone, tendon, and skin are recovered from deceased donors after there has been complete cardiac and respiratory cessation for some time period. The collection of tissue allografts from the deceased donor should begin as soon as possible after death to reduce the risk of endogenous or exogenous bacterial contamination and to maintain functional characteristics or, in some cases, viability of the tissue. Professional standards generally require bone, tendon, and heart valve recovery to be performed within 12 hours of death if the body is not refrigerated or within 24 hours of death if the body is refrigerated. There is, however, variation in practice in different parts of the world, with some tissue facilities undertaking tissue recovery up to 48 hours after cessation of heartbeat, or even longer. This represents a risk of postmortem translocation or transmigration of bacteria from the intestines or respiratory system to other parts of the body prior to the tissue being removed for transplant purposes. It is recommended that the recovery procedures employed by tissue banks minimize the risks associated with translocation and transmigration of bacteria, including with regard to cooling of the deceased's body after death. As body cooling after death can be affected by numerous factors, limitations on the interval from the time of death to the time of tissue recovery, should be established and strictly followed.

Reducing the risk of bacterial and fungal contamination of tissue at the time of tissue recovery includes methods to cool the body and then taking specific steps to prevent contamination and cross contamination. Methods have been described to accomplish this, including the following: isolation draping of body areas with trauma; use of zone recovery techniques that utilize frequent sterile glove changes and sterile instruments dedicated to use with preestablished, specific body zones; and documenting the sequence of recovery so culture results for individual tissues can be better evaluated [20]. It is considered by many to be best practice to procure tissues before postmortem (autopsy) examination if the latter does take place.

The environment in which the tissue allograft is removed can also have an impact on microbial contamination. Tissues are removed at various environmental sites: hospital operating rooms, autopsy suites in hospital morgues, regional forensic medical examiner facilities, funeral homes, in dedicated tissue procurement facilities, at medical examiner facilities or tissue banks. Contamination by bacteria of low and high virulence is a common finding in tissues freshly removed for purposes of transplantation and is a common reason for not using donor tissue. This risk may be reduced by ensuring that the recovery site is as clean as possible. The cleanliness of the site where a tissue recovery takes place can be controlled by establishing site suitability requirements [20].

Bacterial testing should be performed on all tissues when first obtained from the deceased donor prior to temporary storage, exposure to antibiotics, or further processing. Sampling should, as a minimum, include swabbing the entire surface of a recovered tissue. For tissues that cannot be terminally sterilized, preprocessing bacterial testing is an essential first step to enable the tissue bank to detect and identify contaminants and discard tissues with virulent organisms. Tissue banks need policies to define which organisms found on the tissue prior to contamination are a reason to discard the tissue or to subject it to sterilizing techniques.

Tissue allografts can also become contaminated during processing at the tissue bank from environmental surfaces, air, personnel, contaminated reagents, surgical instruments, supplies, and processing equipment. Monitoring of trends in microbiological findings in tissue facilities and their environment, as well as in the donations themselves, is also needed to provide early warning of sources of potential contamination. Examples might include contaminated water supplies, other reagents, or environmental contaminants. Tissue establishments are expected to develop in-process controls that monitor the potential for contamination and cross-contamination during processing steps.

Testing for bacterial and fungal contamination by standard culturing techniques has its limits, and new, more sensitive methods with more rapid turnaround times are being developed. The use of PCR has promise for improved testing, and test kits are being developed, e.g. for mycobacterium. Amplification technology can also be used to target commonly shared bacterial 16S rRNA genes (via pan-bacterial primers), and subsequently, direct sequencing is used to detect and differentiate bacteria. These techniques could eventually be further developed and would represent an added benefit to conventional cultures to screen for bacteria that may contaminate tissues.

Mycobacterium infection has been transmitted by the use of frozen bone allograft. About 50 years ago, several cases of tuberculosis of the bone developed from the use of frozen rib allografts. The source of bone allograft was the rib resected during chest surgery in patients with active pulmonary tuberculosis, and this was not detected by swab and culture, demonstrating the need for validation of sampling techniques. Cases of miliary tuberculosis developing after receiving a human heart valve allograft have also been reported. There was suspicion that the source of the infection came from the implanted valves, and there was evidence that these cases arose from contamination during processing. Current donor exclusion criteria used by tissue banks include active or previously treated tuberculosis [21]. This exclusionary criterion is important because there is no blood screening test for tuberculosis with a good predictive value. Current requirements for final testing of human heart valves after processing include testing for contamination by mycobacterium and fungus.

Other communicable diseases and emerging infections

Infectious risks of tissue transplantation have usually been identified after first being recognized as blood transfusion transmitted infections. The American Association of Blood Banks (AABB) has compiled a list of 66 agents, including viruses, prions, rickettsia, protozoa, and nematodes, for which transfusion safety may be of concern. Several diseases that can be transmitted by transfusion and transplantation are prevalent only in limited geographic areas of the world and others have been spread to distant areas. Whether a communicable disease is relevant and tissue donors need screening depends on whether the infection causes disease, whether the disease is a threat in that specific geographic area, and whether tests are available. Global travel has resulted in infections usually prevalent in some parts of the world becoming transported to other unexpected areas.

Most recently, West Nile virus (WNV) infection has swept through the United States, with nearly 4,000 human cases identified and 254 deaths in 2002. In addition to being mosquito borne, WNV has been transmitted through organ transplantation, blood transfusion, transplacental intrauterine spread, and percutaneously from laceration and needlestick. No case of WNV transmission through tissue transplantation has been reported, and to date, donor risk assessment is based on gathering recent medical and clinical history. Nucleic acid testing for WNV RNA has been recently licensed for use in living and deceased cell and tissue donors, but donor testing has not become a requirement.

Malaria, babesia, and *Trypanosoma cruzi* transmissions have all been reported from parasitemic blood donors, but testing is not routine for tissue donors. Testing may be performed depending on whether there are increased risks in certain geographic regions with a high prevalence of the disease. Chagas' disease is caused by the trypanosome *T. cruzi*, is prevalent in Central and South America, and has been transmitted by transfusion and organ transplantation in the United States but not by tissue transplantation. The US FDA has announced its approval of an infectious disease test kit for screening certain donors for Chagas' disease. Its application for organ and tissue donors has been evolving and is used by some only when the donor has traveled to or lived in a geographic area where the disease is prevalent.

Quality of deceased-donor blood samples

Deceased donors are the principal source of tissues for transplantation. Assuring the microbiological safety of deceased donors is different from that of living donors, as a comprehensive medical and behavioral history cannot be obtained directly from the deceased donor and must be obtained from others. The role of blood testing, tissue processing, and disinfection is greater for ensuring safety of tissues derived from deceased donors.

When tissues are obtained from living donors or brain-dead, heart beating organ donors, the blood sample used for infectious disease testing may be of better quality than blood samples obtained postmortem from a deceased donor following complete cessation of the circulation. Postmortem samples may be hemolyzed and can contain substances that diminish with the accuracy of infectious disease testing. The testing of deceased tissue donors for evidence of blood- or tissue-borne viral infections raises two concerns: false-negative results with the possibility of transmission of undetected viral disease (lack of sensitivity) and false-positive results (lack of specificity), which render donated tissues unsuitable for use although they are not infectious. The testing of deceased-donor blood for viral markers may be complicated by false-positive tests when sampling is delayed after death or when there is hemolysis. False-positive results for hepatitis B surface antigen (HbsAg) as a result of hemolysis may be found, depending upon which manufacturer's test kit is used [22].

Postmortem degradation of the viral genome and the presence of hemoglobin and possibly other factors can cause false-negative results when testing for HIV, HBV, and HCV by NAT. Internal controls are provided to determine inhibition by these factors. Nucleic acid extraction methods can reduce this risk. A simple 1:5 dilution step of the blood sample appears to overcome this inhibition without significantly compromising sensitivity. Therefore, the recommended protocols include the use of a dilution step if the initial undiluted sample yields an inhibited result. In the case of PCR or TMA, a 1:5 dilution is suggested from the start on all samples [23,24]. Frozen storage and multiple freeze–thaw cycles do not have a major effect on the detectability of antibodies to infectious agents in serum but may reduce the reliability of NAT.

The testing of deceased tissue donors for viral markers in Europe is, in principle, the same as that applied to living tissue and blood donors [25]. However, commercial test kits for the detection of HBsAg, anti-HCV and anti-HIV 1 and 2, which are used for testing samples from cadavers, have generally not been evaluated for this purpose. Many kits are currently licensed for use with deceased-donor blood specimens by the US FDA, but these are not available in Europe [26].

Hemodilution of donor blood sample

Hemodilution of the blood sample as a cause of false-negative test results must be considered in deceased tissue and organ donors dying with blood loss and transfusion of blood products or infusion of colloids and crystalloids. Massive blood loss followed by intravascular volume replacement can cause hemodilution and result in unreliable donor test results for infectious diseases [27].

In 1993, US federal regulations were first published by the US FDA, with subsequent modification, requiring quarantine of tissue from adult donors who had blood loss and received greater than any combination of two liters of either blood and colloids within 48 hours of blood sampling or crystalloids within one hour of sampling. The donated tissue was not to be used unless a pretransfusion sample was available for testing or an algorithm was used by the tissue bank to evaluate the degree of haemodilution caused by blood, colloid, and crystalloid volumes administered prior to blood sampling. This was done to ensure that plasma dilution sufficient to alter test results had not occurred.

An algorithm can guide and simplify making a decision whether to accept a diluted blood sample for testing [5,27]. The algorithm should include decision making regarding whether blood loss had occurred. Regardless of the amount of blood, colloid, or crystalloids infused, the sensitivity of the donor testing should not be affected unless there is blood loss requiring the transfusion or infusion. The evaluation of the effects of dilution is based on the volume of blood, colloid, and crystalloid transfusions that were received in comparison to the donor's estimated blood volume. No one algorithm can be comprehensive enough to cover all possible variations of donor blood loss, transfusions, and sample testing. The AATB standards require tissue banks to follow written procedures setting hemodilution limits to prevent acceptance of false-negative results when testing posttransfusion blood samples for infectious disease. Acceptability limits must be part of written procedures. The tissue bank physician has a very important role in making final interpretations about the acceptance of blood samples from prospective donors, if there potentially has been blood loss. Determining tissue and organ donor suitability is an inexact science requiring physician judgement.

Testing of newborns

Testing of newborns less than one month of age for viral antibodies is not reliable because of the newborn's immature immune system, which is not capable of rapidly developing antibodies when exposed to infection in the uterus. Although some maternal IgG antibodies can pass through the placenta into the newborn's circulation, IgM antibodies, which develop first during early infection, are larger molecules and do not pass into the fetal circulation from the mother. For these reasons, if a prospective tissue donor is one month of age or younger, a blood sample from the birth mother must be collected, within seven days of donation, and tested, instead of or as well as testing the newborn donor's blood. If a blood sample from the birth mother of a donor one month of age or younger is unavailable, the donor is ineligible. Samples collected for evaluating an infant donor more than one month of age should be collected from the donor rather than the birth mother. Special consideration for testing any infant who is being breast-fed may still require testing of the mother.

Sample and donor identification issues

Accurate identification of tissue allografts is important to ensure full traceability and that the results of donor blood and tissues relate to the correct donor. Errors in blood sample, or other analyte, labeling can also result in erroneous blood testing, including ABO typing. The ABO compatibility between the donor and recipient is important in transplanting organs, but it is of uncertain importance in transplanting fresh tissue grafts or cryopreserved cardiovascular tissues. One of the most common causes of transfusion-related fatalities is a hemolytic reaction as a result of transfusion of the wrong blood to the wrong patient. Erroneously transplanting organs of incompatible ABO blood types has also caused fatalities.

Accuracy in blood sampling of the deceased donor first depends on being certain that the person being tested is indeed the actual donor. Blood samples should be labeled immediately after obtaining the sample and while in the presence of the donor to reduce the risk of mislabeling. The label must contain a unique identifier that will be applied to blood samples and tissues from the same donor. This unique identifier also permits traceability of tissues to the final recipient and backwards from the recipient to the donor. Tissues must be traceable by using a distinct identifier code and must indicate that tissues are quarantined during storage or shipment that occurs prior to the determination of donor eligibility. Tissue samples that are not fully identified on the label are discarded but, in some cases, have been linked to the index donor by molecular techniques [28].

A distinct identification code assigned by another establishment engaged in the manufacturing process can be used, or a new code can be assigned. If a new code is assigned, there must be procedures established and maintained for reliably mapping the new to the old code. To prevent mix-ups, identification methods should be used and recorded which verify that distinct identifier codes and dates are properly documented and indicated on recovered tissues and related donor specimens and on all forms that will be used as manufacturing records. This can be accomplished by verification methods (double checks) involving more than one person, or if not possible, accuracy and content can be verified by one person using a procedure that reduces the chance for identification errors (e.g. clerical errors). Discussions are ongoing in both Europe and the United States concerning the use of a standardized bar code system, e.g. ISBT 128, to provide unique donor identification to facilitate traceability.

Summary

Tissue-banking organizations have introduced various donor and tissue testing procedures to reduce the risk of the transmission of viral, bacterial, and fungal infections by tissue grafts. Currently, the measures used to assess tissue donor suitability include the following: a review of the donor's medical history and an assessment of the behavioral risk; the testing of donor blood samples for HBsAg and for the antibodies against HIV, HCV, HTLV, and syphilis; and testing tissues for bacteria and fungus. Donor blood testing and requirements to reduce tissue contamination are very similar among various countries but have minor variations, as spelled out by the AATB [2], EBAA [3], EATB [4], US FDA [5,6], Canadian standards [7], European Commission Directives [8], and Australian TGA [11].

The recent implementation of NAT for tissue donors in some countries has further reduced the residual risk of viremia and tissue-transmitted infection in proportion to the decrease in the window period. The use of both antigen and antibody detection combined with NAT add to safety, albeit at extra cost, and bring testing of tissue donors into line with testing of blood donations. Nucleic acid testing continues to improve dramatically and may come to be applied in new ways, thereby potentially increasing the safety of tissue transplantation. Testing of the donor's blood, even with use of NAT, and tissue testing for bacteria and fungi are not sufficient to detect all contaminated tissues, and other steps taken to prevent tissue-transplant-transmitted disease continue to be important, i.e. safe selection of donors, tissue disinfection and sterilization steps, and sterility testing.

KEY LEARNING POINTS

- Viral, bacterial, prion, and fungal infections have been transmitted via tissue allografts such as bone, skin, cornea, and heart valves. Donor testing has prevented many of these diseases from being transmitted.

- During the past two decades, the disease transmission risk associated with tissue transplantation has been greatly reduced by improvements in existing donor tests and added testing required by standards set by professional organizations and governmental regulations.

- Donor testing has limits and cannot replace safe donor selection and tissue disinfection, sterilization, and testing. Viral infections can be transmitted through tissues if the donor has a viral infection and the viral levels are too low for detection.

- The testing of deceased-donor blood for viral markers may be complicated by false-positive or false-negative tests when sampling is delayed after death or when there is hemolysis or hemodilution.

- The addition of HIV and HCV NAT of donors is an important new step for tissue safety, albeit at extra cost, and its application can bring testing of tissue donors into line with testing of blood donations.

References

1. Eastlund T, Strong DM. Infectious disease transmission through tissue transplantation. In: Phillips GO, editor. Advances Tissue Banking, Volume 7. Singapore: World Scientific; 2004. p. 51–131.
2. Pearson KA, Brubaker SA, editors. Standards for Tissue Banking, 11th edition. McLean, VA: American Association of Tissue Banks; 2006.
3. Eye Bank Association of America. EBAA Medical Standards. Washington, DC: EBAA; 2002. https://www.eyebankassociation.org/eweb/docs/members/standards/medstandards1106.pdf (accessed January 25, 2007).
4. European Association of Tissue Banking. Common standards for tissue and cell banking. http://www.eatb.de/html/standards.htm (accessed January 5, 2007).
5. US Food and Drug Administration. Guidance for Industry. Eligibility determination for donors of human cells, tissues, and cellular and tissue-based products (HCT/Ps). http://www.fda.gov/cber/gdlns/tissdonor.htm (accessed January 5, 2007).
6. US Food and Drug Administration. Guidance for industry: donor screening for antibodies to HTLV-II. August 1997. http://www.fda.gov/cber/guidelines.htm (accessed January 5, 2007).
7. National Standards for Cells, Tissues and Organs for Transplantation and Assisted Reproduction. Canadian Standards Association, National Standards of Canada CAN/CSA-Z900.1 (general standards) and CAN/CSA-2900.2.2 (tissue standards). http://canadagazette.gc.ca/index-e.html (accessed January 5, 2007).
8. Commission Directive 2006/17/EC. Implementing Directive 2004/23/EC of the European Parliament and of the Council as regards certain technical requirements for the donation, procurement and testing of human tissues and cells. Official Journal of the European Union. 2006 Feb 9.
9. Commission Directive 2006/86/EC of 24 October 2006 implementing Directive 2004/23/EC of the European Parliament and of the Council as regards traceability requirements, notification of serious adverse reactions and events, and certain technical requirements for the coding, processing, preservation, storage and distribution of human tissues and cells. Official Journal of the European Union L. 2006 Oct 25;294/32.
10. Directive 2004/23/EC of the European Parliament and of the Council of 31 March 2004 on setting standards for quality and safety in the donation, procurement, processing, preservation, storage and distribution of human tissues and cells. Official Journal of the European Union L. 2004 Apr 7;102/48.
11. Australian Code of Good Manufacturing Practice – Human Blood and Tissues. http://www.tga.gov.au (accessed January 5, 2007).
12. Zou S, Dodd RY, Stramer SL, Strong DM for the Tissue Safety Study Group. Probability of viremia with HBV, HCV, HIV, and HTLV among tissue donors in the United States. N Engl J Med. 2004;351(8):751–9.
13. Conrad EU, Gretch D, Obermeyer K, Moogk M, Sayers M, Wilson J, et al. The transmission of hepatitis C virus by tissue transplantation. J Bone Joint Surg. 1995;77-A(2):214–24.
14. Eastlund T, Tomford W. The effect of long term frozen storage and freeze thaws on tissue donor serum infectious disease test performance. Tissue Cell Rep. 1995;2(1):18–19.

15. Busch MP, Wilbur JC, Johnson P, Tobler L, Evans CS. Impact of specimen handling and storage on detection of hepatitis C virus RNA. Transfusion. 1992;32(5): 420–5.
16. José M, Gajardo R, Jorquera JI. Stability of HCV, HIV-1 and HBV nucleic acids in plasma samples under long-term storage. Biologicals. 2005;33(1):9–16.
17. Sanzen L, Carlsson A. (1997) Transmission of human T-cell lymphotrophic virus-type I by a deep-frozen bone allograft. Acta Orthop Scand. 1997;68(1):72–4.
18. Warwick RM, Eglin R. Should deceased donors be tested for vCJD? Cell Tissue Bank. 2005;6(4):263–70.
19. Eastlund T. Bacterial infection transmitted by human tissue allograft transplantation. Cell Tissue Bank. 2006;7(3):147–66.
20. American Association of Tissue Banks. Guidance Document No 2; Prevention of contamination and cross-contamination at recovery: practices and culture results. http://aatb.timberlakepublishing.com/files/2007bulletin46attachment1.pdf (accessed January 6, 2007).
21. Warwick RM, Magee JG, Leeming JP, Graham JC, Hannan MM, Chadwick M, et al. Mycobacteria and allograft heart valve banking: an international survey. J Hosp Infect. 2008;68(3):255–61.
22. Heim A, Wagner D, Rothamel T, Hartmann V, Flik J, Verhagen W, et al. Evaluation of serological screening of cadaveric sera for donor selection for cornea transplantation J Med Virol. 1999;58(3):291–5.
23. Padley DJ, Lucas SB, Saldanha J. Elimination of false-negative hepatitis C virus RNA results by removal of inhibitors in cadaver-organ donor blood specimens. Transplantation. 2003;76(2):432–4.
24. Strong DM, Nelson K, Pierce M, Stramer SL. Preventing disease transmission by deceased tissue donors by testing blood for viral nucleic acid. Cell Tissue Bank. 2005;6(4):255–62.
25. Guidelines for the blood transfusion services in the United Kingdom http://www.transfusionguidelines.org.uk (accessed January 16, 2008).
26. US Food and Drug Administration. Donor screening tests for testing HCT/P donors. http://www.fda.gov/cber/tissue/prod.htm (accessed January 16, 2008).
27. Eastlund T. Hemodilution due to blood loss and transfusion and reliability of cadaver tissue donor infectious disease testing. Cell Tissue Bank. 2000;1(2):121–7.
28. Warwick RM, Rushambuza FG, Brown J, Patel R, Tabb S, Poniatowski S, et al. Confirmation of cadaveric blood sample identity by DNA profiling using STR (short tandem repeat) analysis. Cell Tissue Bank. 2008;9:323–8.

7 The Management of Donor Test Results

Patricia Hewitt,[1] Chris Moore,[1] and David M. Smith[2]

[1] National Health Service Blood and Transplant, London, UK
[2] Community Blood Center Community Tissue Services, Dayton, Ohio, USA

Introduction

In this chapter, we describe the management of microbiological test results for tests performed on samples from both living and deceased tissue donors. The chapter is written from both the UK and the US perspective, and, for clarity, differences in practice are noted as each policy and procedure is described. The principles described will be applicable in many other settings as well as in the two countries described.

In the United Kingdom, aside from locally organized hospital-based bone banks, including some hospitals working together in consortia for bone banking, there are a number of large tissue-specific banks that deal with ophthalmic tissue donation and heart valves and that are based in hospitals. The largest multitissue banks have developed in various UK national blood services. National Health Service Blood and Transplant (NHSBT) includes the (English) Tissue Services (TS), which accepts donations from both deceased and living donors. The TS femoral head program has about 60 participating hospitals. Approximately 30% of the deceased tissue donors are also donors of organs, and many are also cornea donors. In the Scottish National Blood Transfusion Service, tissue donations are from deceased donors referred by organ donor coordinators, and there is also a femoral head donation program. All of these programs fall under the jurisdiction of the Human Tissue Authority, which is the Competent Authority for England and Scotland for the European Commission Tissues and Cells Directive, and are required to be licensed accordingly.

Tissue and Cell Donation: An Essential Guide. Edited by Ruth M. Warwick, Deirdre Fehily, Scott A. Brubaker, Ted Eastlund. © 2009 Blackwell Publishing, ISBN: 978-14051-6322-4.

Tissue banking practice in the United States differs substantially from that in the United Kingdom from many perspectives. As one of few exceptions in the developed world to governmental mandated universal health care, tissue banking in the United States comprises hundreds of entities engaged in the recovery, processing, and distribution of tissues and cells from both living and deceased donors. All of these organizations fall under the regulatory jurisdiction of the United States Food and Drug Administration (US FDA). Some individual states, such as New York and Florida, also have mandatory regulations that can differ substantially. However, banks are not currently required to adopt other standards such as those promulgated by the American Association of Tissue Banks (AATB), which provides additional guidance on best practices for the industry.

In both the United Kingdom and the United States, much of current practice has emerged as a result of experience in the management of the results of infectious disease tests performed on blood samples from blood donors, in relation in particular to mandatory tests, which include serological tests for syphilis, hepatitis B, hepatitis C (plus nucleic acid testing [NAT] for hepatitis C virus [HCV]), HIV, and Human T cell Lymphotropic virus (HTLV) infection. In NHSBT, all test kits have been approved by the advisory body on the use of such kits and are required to meet standards of sensitivity and specificity required for blood donor testing. The validation for use of tests on deceased-donor samples is best practice and should be undertaken both for mandatory tests and discretionary tests. (The issues around testing are described more fully in Chapter 6.) As in the United Kingdom, the US requirements are similar to those defined for blood donors, though only a few of the tests are currently licensed by the US FDA for use with deceased-donor specimens (hepatitis B surface antigen [HBsAg], antibody to HIV-1 and 2, antibody to HCV, and NAT for HIV-1, hepatitis B virus (HBV), and HCV ["Donor screening tests for testing human cells, tissues, and cellular tissue-based produces (HCT/P) donors," 2007]). NAT for the West Nile virus (WNV) is also US FDA licensed and used by some tissue banks.

The need to inform donors of test results of significance to their health is accepted [1]. The AATB's standards make specific reference to this in D4.356: "The donor's next of kin (NOK) or a physician who will counsel the NOK shall be notified of confirmed positive results that may be medically relevant as determined by the Medical Director or licensed physician designee. The state or local health department(s) shall be notified of positive test results as required by state and/or local rules and/or regulations" [2]. However, a decision has to be made about whether donors should be told about results that prevent the use of the donation but are not relevant to their health. Blood donors in the UK are notified when their donations cannot be used, as it is considered unethical to continue to take donations in this situation. For tissue donors, however, there are notable differences. Tissue donors are less likely to give repeat donations, although it is not uncommon for individuals to have, for example, a hip replacement on one side followed later by a similar operation on the other hip. The health of the donor is not a concern for deceased donors, but there may be health implications for family members. Issues may arise with the donor family when donated tissue from a deceased family member cannot be used, and there should be careful consideration of when and why donor families may need to be informed about test results.

In NHSBT TS, practice is set out for living donors in accordance with the policy for blood donors [3]. This includes the interpretation of test results with the aim of notifying donors of those results considered of significance to the donor's health. NHSBT policy recommends explaining the implications of the results to the donor, from both the medical and the social standpoints, and arranging referral for further clinical assessment and treatment as appropriate. For deceased donors, a decision is made in each case about the relevance of the test result to family members or sexual partners, and those individuals are currently notified only of those results considered to be of significance to their health. The individual can then be offered testing for the infectious agent and clinical follow-up as necessary.

In the United Kingdom there is no requirement to notify other agencies of test results, but the blood services operate a voluntary system of reporting test results (without patient identifiers) to a centralized surveillance scheme, where the results are collated and can then be used to calculate residual risk for tissue-transmitted infections.

In the United States, Medical Directors of tissue banks are responsible for the notification of confirmed positive test results. It is implicit for living donors to be notified of confirmed reactive test results according to applicable federal, state, and local laws and regulations. In the case of deceased donors, the NOK or physician who will counsel the NOK is required to be notified of "medically relevant" results unless laws and regulations state otherwise. The Medical Director determines what is medically relevant. In addition, test results must be reported to local and state agencies as required in these jurisdictions. It can be challenging to develop notification policies when organizations involved in banking of tissues and cells operate in multiple states and localities. As shown in the following outline, many issues and questions need to be considered in the course of notification, whether in the United Kingdom or United States.

The key issues are:

1 interpretation of test results;
2 informing living donors;
  • Which results?
  • Who should inform?
  • How to inform?
  • What to tell?

3 informing families;
- Which results?
- Who to inform?
- How to trace?
- Who should inform?
- What to tell?
- Who will test?

Another important consideration arises as the science and industry of human-derived biologics continues to develop. New technologies now allow the collection of a broader range of tissues and cells, expanded use of tissues for new applications, and the combination of allograft materials with synthetics and other biologics and autogenous tissues, cells, and blood-related components. These other organizations who share tissues and cells must be notified in a timely manner as well.

Other dilemmas arise in relation to emerging infections and their significance. There is the challenge of Creutzfeldt–Jakob disease (CJD) and variant Creutzfeldt–Jakob disease (vCJD), especially in relation to deceased donors and implications for the family. There are currently no blood screening tests that can be used to determine whether CJD/vCJD infection is present. Immunohistochemical tests, such as immunoblots, can be applied to tissues, and a pilot study of such screening has been carried out within NHSBT TS. The test is currently used only in deceased donors who have not been organ donors, so that a "reactive" test result will only be relevant to donated tissue that has not been transplanted. The potential difficulties in interpreting a "reactive" test result are somewhat mitigated by the fact that there is currently believed to be no implication of such a result on other family or household members. The need for consent for further study cannot be ignored. Other emerging infections and additional testing for diseases related to travel history or seasonal transmissible viral infections must also be taken into account. This applies in the United States as well, along with questions about the relevance of testing for diseases such as WNV and Chagas' disease. Currently, testing for these is not required, though screening in the medical and social history is.

Nature of infectious disease screening tests

Screening tests by definition are designed to be highly sensitive for the disease agent, but may not have as high a specificity. This fact often leads to a higher than desired false-positive rate, where false-positive results outnumber true positives by a large margin. Numerous tissue donors in the United States are lost to false-positive hepatitis B core antibody test results. Another complicating factor is that tests are frequently performed on deceased-donor blood samples with their inherent heterogeneity, contamination, and frequent varying degrees of hemolysis. The changes in the milieu of chemistries, coagulation factors, and physical characteristics, along with effects on clinical blood test results, have been extensively studied and addressed in the forensic pathology literature (see Chapter 6).

Interpretation of test results

The interpretation of the test results and their implications for the donor and the donated tissues are the necessary first stage in managing results [2]. In the United States, to minimize the possibility of discrepant test results, it is the standard of practice for cooperation among recovery agencies to arrange for a single panel of infectious disease tests that is shared among all agencies. This would be an ideal to aim for in the United Kingdom, but currently, although there is cooperation among agencies, there is not as yet the infrastructure to perform only one test panel for all agencies recovering tissue or organs from a single donor, and there remains the possibility for there to be conflicting results, albeit with agreement to notify all agencies as soon as a test result is found to be reactive.

Possible Interpretation of Test Results Test results can be:	
Negative on screening	Tissue suitable for release
False positive	Repeatedly reactive on screening; unconfirmed on further testing
Confirmed positive	Repeatedly reactive on screening and confirmed on further testing – may include genomic testing
Indeterminate	Repeatedly reactive on screening; further testing unconfirmed, but reactivity present, requiring further interpretation
Inhibitory	Genomic testing not done – test failed
Screen positive	No sample for further work

A substantial number of initially reactive results will be shown to be falsely reactive, negative on further confirmatory testing. These results are of no significance to the health of the donor, but pose problems for the management of tissue allografts. The system in place in NHSBT TS ensures that tissue associated with repeatedly reactive blood samples for any of the mandatory tests is discarded. This is consistent with the practice for blood donations, where the Information Technology (IT) system will block the issue of the (repeatedly reactive) donation. However, there are grounds for considering quarantine as an alternative to discard for tissues associated with repeatedly reactive results that are confirmed to be negative on reference testing. This could be particularly valuable for tissues from deceased donors, where up to 40 recipients may benefit from the tissue, and for scarce lifesaving tissues such as skin. In order for this policy to be implemented, a specially designed quarantine facility would need to be introduced into current IT systems, which would need to have the agreement of the regulatory authority – the Human Tissue Authority in the United Kingdom. In the United States, there is a similar practice of not notifying the NOK when there are false-positive or unconfirmed results. However, there are no current mechanisms or algorithms in place to allow for the clinical use of any tissues derived from these donors. The only exception is when an initially reactive serological test for syphilis can be overridden by a treponemal-specific test such as Fluorescent Treponemal Antibody test (FTA).

At present, TS living tissue donors with falsely reactive test results are not informed, as the results are of no significance to their health. This practice contrasts with that for blood donors, who are informed so that further donations that must be discarded are not taken, as this is thought to be unethical. The majority of blood donors with false-positive test results are able to continue to donate once the algorithm in the "Guidelines for the Blood Transfusion Services in the UK" [4] has been followed, but as very few living donors give more than one tissue donation, the need to explain the results to prevent discard of future tissue donations does not apply. However, issues about the discard of the donation can be raised by family members or by the donors themselves, and these are discussed later in the chapter.

Indeterminate test results require further interpretation. In the United Kingdom, they apply almost exclusively to tests for hepatitis C antibody. Deceased-donor samples are subject to additional testing for genomic material; if such results are available, this adds greatly to the information available for interpretation, a positive result confirming infection in the donor. For living donors, doubt may be dispelled by arranging a further blood sample, having first spoken to the donor about the possibility of infection and exploring possible exposures. For deceased donors, a view will need to be taken about informing family members and contacts on the basis of one unconfirmed result, unless another sample or result is available from another bank, such as an eye bank, to which tissue has also been referred. Decisions about indeterminate test results center around whether they are false-positive reactions or of clinical significance – possibly related to past infection. These can be the most difficult decisions to be made. On the one hand, there is the potential for anxiety generated by raising the issue with family members at a difficult time, and on the other, the possibility of neglecting to inform a person who may have been at risk of a transmissible and probably treatable infection. Similar dilemmas exist where a screening test is positive but no further confirmatory testing is possible, because there is insufficient sample and a further sample is impossible to obtain. Again, a view needs to be taken about the likelihood of the result being "real." In these instances, the details of the results, such as ratios or optical densities can be considered. Experience in the interpretation of the results of the relevant assays is invaluable in these cases. In the United States, notification does not occur for indeterminate or "inhibited" results. In most instances, there is concern that testing another specimen or accepting another organization's results might be considered "testing into compliance" (use one test result instead of another one that is discordant) by regulatory and/or state agencies. While sharing of test results (donor testing or tissue culture results) is commonplace in the United States and is described by the US FDA in two places in the regulations, testing "into compliance" is not permitted. Sharing of results is described in the US FDA's Good Tissue Practice Final Rule at the part that is titled "1271.160 Establishment and Maintenance of a Quality Program." At "1271.160(b) (2)," it generally states that relevant organizations must "share any information pertaining to the possible contamination of the HCT/P or the potential for transmission of a communicable disease by the HCT/P." This is commonly done and expected.

The second place that sharing of results appears in US FDA's Final Guidance for HCT/P Donor Eligibility is at "1271.85," where it states that "if you are aware that other establishments are performing such (infectious disease) tests and the test results are available, such test results must be included in the donor's relevant medical record (see § 1271.3). Because these test results are part of the medical record, you must consider any results from those tests when you make a donor eligibility determination."

In AATB's *Standards for Tissue Banking* at "D4.500 Information Sharing," it goes further in describing that preprocessing culture results must be shared by the tissue bank performing the recovery with all other tissue banks that received tissue from that donor, and if a donor is determined to be unsuitable by any tissue bank for any reason (this might include testing, cultures, behavioral history, or autopsy results), that information must be shared with all tissue banks involved with that donor. In the United States, with regard to consideration of a "superior sample" or test methodology in deciding which sample or test result is used to determine the suitability of the donor, all results must be considered when determining final donor suitability for release of tissue for transplantation. There is no provision that the use of a better test or better sample proves the other test results were not accurate or the sample used was not acceptable.

Having discordant test results from different specimens is a potential recipe for disaster in the industry. This underscores the importance of performing a single set of tests and sharing results among all tissue or cellular agencies.

In contrast, confirmed positive test results are relatively easy to deal with. Positive tests for HIV, HBsAg, and HTLV are straightforward, and interpretation is restricted to whether positive HCV and syphilis test results reflect current or past infection. For hepatitis C, genomic testing results will often be available; if not, the supplementary test results, such as antibody reactivity and strength of bands in the Recombinant Immunoblot Assay (RIBA-III) provide good information. The interpretation of antibody results of assays for treponemal infection will also depend largely on experience. However, the results are unlikely to determine whether the infection was syphilis or another treponemal disease such as yaws or pinta. Demographic data on the donor may sway the balance of probability, but in our experience, results for treponemal antibody are almost always indicative of infection from the distant past, which may or may not have been treated. The implications for family members are most probably negligible, but in cases of doubt, it may be pertinent to inform family members who may have been at risk, who can then be tested. For living donors, a further blood sample (in the case of hepatitis C, subjected to genomic testing, if a result is not already available), as well as serology, will usually provide the answer. In our experience, informing elderly donors about treponemal antibodies indicative of infection many years previously causes unnecessary distress, and as clinical assessment is almost always refused, we would only rarely now notify an elderly donor of these results.

Where there is a mandatory requirement for a negative result before tissue can be issued and the results in a test for viral material indicate inhibition, which means that the test was not completed, then these can present difficulties for the use of the tissue. In NHSBT TS, there is an obligation to discard donations from deceased donors if this occurs, but a concessionary issue system allows the responsible clinician to override this requirement for emergency material, almost exclusively skin. In the United States, no such provision exists. Even lifesaving tissues, such as skin, are discarded in these circumstances.

Donor notification

In NHSBT TS, living donors are notified of the results of significance to their health (confirmed positive results, and results thought to reflect past infection) in accordance with the clinical policy for blood donors, as described elsewhere [3].

In TS, in contrast to blood donation, part of the consent for tissue donation includes the agreement to communicate with the donor/patient's primary general physician (GP) if necessary; if contact with the donor fails, the GP will be informed of the findings and advised to see his or her patient. As mentioned earlier, in the United States, regulations, laws, and standards define notification and not the consent. In the United States, it is not the federal regulator (US FDA) that is notified but the local departments of health, i.e. regulators at state level. The AATB standards require notification

Aims of the living donor post-test discussion

1 to explain the meaning of the test results and why (further) donation is not possible, bearing in mind the context that most living donors do not have the opportunity for additional donations in the future as such donors are usually femoral head or amnion donors;

2 to repeat the tests on a further blood sample;

3 to explore the consequences for the donor's future health and circumstances;

4 to arrange appropriate medical referral;

5 to reduce the risk of onward transmission;

6 to obtain information about the source of infection;

7 to maintain confidentiality.

of living donors and the NOK of deceased donors or the physician who will undertake the counseling of those individuals. In addition, the notification of state or local health departments must be undertaken. All states have laws and regulations requiring that doctors notify donors about a wide range of infectious diseases that are newly diagnosed, including HIV, HCV, HBV, WNV, and syphilis.

Positive or significant test results on samples from deceased donors present a very different challenge. As well as interpretation of results, each case must be assessed in order to decide who should be informed about the results. NHSBT IT systems ensure that no product is issued, but the results pertain to an individual who cannot be notified. There are issues of confidentiality, even for a deceased donor, and in practice, the decision to inform is made on the basis of "who is at risk." In some cases, there is insufficient information available to identify anyone at risk; in others, several family members may need to be informed, resulting in a lengthy notification process. In the United States, federal laws regarding confidentiality (the Health Insurance Portability and Accountability Act, which includes provisions for health insurance portability, fraud and abuse control, tax-related provisions, group health plan requirements, revenue offset provisions, and administrative simplification requirements. Additionally, the Act creates national standards to protect individuals' medical records and other personal health information) do not extend to deceased individuals, though many hospitals and healthcare agencies require acknowledgement of the need for confidentiality before releasing medical records for review. These records, including private physician records, sometimes can clarify the disease process and the likelihood of risk to exposed individuals. The following case histories illustrate various scenarios common to both countries and the process of notifying the NOK or persons at potential risk.

CASE 1

Treponemal antibodies

1 Deceased donor, male, born 1958
2 Consent for skin, bone, tendons, meniscus, heart valves, and corneas
3 Blood sample confirmed positive for treponemal antibodies; consistent with past/treated infection
4 Donor born in Vietnam
5 Sister had given consent
6 No known sexual partner or children

Conclusion: **1** In the United Kingdom, no notification because no recognized risk to family.
2 In the United States, AATB standards require notification of NOK and regulatory standards require state departments of health to be notified.

CASE 2

Sample confirmed anti-HIV positive

1 Deceased donor, male, aged 45 years
2 Found unconscious at home when he failed to go to work
3 Died of subarachnoid hemorrhage
4 Consent had been given for skin and bone, but skin not taken as "too thin"
5 Consent given by sister
6 Blood sample confirmed anti-HIV positive
7 No evidence of a sexual partner; donor lived alone

Conclusion: notification of contacts not possible.

CASE 3

Hepatitis C infection confirmed 1

1 Male, born 1944
2 Died of myocardial infarction
3 Donated skin
4 Blood sample confirmed positive for anti-HCV and HCV RNA
5 Consent given by wife
6 Low but real risk assessed
7 Wife's GP traced and informed

8 Wife offered testing

9 Told GP at interview that husband had used drugs "in the 1960s"; information not elicited at selection interview

10 Wife tested, but NHSBT TS not informed of result

Conclusion: successful notification.

CASE 4

Hepatitis C infection 2

1 Female donor, aged 45, referred by organ donor coordinator

2 Confirmed positive for hepatitis C antibodies; results consistent with infection, but polymerase chain reaction test inhibitory

3 Donor's mother had given consent

4 Donor known to have 13-year-old son

5 Low but real risk to son

6 Child under care of grandmother

7 Organ donor coordinator familiar with family

8 Boy's GP contacted and coordinator kept informed

9 Grandmother contacted by GP

10 Coordinator spoke to grandmother and confirmed boy will be tested

Conclusion: successful notification.

CASE 5

Probable HIV infection

1 Male donor, aged 60

2 Donated skin and bone

3 Anti-HIV repeatedly reactive in two assays, reported by public health laboratory as "probable HIV infection"

4 Son had given consent – NHSBT TS contact

5 Discussed findings with son

6 Details of donor's second family revealed, including current partner who could not speak English

7 All family members traced through GPs, so testing could be offered

8 Individual outcomes not known to TS, but those at risk informed

9 Tracing took more than six months

Conclusion: successful notification and follow-up.

In each case, a decision was first made about the need to inform family members based on the risk to those individuals. In cases 1 and 2, individuals at risk could not be identified, so no notification was possible or necessary. In the United States, tissue bank Medical Directors would be required by AATB to notify the NOK and by regulations to notify state departments of health.

For the other cases, the primary point of contact was the individual who gave consent for the donation. In case 5, sufficient information was provided by this person to be able to trace several persons potentially at risk. In cases 3 and 5, the tissue bank organization was already aware of some individuals at risk, but not that there were potentially so many individuals in the latter case. Collaboration with the organ donor coordinator from a sister organization was invaluable in case 4 as the sister organization had spoken to the family and knew the family relationships. In the United States, it is usually the organization which obtained consent that is responsible for notification, except when defined elsewhere by laws and regulations. As in England, this organization is also responsible for informing other agencies receiving biologic materials from the donor. If the donor was an organ, tissue, and eye donor, it is usually the organ procurement organization that notifies the tissue bank and eye bank of test results. If the tissue bank shared tissues with another processor or processors, it is the tissue bank's responsibility to inform these organizations. In the event that results become available after the release of tissues (such as fresh skin), it is the releasing bank's responsibility to notify.

In the United Kingdom, it is considered good practice that the NOK notification of possible risk in a deceased donor is best done by a clinician who already knows the person concerned. It is NHSBT practice to first approach the primary GP to explain the circumstances and the test results to this clinician and offer support, as required. In England, it is possible to trace an individual's GP from a national database to which NHSBT has access. Without this tool, or if the person does not have a GP, NHSBT would approach the organ transplant coordinator who had contact with the family member(s) before donation, to determine whether contact may appropriately be made through this route. As a last resort, NHSBT would approach the person directly, but would not then have the advantage of knowing his or her circumstances, such as current health, before doing so. Any testing which might be necessary can usually be arranged by the GP, and it is considered that there is no obligation to inform NHSBT of results, as these are confidential and are of no relevance to TS.

In the United States, tissue banks must have processes in place to meet legal and regulatory requirements. Notification of the NOK about positive test results is a professional standard rather than a law. Tissue banks are required to inform the NOK or a physician who will provide counseling for the NOK. Tissue bank Medical Directors are available to answer questions for individuals and physicians who may not be familiar with the interpretation of the test results or the health implications for exposed persons. Notification of the state department of health about confirmed positive infectious disease test results is a requirement of state law and of the AATB standards and functions as a public health protection measure.

Discarded tissue

NHSBT TS's living donors whose bone has been discarded are given a full explanation if they ask, and this information will be given by the TS staff. Donor families (of deceased donors) are often keen for reassurance that the tissue they agreed to donate has been useful, and this desire for information can present problems where tissue has been discarded. As a matter of principle, the organization will not lie to families about the fate of tissues, but on the other hand, there is the matter of confidentiality, especially pertinent when infectious disease test results are to be considered. NHSBT TS have taken the view that they will not discuss in detail with donor families, even if they ask, the reason for tissue discard and find it important to mention this policy from the beginning, during the consent discussion with the family. It is explained that various medical or technical factors may make the tissue unsuitable for use, but for reasons of confidentiality, exact details will not be given. Consent for research use is always requested, and if this has been agreed, its usefulness can be emphasized should the need arise. In the United States, there is no consensus about telling families when donor tissues are discarded. Opinions vary from full prospective disclosure to not disclosing at all. Most banks will disclose the outcome if asked by the NOK, but this can cause significant grief and anger for families who have envisioned people's lives being changed by their loved one's tissues. Some are angered that they were not offered the opportunity to bury or cremate the unused tissues and threaten legal action. The nature of the reason for discard is sometimes difficult to address. When the ineligibility is because of an obvious false-positive blood test result, prohibited medical social behavior, medical information derived from hospital records, or other similar circumstance, it is relatively easy to explain. However, when the discard of tissue is because of a recovery error, mislabeling of tissue or a tissue donor blood sample for testing, or accidental commingling of tissues with another donor during processing, it can be devastating to a family and can lead to the potential of legal liability. However, in the United States, it is very common for tissue banks to share with the NOK the outcome of the donation in general terms with regard to the type of grafts and types of recipient. An explanation is given if tissues are discarded.

KEY LEARNING POINTS

- It is important to notify living tissue donors and the NOK of deceased tissue donors of confirmed positive infectious disease test results. This requires careful evaluation of the relevance of the results to the health of those involved. In the United States, there are laws regarding notification of health authorities.

- The notification of the donor or NOK is an important public health measure because knowledge of a previously undiagnosed disease can enable treatment when warranted and can prompt evaluation and testing of the donor's close contacts.

- Infectious disease testing and notification of results carry ethical implications, including protection of privacy, maintenance of confidentiality, duty to warn, and freedom to make choices through informed consent including whether to donate and be tested with its subsequent potential impacts.

References

1. Barbara J, Contreras M, Regan F, editors. Transfusion Microbiology. Cambridge: Cambridge University Press; 2008.
2. Standard D4.356. In: Pearson KA, Brubaker SA, editors. Standards for Tissue Banking, 11th edition. McLean, VA: American Association of Tissue Banks; 2006. p. 35.
3. Miller R, Hewitt PE, Warwick R, Moore MC, Vincent B. Review of counselling in a transfusion service; the London (UK) experience. Vox Sang. 1998;74(3):133–9.
4. Guidelines for the Blood Transfusion Services in the UK, 7th edition. London: The Stationery Office; 2005.

8 Case Studies from Diverse Cultural, Religious, and Economic Situations

Aziz Nather,[1] Li Baoxing,[2] Muhammed Cassim,[3] Hamid Reza Aghayan,[4] Arieh Eldad,[5] and Ján Koller[6]

[1] Department of Orthopaedic Surgery, Yong Loo Lin School of Medicine, National University of Singapore, Singapore
[2] Shanxi Provincial Tissue Bank, Taiyuan, Shanxi Province, China
[3] Sri Lanka Eye Donation Society, Dr Hudson Silva Eye Donation Headquarters, Colombo, Sri Lanka
[4] Tehran University of Medical Sciences, Tehran, Iran
[5] Hebrew University School of Medicine, Jerusalem, Israel
[6] University Hospital Bratislava, Ruzinov Hospital, Bratislava, Slovakia

Introduction

The level of development of tissue banking in each country is largely dependent on the religious, cultural, and legal context prevailing in that country. These issues vary from one region to the next and, indeed, even in different countries in the same region.

While tissue donation and transplantation in the United States and in Europe are well described in the literature, little is written about the status of tissue banking in the Asia Pacific region, Australia, Latin America, the Middle East, and Africa. In Africa, apart from banks in South Africa and one in Zambia, there is little tissue-banking activity, although interest has been shown by Algeria, Egypt, Libya, Nigeria, and Ghana. This chapter focuses in particular on the religious, cultural, legal, and other issues that impact on these activities in a selection of countries where these influences are strong.

Tissue and Cell Donation: An Essential Guide. Edited by Ruth M. Warwick, Deirdre Fehily, Scott A. Brubaker, Ted Eastlund. © 2009 Blackwell Publishing, ISBN: 978-14051-6322-4.

Ethical issues

Ethical principles should not differ from country to country or from region to region; our set of core moral values must, after all, remain the same.

Tissue donation is an act of humanity enabling one to alleviate the sufferings of fellow human beings. It is therefore sacrosanct that tissue banks must not sell or make profit from the act of donation but instead must provide tissue grafts on a noncommercial basis without any profit motive [1,2]. Despite this, many for-profit organizations now operate, particularly in the United States. The American Association of Tissue Banks publishes standards to help ensure that tissue banks conform to ethical practices in addition to meeting acceptable technical norms. In the United States, tissue banks fall into two categories: "for-profit" organizations, where any surplus or income of the organization may be shared among its shareholders, and "not-for-profit" organizations, where any surplus is not distributed to shareholders but may be plowed back into the organization for research and development. "For-profit" organizations may be in conflict with some ethical principles though the argument made is that the profit is earned from the technology developed by the company and not made on the donated tissue itself. In Europe, tissue banks are encouraged to comply with the Ethical Code of the European Association of Tissue Banks (EATB).

In the Asia Pacific region and in Latin America, there is no formal ethical code for the regions. Nevertheless, tissue banks in both regions comply with all the principles described in the Ethical Code of EATB. The guiding principle followed by all tissue bank operators is enshrined in the "Hippocratic Oath" requiring doctors and health workers to "non nocere" (not to injure or harm).

In the day-to-day running of the tissue banks, we note that costs are incurred during tissue donation, processing, and distribution. It is therefore not unethical that tissue banks be allowed to charge "processing costs," provided that there is a provision in the law of that country (if a law exists) to allow the tissue bank to do so. A common, acceptable practice in institutional tissue banks is to work out the total costs incurred, including manpower costs, equipment maintenance costs, costs of electricity and water, and costs of other consumables. Such "processing costs" could be charged to the recipients of the tissues. Countries in the Asia Pacific region charging processing costs include Japan, Singapore, Malaysia, India, and Sri Lanka [1,2].

Tissue banking helps to reduce the healthcare costs in a country [3]. Tissue allografts are generally less expensive than custom-made prostheses or ceramics. In many countries, bone and other allografts are produced by noncommercial or institutional tissue banks and are either provided free of charge (funded by the health service) or at nominal costs ("processing costs only") to ensure equal patient access.

Religious and cultural issues

Tissue donation is a sensitive subject as it involves important issues regarding ownership and dignity of the deceased and living – the concept of brain death and the concept that tissue donation is the ultimate gift one may bestow upon his or her fellow human being after one's death. Such issues are strongly linked to the dominant religious and cultural mind-sets in each country. It should be recognized that the culture of an ethnic group is often inseparable from the religion practiced by that group. Religion plays a major role in influencing the development of tissue banking in each country.

Buddhism

Buddhism is a predominant religion in several countries in the Asia Pacific region, including Thailand, Vietnam, Cambodia, Laos, and Sri Lanka. The attitude of Buddhism is in perfect agreement with tissue donation [1,2]. Buddhism strongly advocates the practice of "Dana" or giving (donation). Donation is one of the most important and basic tenets of the religion. It is the first practice that one should cultivate in order to purify and develop an ordinary mortal's mind. It is in the one who gives that the qualities of kindness and of being free of greed and selfishness can grow. The one who steps upon the Buddhist path to liberation through complete nonattachment should practice donation methodically and well. Buddhism teaches that the practice of giving should be cultivated continuously throughout the cycle of rebirth.

Giving can be in the form of physical objects, e.g. money. It can also be by giving one's labor or intellect – sharing knowledge and experience. It could also be in the form of giving one's body, e.g. blood and tissues for the benefit of others. The highest form of giving is to give one's life. There are thus three levels of donation "Dana Paramitha:"

1 Dana Paramitha: the giving of physical possessions (first step);
2 Dana Upaparamitha: the giving of blood, eyes, and tissues of the body (second step);
3 Dana Paramatta Paramitha: giving one's life for the good of others (third and final step).

In Buddhist scriptures in the "Sivi Jatakaya," King Sivi gave away one of his eyes with the help of the royal eye surgeon to help a blind man to see. It is these principles that strongly influence a very large number of Buddhists to donate parts of their body.

Buddhism is also one of the major religions in several countries in the Asia Pacific including Korea (30%) and Singapore (also about 30%). In both countries, tissue donors are predominantly Buddhists – more than 95% in Singapore. Indeed, the success of the National University Hospital Tissue

Bank in Singapore is largely a result of the strong support given by the Buddhist community to donate all tissues including eyes, musculoskeletal tissues, and skin [1,2].

CASE 1

Eye donation in Sri Lanka

In Sri Lanka, the clergy plays an important role in the lives of Buddhists. Buddhist monks talk about body donation in their regular services. Buddhists who flock to the temples, especially on the days of the full moon, are encouraged to pledge their eyes and other parts of their body. It is in such an environment of strong Buddhist influences, and the notability of eye donation, that the late Dr. Hudson Silva conceived the concept of human eye donation and developed a public education program based on Buddhist philosophy. The Sri Lanka Eye Donation Society was set up in 1961 with its Central Eye Bank in Colombo and Regional Banks covering the whole island. Trained personnel perform eye procurement in all banks. Eye donation campaigns were carried out in various temples on the island with the help of priests and members of the Eye Society. The society runs meetings with the public twice a month. Direct contact with the public has been found to be more effective than communication with the public through the media. Indeed, the Eye Donation Programme in Sri Lanka is the most successful eye donation program in the world. A total of 40,000 eyes have been procured for the benefit of all mankind – a target Dr. Silva set and proudly achieved by May 1999. To date, over 850,000 pledges for eye donation have been received.

On the basis of the renowned success of eye donation in Sri Lanka, the International Atomic Energy Agency (IAEA) supported the establishment of a "Model Human Tissue Bank." An agreement was signed in 1993 between the IAEA and the Ministry of Health in Sri Lanka, in which the government gave a big piece of land for the development of the tissue bank. The IAEA provided several pieces of equipment, including a Gamma Cell 200 to be housed in the tissue bank itself. The bank was inaugurated on May 8, 1996 by the prime minister of Sri Lanka [4].

Hinduism

Hinduism is predominant in India, a secular country in the Asia Pacific region. It is also an important religion in a number of other countries in the Asia Pacific region, namely Sri Lanka (about 10%), Malaysia (about 10%), and Singapore (about 10%).

With regard to tissue donation, the religious dogma of Hinduism is parallel to that of Buddhism in many ways; there is no objection to tissue donation. Devotees of both religions practice cremation of the deceased – an act of destruction of the body in front of and with complete knowledge and acceptance by all the relatives [1,2].

Islam

Islam is the predominant religion practiced in most countries in the Middle East, including Saudi Arabia, Jordan, Kuwait, United Arab Emirates, and in Egypt, Iran, and Iraq. It is also the predominant religion in several countries in the Asia Pacific region, including Bangladesh, Pakistan, Malaysia, and Indonesia. In all these countries, Islam is the official religion except in Indonesia. Indonesia is a secular country that follows the five principles of Pancasila. It is very important to point out that there are about 200 million Muslims in China – another secular country. Islam also plays an important role in Singapore (about 20% are Muslims) and in India (about 40%) [1,2].

As in all religions, the Koran respects life and values the needs of the living over the dead. It allows organ donations in situations where it can save a person's life. However, it is important to point out that there is no mention made concerning permitting organ and tissue donation to improve the quality of life of another human being. Therefore, Muslims are more likely to allow kidney donation and less likely to allow tissue donation as the latter is perceived as improving quality of life and not saving another person's life. The interpretations of the Koran vary according to the interpretations of different "ustazs." Ustazs are the religious leaders who teach the practice of Islam to their own group of followers. In general, the members in each group will not follow anything their own leader does not endorse or practice in the interpretation of the texts written in the Koran, regardless of what is the national stand on that issue by the "mufti" – the overall religious leader appointed by the government to represent all issues in Islam for the country. Tissue donation is not explicitly forbidden in the Koran; however, some ustazs interpret it differently and their followers would not donate.

In Islam, there are religious rulings on the issue of organ and/or tissue donation; these are called "fatwas." These are official positions taken by the religious committee appointed by the government and chaired by the "mufti." Although they are not, strictly speaking, legally binding, they are almost equivalent to law in terms of guiding the actions of citizens. A "fatwa" was passed in Saudi Arabia in 1985 sanctioning both living related and cadaveric donation of organs. Likewise in 1998, a fatwa was passed in the United Arab Emirates sanctioning living and cadaveric organ donation and organ donation from Muslims to non-Muslims and accepting the concept of brain death [5].

The first "fatwa on bone, skin, and amnion" was passed in Malaysia in September 1995. This was followed in June 1997 by a "fatwa on bone, skin, and amnion" passed in Indonesia – a good leap forward as "The Indonesia 1992 Health Regulation" had allowed tissue procurement from living donors only. In Singapore, a "fatwa for cornea" was passed in 1999 – a first "fatwa" for tissues – but attempts to make a "fatwa for bone and skin" did not succeed [1,2].

Despite having or not having "fatwas," the decision to donate tissues remains very much the prerogative of the individual and his or her family with their "ustazs," depending on the latter's interpretations, exerting a very strong influence.

An important factor in the organization of tissue procurement in Muslim communities is to recognize the religious necessity among Muslims to bury the body of the deceased as soon as possible. Tissue procurement takes time and will delay the burial and is therefore not widely accepted.

Culturally, Muslims believe strongly that God created them whole, and they want to return to him whole. They practice burial of body parts such as amputated limbs and even foreskins from circumcisions and the placenta following childbirth. Muslims are therefore culturally reluctant to allow tissue donation.

In Islam, the opinion of the next of kin, or "waris," is very important. When a person dies, the "waris" is responsible for taking care of what can happen to the body of the deceased. Consent is needed not only from the deceased before his death but also from the next of kin after death [2].

As a group, Muslims constitute a religious group where there is a great deal of controversy regarding donation after death and where many are not likely to agree to tissue donation because of their religion. Countries with predominantly Muslim populations all face great shortage of donors in both their organ and tissue transplantation programs. However, successful donation programs have been achieved in Muslim countries, as we see in case 2.

CASE 2

Tissue donation in Iran

The Islamic Republic of Iran is located in the Middle East with 98% of its 68 million population being Muslims. Transplantation has a long history in Iran. Avicenna, the great Iranian physician, performed the first nerve repair in 11th century. Cornea was the first tissue transplanted in 1935 [6]. The Central Eye Bank of Iran was established in 1991 and the Iranian Tissue Bank (ITB) in 1994.

The ITB is the first and unique multitissue bank in the country that processes bones, soft tissues, cartilage, heart valves, and amniotic membrane. As in other Muslim countries, Islam is an important arbiter in the daily life of many people. Social attitudes and ethical principles are closely intertwined with Islamic tradition, teaching, and heritage.

In the beginning of ITB's activity, a lack of legislation was the main problem. Fortunately, in response to an *istifta* (religious question), most of the prominent scholars have given a positive opinion (*fatwa*) regarding *organ and tissue* donation. These religious rulings helped the establishment of tissue donation before legislation was in place.

The Act of "Deceased or Brain-dead Patient Organ Transplantation" was passed on April 6, 2000 by the parliament and an executive bylaw passed by the Cabinet Council on May 2002. There is no separate legislation for tissue transplantation, but the legal framework is the same as for organ transplantation. According to the law, the deceased person's will with respect to organ or tissue donation could be either in oral or in written form and can be approved by written notice of an heir apparent. If the original will is not available, a special consent form designed by the Ministry of Health can be signed by informed heirs [7].

Despite the importance of religion and legislation, it seems that the main barriers against organ and tissue donation are sociocultural factors, family relations, lack of knowledge, and filial obligations. So ITB has conducted many educational programs and campaigns with the support of mass media. The result has been a considerable growth in the number of tissue donors. From 1994 to the end of 2006, the number of tissue donors increased to more than 2,600 of which 2,100 (80%) of the cases were after the introduction of legislation. Iran is certainly a "success story" of tissue donation in a Muslim country following the introduction of a law for tissue donation. No other Muslim country has experienced such a success after the enactment of a similar law.

Christianity

Christianity is the predominant religion in most countries in Europe and Latin America (about 85%), in the United States, and in Australia. In the Asia Pacific region, it is predominant in the Philippines [1,2]. It is one of the major religions, though not predominant, in two other countries, namely Korea (about 30%) and Singapore (also about 30%).

Tissue donation is consistent with the religious Christian dogma of loving thy neighbor as thyself, as an act of genuine altruism that involves giving up something to save the lives of others. Indeed, the support of the church for tissue donation was reiterated by the late Pope John Paul II while he was attending the Congress of the Society for Organ Sharing in an audience on June 20, 1991. He quoted the words of Jesus Christ as narrated by the apostle Luke, "Give and it will be given to you; good measure, passed down, shaken together, running over, will be put into your lap (Luke 6:38). We shall receive our supreme reward from God according to the genuine and effective love we have shown to our neighbour," in full support of organ and tissue donation.

Christian communities in Europe, Latin America, and the United States support tissue donation. In Latin America, all countries are active in organ and tissue transplantation activities, including Argentina, Brazil, Cuba, Chile, and Mexico, which have well-established laws. It is interesting to note that all these laws not only refer to organs but specifically mention tissues.

Although the majority of the people in the Philippines are Catholics, culturally the Filipinos consider that God created them whole and they prefer to return to Him whole. Filipinos are generally against their physical nature being altered in any way by the act of tissue procurement. There is therefore an acute shortage of donors in the Philippines. Likewise in Korea, Catholics are reluctant to donate their tissues because of the same cultural beliefs [1,2].

CASE 3

Skin donation in Slovakia

Slovakia is a small country situated directly in the middle of Europe with approximately 5.5 million inhabitants. Slovakia was part of Czechoslovakia but became an independent state in 1993. The religions represented in the country include mostly Catholics (71%), Protestants (9%), and others (3.5%). Atheists represent 16.5% of the population.

The procurement of tissues and cells for transplantation purposes has been regulated since 1966, when it was first included in the healthcare law (Law 20/1966). After Slovakia became independent, this law was replaced in 1994 by a new one (277/1994). In 2004, six new laws for health care were adopted, and donation and transplantation issues were included in Law 576/2004 Z.z. After Slovakia became a Member State of the European Union, the new European Directive 2004/23/EC was implemented by Law 282/2006 Z.z. and Governmental Decree 20/2007 Z.z.

All the regulations mentioned include the principle of *presumed consent* for donations (opt-out system). The attitude of the Slovakian population toward donations is more or less neutral. In 1997, there occurred in the eastern part of the country a case of skin procurement from an elderly deceased lady, which was publicized in a negative way, and it raised negative emotions in the population. Although the procurement was in accordance with the regulations, it was misused in a competitive debate between two funeral companies and was presented as a scandal in the press. Its negative impact on the donation rate was very strong. Following the incident, a new central register of people who refused donation was established at the Slovak Center for Organ Donations in Bratislava. At the present time, all potential donors must be checked by the organ procurement coordinators and tissue banks in this register, and if their names are in the list, the procurement cannot proceed.

Allogeneic skin procurement and banking was started in Slovakia in the year 1988 in the Central Tissue Bank of the University Hospital, and later in the Kosice-Saca hospital skin bank in 1996. Skin grafts are used mostly to treat extensively burned patients [8]. With the introduction of the new law in 2004 and the reorganization of the autopsy rules, allogeneic skin donations in Slovakia ceased completely. It is expected that these problems will be solved soon and that skin donations will resume.

Judaism

In the Yom Kippur War of October 1973, Israel experienced a high percentage of burn casualties among war injuries, and one of the lessons of this war was the need to establish a national skin bank. The objection to autopsies by Orthodox Jews is well known, but when the burn surgeons consulted rabbinical authorities about skin transplantation, they had a very positive response and efforts were made to permit it within the framework of religious law. It is a well-established obligation (a mitzvah, religious obligation) for every Jew to save life. So there was no question about the permission to use skin from a cadaver to save a specific patient whose life was at risk at that given moment. The debate was whether the establishment of a skin bank should be allowed to serve potential future recipients as opposed to the use of donated skin for a specific individual who is a current burn casualty. Another concern was the possibility that the tissue donation might not be used at all within the time frame that it could be grafted before expiry. The Chief Rabbinical (Orthodox) Institute in Israel discussed these issues in 1985 and decided that because of the unique security and military situation in Israel, the context is identical to when a specific patient's life is in danger. The rabbis understood that in a war or a mass casualty situation, medical staff would not be able to allocate professional teams to harvest skin as they would all be busy treating the casualties. They therefore permitted skin banking on a large scale, sufficient to treat 100 severe burn cases. They ordered that unused expired homograft should be buried according to the Jewish halacha (law). Once this was allowed by the supreme institutes of the Orthodox Jews, it was accepted by other groups, such as the Conservative and the Reform Jews, which in Israel constitute smaller groups.

The fact that tissue and organ donation after death, designated for lifesaving, is not only allowed in Judaism but considered as a mitzvah (religious obligation) made tissue transplantation and banking possible, but did not necessarily make it easy to obtain the donations. Only about 20% of the Jewish population in Israel define themselves as "religious" and other cultural factors play a role in tissue and organ donation in Israel. Large-scale campaigns were organized among the general population in a bid to bridge the gap between large needs and the small number of offers of organs. The situation with tissue donation is a little better, and in the case of skin homografts, all clinical needs can now be met.

Until recently, government regulations for donation after death were within the framework of "the law of anatomy and pathology" that regulates autopsies. A subcommittee of the Knesset (the Israeli Parliament) wrote a new bill that will regulate all aspects of organ and tissue transplantation, from live and deceased donors, in an effort to encourage organ donation and to fight trafficking. The wide gap between demand and supply of organs in Israel made many Israelis in need of organ transplantation travel abroad to countries where it is easier to get organs, but the Ministry of Health, the Israeli Medical Association, and various organizations became increasingly concerned about the involvement of Israelis in organ trafficking. The new bill was created with the full cooperation of the rabbinical authorities, the

Israeli Medical Association, the ethics committees, and the Ministry of Health. When finalized, it will allow some compensation for donors and families for organs and tissues that will be harvested after death, as well as recovery of expenses and medical and life insurance and recognition for live donors.

Tissue banks in Israel supply for all patients: Jews, Muslims, or Christians, and during mass casualty terror events, they were all treated together, side by side in the same emergency room or in the hospital wards, and often, the terrorists and their victims were hospitalized together.

CASE 4

The National Skin Bank in Jerusalem

Following the attacks in Israel by Muslim terrorists against the Jews, the National Skin Bank of Haddasah Ein Kerem University Hospital in Jerusalem over the past 20 years has allocated about 25% of the skin procured by the bank for transplantation to terror victims, mainly of suicide bombings. On several occasions, the bank allocated allograft skin to terrorists that were not killed by their suicide attacks in their attempt to kill many others. Such situations did cause stress to some of the victims treated in the same unit and at the same time inviting severe criticisms from the families of victims. Yet, the bank has not encountered any refusal from the medical team to treat such terrorists, not even in one situation where one of the bank's own nurses lost her father in such a bombing attack and one of the terrorists responsible for that attack was severely injured and required skin allografts. The decision to allocate allografts from the National Skin Bank is taken solely on the basis of medical criteria.

Chinese culture

Chinese culture, one of the oldest civilizations in the world, has its unique concept about life and its "carrier" – the body. In the Chinese incunabulum LiJi (206 BC), the Chinese hold the body in the highest regard. Because our body comes from our parents, to express the utmost respect to our parents, we must take good care of it and any procedure that destroys the human body is unacceptable. Tang LuShuYi (AD 652), in criminal law, regarded the act of damaging the human cadaver as felony, and the offender would be subjected to rigorous punishment. For this reason, most Chinese prefer to place their bodies in tombs instead of donating them. This custom has been passed down from generation to generation for centuries.

With the modernization of China over the last 30 years, this ancient custom and philosophy has slowly undergone change. Little by little, changes have taken place to make the public more open to tissue donation. In Shanghai, more than 27,000 have registered to pledge donation of their body posthumously. The Chinese Middleware Documentation Project has registered over a million bone marrow donors. Frequent reports of organ or tissue donation (e.g. kidneys, liver, cornea) have appeared in the media.

A survey of 560 adults revealed that public awareness of tissue donation is related to the educational level; the higher the educational level, the higher the percentage of people who agree to donate.

The role of tissue transplant coordinators

In the United States, Australia, and countries in Europe, tissue transplant coordinators are employed to increase the donor pool. Unfortunately, this is not the case in most countries in other regions, including the Asia Pacific region, Latin America, and Africa. In these regions, some countries employ eye transplant coordinators for eye banks, including Myanmar, Singapore, Malaysia, and Sri Lanka. For the donation of other tissues such as bone, ligaments, tendons, and skin, bone banks and skin banks rely on the support of kidney transplant coordinators to seek consent from donor families, including countries such as Singapore, Malaysia and Indonesia, Korea, and Japan. This situation is not always satisfactory. Until tissue banks can employ their own tissue transplant coordinators, no amount of public awareness campaigns can be successful in increasing the tissue donation pool substantially.

Standard of primary health care achieved

The support given by the government is an extremely important factor in the development of tissue banking in each country. This is, to a large extent, affected by the standard of primary health care achieved by that country [1].

In developing countries, where the standard of primary health care achieved is not high, governments cannot be expected to give priority to tissue banking and are not likely to support tissue banks with substantial financial grants. Their health budgets will go mainly to improving primary health care first. On the other hand, in the better developed countries, where high primary healthcare standards have been achieved, tissue banks are more likely to succeed in procuring bigger grants from their governments for the development of their activities [1].

Conclusions

In planning public awareness programs to promote tissue donation and transplantation, one must take into account the various religious, cultural, socioeconomic, and legal frameworks that apply in each country. Only then can these programs achieve a good outcome. Consideration must also be given to the availability of tissue transplant coordinators in that country and the standard of primary health care achieved by that country. History shows that religious barriers can be overcome and, in some cases, that religion can be a driving force for tissue donation.

References

1. Nather A. Ethical, religious and cultural factors, legal and other regulatory aspects. In: Phillips GO, editor. Radiation and Tissue Banking. Singapore, New Jersey, London, Hong Kong: World Scientific; 2000. p. 217–35.
2. Nather A, Zulkifly AH, Sim YL. Ethical, religious, legal and cultural issues in tissue banking. In: Nather A, Yusof N, Hilmy N, editors. Radiation in Tissue Banking. New Jersey, London, Singapore, Beijing, Shanghai, Hong Kong, Taipei, Chennai: World Scientific; 2007. p. 55–66.
3. Hachiya Y, Sakai T, Nanta Y, Izawa H, Yoshizawa K. Status of bone banks in Japan. Transplant Proc. 1999;31:2032–5.
4. Nather A, Khalid KA, Sim YL. Tissue banking in the Asia Pacific region – Past, present and future. In: Nather A, Yusof N, Hilmy N, editors. Radiation in Tissue Banking. New Jersey, London, Singapore, Beijing, Shanghai, Hong Kong, Taipei, Chennai: World Scientific; 2007. p. 25–53.
5. El-Shahat YIM. Islamic viewpoint of organ transplantation. Transplant Proc. 1999;31:3271–4.
6. Larijani B, Zahedi F, Taheri E. Ethical and legal aspects of organ transplantation in Iran. Transplant Proc. 2004;36:1241–4.
7. IR Iran Parliament. Deceased or Brain Dead Patients Organ Transplantation Act. H/24804-T/9929. June 4, 2000.
8. Koller J, Orság M. Skin grafting options at the Burn and Reconstructive Surgery Department of the Faculty Hospital in Bratislava. Acta Chir Plast. 2006;48(2):65–71.

9 Facilitating Donation – The Role of Key Stakeholders: The Medical Examiner, the Coroner, the Hospital Pathologist, and the Funeral Director

Charles V. Wetli,[1] Diego Ponzin,[2] Christopher Womack,[3] and George McCann[4]

[1] Department of Health Services, Division of Medical Legal Investigations and Forensic Sciences, Suffolk County, New York, USA
[2] Fondazione Banca degli Occhi del Veneto, Venice, Italy
[3] Histologix Ltd, Nottingham, UK
[4] Musculoskeletal Transplant Foundation, Edison, New Jersey, USA

As we have seen in Chapter 2, many different professionals participate in making tissue donations happen. This chapter focuses on the professionals who would not consider that their core purpose is to facilitate donation after death but whose contribution to making tissue donation a reality can be hugely significant. The support of hospital pathologists, funeral home directors, and medical examiners and coroners can be crucial to ensuring that the option of tissue donation can be offered outside of the intensive care unit. The public perception of these professionals is associated with the negative aspect of death and their role in facilitating transplantation can be conveyed as a positive opportunity for improving and broadening that impression.

The supply of donors can, in general, be considered to be dependent on the following factors:

1 willingness of the public and professionals to support organ and tissue donation
2 detection of potential donors

Tissue and Cell Donation: An Essential Guide. Edited by Ruth M. Warwick, Deirdre Fehily, Scott A. Brubaker, Ted Eastlund. © 2009 Blackwell Publishing, ISBN: 978-14051-6322-4.

3 clarity regarding the wishes of prospective donors and their surviving relatives who may be required to give/withhold consent

4 the scope for, and willingness of, doctors and medicolegal personnel to initiate donation procedures in a timely fashion

5 the cooperation among all parties involved in the collection of information useful for donor screening in order to prevent donor to recipient transmission of diseases via tissue transplantation

Medical examiners and coroners, hospital pathologists, and funeral directors all have legitimate and fundamental roles to play in facilitating donation. Their active intervention and collaboration, by taking into account the wishes of donors and their families, identifying potential donors, verifying donor suitability for recovery and subsequent surgical use, and initiating donation procedures can help to increase the availability of prospective donors.

The role of the medical examiners and coroners

Medicolegal death investigation is the responsibility of the medical examiner and/or coroner. Historically, in the ancient Roman Code, the coroner was a judicial officer acting on behalf of the monarch (as in England). The later Napoleonic Code became the forerunner of medicolegal death investigation systems that exist today to investigate deaths in the United States and many European countries. Nowadays, a medical examiner in the US is typically a physician with a specialty in pathology who has undertaken additional training and, ideally, certification in forensic pathology. A coroner in England or a procurator fiscal in Scotland is a doctor and/or lawyer of five years' standing or more and is appointed by the government. A coroner in the US, however, is often a lawyer, a funeral director, or an administrator who occupies a political position, either having been appointed or elected. In the United States, a coroner may be a certified Forensic Pathologist or, alternatively, may have had little or no training in death investigation. Tissue procurement organizations and/or transplant coordinators[1] may therefore be required to interact with both entities or with only one,

---

[1] In many parts of Europe the progressive incorporation of organ transplants as a therapeutic resource resulted in an organizational adaptation of overall transplant management by tissue procurement organizations, leading to the emergence of tissue coordinators. In Spain, for example, the National Organization of Transplants (*Organizacion Nacional de Transplantes*) was created in the mid-1980s, establishing a system called the "Spanish model" based on a network of coordinators at three levels: national, the autonomous community, and the hospital. For the purposes of brevity, the term tissue procurement organizations will be used throughout the chapter to cover the activities carried out by tissue procurement organizations and tissue coordinators.

depending on the local jurisdiction and its political and professional structure.

Regardless of the political structure, medical examiners and coroners are responsible for determining the cause and manner of death (i.e. natural, accident, suicide, or homicide) of those cases that come under their jurisdiction. In broad terms, the jurisdiction includes all deaths that occur suddenly and unexpectedly while the individual is in apparent good health and when there is a suspicion for an unnatural death. Some jurisdictions may also include deaths that occur during diagnostic or therapeutic procedures and cases where there is a potential threat to public health (e.g. suspected smallpox or anthrax). Although the law defines the responsibilities and purpose of medical examiners and coroners rather narrowly, the reality is that the investigation, which most often includes the performance of an autopsy and ancillary studies, has a confirmatory and an evidentiary function as well [1]. Thus, the cause of death may appear obvious (e.g. a gunshot wound of the head), yet the medical examiner and coroner investigation will yield information about the range of fire, the direction of the projectile, whether it could have been self-inflicted or not, the role of drugs and natural disease, and a host of other considerations that may have profound medicolegal implications for both criminal and civil proceedings. Most perceive medical examiners and coroners to be involved predominantly with homicides, suicides, and accidents. However, in most medical examiner jurisdictions in the US, about two-thirds of the cases investigated and autopsied are sudden natural deaths. Although relatively few of these natural deaths become involved with civil litigation, the results of the investigation are of interest and consequence to family, acquaintances, and sometimes to the general public as well. Consequently, when a request for tissue donation is made, medical examiners and coroners must evaluate the decision in light of their statutory requirements and their obligations to the civil and criminal justice systems and to the families of the decedent. The decision to allow tissue recovery will be initially influenced by factors such as whether the apparent cause of death is traumatic or natural, an apparent homicide, or potentially high profile (e.g. death in police custody), or if it is a pediatric death. At this point, medical examiners and coroners and their offices have the potential for positive public influence in highlighting the need for tissue donation and educating the public of the benefits of tissue donation for transplantation and other purposes, especially in the context of bereavement, where such knowledge may help ameliorating grief.

In deaths from trauma, the concern of medical examiners and coroners is that the tissue recovery process will interfere with or destroy external signs of important evidentiary value. Some examples include the presence of petechiae of the eyes, which may be supportive evidence for an asphyxial death; deposits of gunshot residue or other trace evidence, which could be removed with handling the body or washing; and pattern injuries, which may provide information about a type of weapon or instrument (needed to reconstruct the terminal event). Internally, the concern is that the removal of cardiovascular tissues and bones may result in artifacts that could make the interpretation of injuries difficult, or even destroy or alter crucial findings. There is also the fear that crucial observations (e.g. hemopericardium, hemothorax) may not be adequately documented. Another concern is that the tissue procurement procedure may preclude the determination of the death as the result of pulmonary thromboembolism, or destroy the source of the embolism if the deep leg veins are removed. For these reasons, some medical examiners and coroners have, unfortunately, ruled that tissue recovery is not permitted in cases of apparent homicide or in deaths in police custody, or when there is the potential for civil litigation. However, such a blanket proscription against tissue donation in the context of a medical examiner and coroner case is currently not considered justifiable when it is possible for medical examiners and coroners to view the body first and document the external and internal evidence needed for criminal and civil proceedings [2].

Although sudden natural deaths do not generally have the potential for legal proceedings that trauma cases do, medical examiners and coroners have an obligation to the family to determine the cause of death. Here the concern is generally the removal of the heart (for valves) as the cardiectomy must occur under aseptic conditions; the heart is then transported to a tissue processing facility where it is examined by experienced technicians and, upon request, can be further examined by another pathologist. In fact, in the US, over 50% of all hearts donated for valve dissection are eventually forwarded to a pathologist who performs a gross and microscopic examination on the heart remains postdissection. However, it is not usually examined by medical examiners and coroners who must determine and certify the cause of death. Consequently, heart-for-valve recovery is often denied in cases of sudden unexpected, apparently natural, deaths. To overcome this obstacle, a dissection technique has been devised so medical examiners and coroners may examine the heart under aseptic conditions, document the cardiac cause of death, and yet permit valve donation [3]. In this algorithm, if the cause of death is not found in the heart, the specimen is refrigerated and the autopsy is completed. If the cause of death remains undetermined and there is the likelihood that a cardiac conduction system study is needed (a relatively rare circumstance), the valve donation is denied. The reality is that this denial almost never occurs.

The third area of great concern to medical examiners and coroners is a pediatric death, as the unexpected death of a child is considered as potentially a homicide until proven otherwise. And if the death is indeed the result of child abuse, the injuries must be carefully documented not only as to their location and nature, but the estimated time of injury as well. Again, the fear and concern are that the tissue recovery procedure will interfere with a criminal investigation and prosecution. In deaths that suggest the possibility of sudden infant death syndrome, it has traditionally been required that a complete autopsy is necessary for the diagnosis and that the procurement of tissue (e.g. the heart for valves) would preclude this determination or eliminate the possibility of diagnosing a congenital heart defect, which could potentially affect other family members. However, studies have now shown that this potential is more theoretical than real [4], and protocols for examining pediatric hearts to allow valve donation have also been established [5].

The concerns of medical examiners and coroners, as noted earlier, are the ones most commonly encountered. Some, such as those concerning homicide, may also be influenced by concerns of police investigators or prosecutors. These issues have been thoroughly evaluated in the United States by the National Association of medical examiners and addressed in a position paper [2] that indicates that tissue donation should never be totally denied regardless of the type of case. However, there may be some restrictions (e.g. the body must be examined first for trace evidence, petechiae, etc.) or denial of the recovery of leg veins in cases of suspected pulmonary thromboembolism.

Efforts to increase the donation rate of transplantable tissues are occurring worldwide and address political, cultural, and ethical issues [6]. These include such concepts as "presumed consent" (opting out) and "required request" (opting in). In the United States, the Uniform Anatomical Gift Act (UAGA) strongly encourages tissue procurement organizations and medical examiners and coroners to jointly develop policies that will satisfy the need for information and documentation for the timely procurement of tissues and establish criteria for selected restriction of tissue recovery. Likewise, national transplantation laws in individual European countries have sought to establish a coherent legal framework for promoting the act of donation as well as its safety. Examples include the regulations regarding organ and tissue retrieval and transplantation, Law 91 of April 1, 1999, in Italy [7], and The Organ Donation Act of 1998 for the Netherlands [8]. Coupled with pan-European legislation and guidelines [9, 10], they formulate the essential requirements and principles regarding the institutional infrastructure and organization, facilities, and training necessary for the retrieval, evaluation, processing, storage, and distribution of donor organs and tissues.

Mutual in-service training is valuable in facilitating the missions of both the tissue procurement organizations and medical examiners and coroners. The tissue procurement organization personnel must be aware of the concerns of the medical examiners and coroners, be willing to document their findings, and perform tissue procurement (e.g. bones and peripheral veins) after the autopsy whenever possible. The recovery of tissue after the completion of the autopsy has one disadvantage because of increased contamination of the tissue as verified by the results of the tissue's preprocessing microbiologic cultures. Whenever possible, if it is feasible that tissue recovery take place before autopsy, this should be considered to keep bacterial contamination low. medical examiners and coroners must be educated as to the necessity of tissue donation, and the tissue procurement organizations should provide information to the medical examiners and coroners and their investigative staff regarding the criteria for suitable tissue donors and how tissues are utilized in a clinical setting. Awareness of time limitations and other criteria for potential tissue donation have enabled some medical examiner and coroner facilities to actually notify the local tissue procurement organization of potential cases when the person is not taken to a hospital first (e.g. suicide, where the time of death is known, or a witnessed death). Some medical examiner facilities now include areas dedicated to on-site recovery of tissue.

CASE 1

Medical examiner support increases donations

The value of cooperation and communication was highlighted when an issue arose concerning heart valve procurement from a man who died shortly after being stung by a wasp. The medical examiner denied approval for the donation of the heart for valves as it was not certain whether the death was related to the wasp sting or to coronary artery disease. This prompted subsequent discussions with the tissue procurement organization and the tissue processing organization and led to the medical examiner developing a procedure whereby the heart could be evaluated under sterile conditions to identify and document the cardiac cause of death and yet preserve the heart valves to allow donation for transplantation. Future cases of sudden unexpected death of presumed cardiac origin could therefore be evaluated and the valves procured for transplantation. The medical examiner's obligation is met, the donor family is satisfied, and recipient lives may be saved or enhanced. As always, with competing agendas, open communication directed toward finding solutions for the common good is preferable to legislation, which forces acquiescence of one party or another.

The role of the funeral home director

After death, the practices of memorializing the deceased vary greatly depending on the country, the culture, and religious practices. In some cultures, tissue donation after death may have an impact because in many countries, funeral services take place after embalming and cosmetic restoration by professionals in the field.

When tissue donation was first introduced into a community, tissue procurement organizations often did not consider the impact of tissue donation and recovery on the funeral director's services. Communication with the funeral professional was sometimes nonexistent to minimal, at best. Sometimes, lack of knowledge of, and appreciation for, their respective roles in death care created conflict between the two professions. In some cases, local funeral home professionals opposed donation, to the point of actively discouraging families from donating. It was not an uncommon scenario for a tissue procurement organization to encounter a family who had initially consented to the donation of their loved one's tissues, but then rescinded that consent after visiting with their funeral home director.

There were several reasons for these conflicts and the need to overcome them. First, the tissue donation process interferes with the usual work of the embalmer and funeral director in that tissue donation can create delays for the funeral service, interferes with embalming by disrupting the arterial system, and can cause disfigurement of the body, making cosmetic restoration more difficult. In addition, the success of funeral homes, often family-run businesses, is based on their professionalism and impeccable reputation of excellent service at the time of need, and a very well-preserved and presentable body at the time of viewing. Anything that jeopardizes that reputation would be detrimental to a funeral home's success, and, therefore, be discouraged.

The recovery process can seriously complicate the funeral director's ability to adequately preserve the donated body, and to his or her ability to restore that body to a viewable condition. For trained embalmers, the "gold standard" of embalming practice is the preservation of tissues through arterial injection of embalming fluids. This provides the most thorough distribution of the embalming chemicals to all tissues, and, therefore, the most complete preservation. Arterial injection is severely compromised by the disruption of the intact vascular system as a result of cardiectomy, recovery of the peripheral vessels, or trauma caused by the recovery of organs, bone, and connective tissue. Other challenges to the embalmer's restoration process include the recovery of such tissues as the mandible, vertebral bodies, whole knees and elbows, the recovery of full-thickness skin (when a dermatome is not used), and ocular tissue.

The working relationship between funeral directors and tissue procurement organizations varies from enthusiastic support and cooperation to being uncooperative, unsupportive, and sometimes outright antagonistic. Anecdotal reports of funeral directors still using their influence to discourage a family from donating are not uncommon. There are also numerous reports of funeral homes intentionally transporting and embalming the body of a potential donor before the donation consent/authorization can be confirmed. Conversely, there are many examples of funeral directors tolerating, supporting, encouraging, and even actively participating in the donation process. This type of support ranges from help with transportation of the body, use or lease of funeral home space for recovery, provision of donation-related literature to families, to actively approaching families for consent and serving as members of recovery teams.

Over the past 10 years, the tissue banks in the United States have made significant progress in improving relationships with funeral home professionals. Many tissue banks have established a "funeral director liaison" position to provide a contact person for the funeral directors within their service area. Those tissue banks with successful relationships develop profiles on each funeral home regarding preferences for types of prosthetics, suturing technique, notification practices, etc. They maintain lines of communication through phone calls with funeral home representatives if the funeral home has been selected. These innovative tissue banks communicate with funeral directors on an individual basis, on a local or county level, and often on a professional, state association level. Another effective tool has been the formation of a tissue procurement organization/funeral director committee, comprising representatives of tissue procurement organizations and regional members of the funeral industry. Such a committee provides an excellent forum to discuss mutually important issues on a regular schedule or on an ad hoc basis.

In 2001, in the United States, representatives from the American Association of Tissue Banks (AATB) and the National funeral directors Association (NFDA) met at the NFDA headquarters in Brookfield, Wisconsin, US to discuss the relationship between the tissue banking and funeral service professions, and to work on improving the relationship between the two groups. The Association of Organ Procurement Organizations (AOPO) was subsequently brought into these discussions. The result of these meetings was the production of a document, "AATB–AOPO–NFDA Best Practices for Organ and Tissue Donation" (see Table 9.1). This document, distributed by the NFDA to its membership and by the AATB and AOPO to their constituencies, outlines a consensus of important issues integral to the improvement and maintenance of a good working relationship between the funeral service profession and the donation community.

Most progressive tissue procurement organizations are following these best practices. They are building bridges with local funeral directors by recommending that the family consult their funeral director on such issues as the timing of the funeral and appropriate clothing for viewing. These tissue procurement organizations are also

1 restricting incisions to areas covered by clothing, and some tissue procurement organizations will limit the recovery of certain tissues based on a family's funeral plans;
2 supplying the funeral home with prosthetics, body bags, protective plastic garments, and a variety of preservatives and drying and sealing agents;

Table 9.1 AATB–AOPO–NFDA Best Practices for Organ and Tissue Donation for 2001

1 Notification: appropriate notification of the funeral home regarding a donation by the tissue procurement organization
  • the tissue procurement organization must identify the funeral director and notify him or her of donation as soon as details are known
  • communicate time lines, location, nature, tissue procurement organization contact information
  • tissue procurement organization staff maintains ongoing contact as donation case evolves
  • tissue procurement organization should facilitate communication between the medical examiner and the funeral home
  • notify funeral director when the body is ready for pickup after recovery is completed

2 Disclosure: disclosure of the potential impact of donation on the donor body and funeral plans
  • the tissue procurement organization should inform the donor family of factors that may affect the timing of the funeral
  • the consent discussion should include explanation of the potential impact of donation on burial arrangements and the appearance of the body
  • consent/authorization should be specific in describing organs/tissues/eyes to be recovered

3 Recovery procedures: a list of recovery techniques considered helpful to the embalmer
  • all major arteries involved should be ligated
  • replace all recovered bones with prostheses
  • consult the funeral director regarding preferred type of incision closure
  • consider a U or Y incision instead of a midline sternotomy
  • elevate the head on a head block
  • no facial bone recovery if viewing is planned

4 Reimbursement: a statement addressing conditions of financial reimbursement to the funeral home
  • tissue procurement organizations should establish a policy for compensation of funeral directors for additional time and materials
  • funeral home should not charge the donor family additional fees resulting from the donation

5 Communication/education: the importance of communication and cross education between the funeral industry and donation field
  • funeral directors and tissue procurement organizations should reach out to each other and establish lines of communication
  • outreach should include visits to each other's place of business

6 Support
  • NFDA will support and encourage its members to support donation
  • the funeral director should respect the family's wishes to donate and should help facilitate the donation recovery process
  • the tissue procurement organization should refrain from telling the family that no change to the donor's appearance is guaranteed
  • the tissue procurement organization should be aware of the timing of the donation and its effect on the funeral service

AATB, American Association of Tissue Banks; AOPO, Association of Organ Procurement Organizations; NFDA, National Funeral Directors Association.

3 promoting cross education between the two professions by organizing educational seminars for local funeral directors that include expert consultation on embalming techniques for the donor body. They are often able to provide continuing education credits for the funeral directors through state licensing boards.

As some funeral directors have become more involved in the donation process, and particularly when reimbursement is obtained for services, it is critical that a clear understanding of the roles and responsibilities within the relationship exists and that the conditions and requirements for reimbursement are well defined and documented. Tissue banking is a highly regulated activity, governed in the United States by the US Food and Drug Administration's (US FDA) regulations via rules and guidance, by state laws that govern gift law (i.e. consent), and by standards-setting organizations such as the AATB and the Eye Bank Association of America. Likewise, in Europe this activity is regulated by the European Union (EU) by means of directives, which must be transposed into national laws; by the national governments, which must verify compliance with these laws; by other laws of individual member states; and standards-setting associations such as the European Association of Tissue Bank and the European Eye Bank Association. This degree of oversight is often underappreciated by funeral professionals. There have been at least two well-publicized situations in which US funeral service personnel and/or funeral home facilities have been involved in tissue donation without adequate adherence to US FDA regulations or state laws (accessed January 25, 2008 http://www.fda.gov/cber/safety/bts030206.htm and http://www.fda.gov/cber/safety/drs083006.htm). This has resulted in significant concern over the safety of that recovered tissue, a criminal investigation into the personnel involved, and much negative media coverage on an international scale, which has been detrimental. Coincidental to these incidents, the NFDA recognized potential legal liability inherent when funeral service professionals work closely with tissue banks, with or without reimbursement. In October 2005, the NFDA, through its general counsel, released a document to its membership titled, "National Funeral Directors Association Best Practices to Reduce Legal Liability of Funeral Homes Participating in Organ/Tissue/Cadaver Donations" (best legal practices). This document was amended in July 2006 (accessed January 25, 2008 http://www.nfda.org/files/AdvComp/OrganTissueLegalGuidelines.pdf) and advises funeral directors of their legal liability when working with tissue banks at a number of different levels. It is too early to determine the impact of this advice on the working relationship between the funeral directors and tissue banks. At a minimum, funeral homes in the United States may require more formal written agreements with tissue banks to define the nature of their relationships.

Two common and basic forms of a funeral home's involvement in the donation process are to contract for the transportation of the donor body on behalf of the tissue procurement organization, and to allow the use of a funeral home space for tissue recovery. These types of limited involvement by the funeral home carry the least amount of liability. A written agreement, describing the roles and responsibilities of each party for these activities, is preferred to minimize the liability as well as to prevent any misunderstandings as the relationship evolves. The NFDA agrees that each of these activities may be billable by the funeral home.

The use of a funeral home facility as a recovery site is a relatively common practice among tissue banks in the United States. The facility should be of suitable size, construction, and location to prevent contamination. There should be procedures in place that address facility cleaning and sanitation, with documentation and maintenance of cleaning records. In general, the tissue procurement organization should ensure that the team is recovering tissue in a controlled environment – one with adequate ventilation and lighting, controlled access, cleaning and disinfecting capability, and isolation from any other activities within the facility. Despite these safeguards, some states are proposing legislation to restrict or eliminate the use of funeral home facilities as potential tissue recovery sites. To further control the environment where tissue recovery may be performed, the 11th edition of AATB's Standards for Tissue Banking was updated in July 2007 to require a documented evaluation of the tissue recovery site. Preestablished criteria are listed as recovery site suitability parameters and appear in standard D5.500 Recovery Environment (accessed January 25, 2008 http://www.aatb.org/files/2007bulletin46.pdf). A thorough description of these parameters and a sample form for documenting the evaluation of the recovery site were concurrently published in an update to AATB's Guidance Document No. 2 (accessed January 25, 2008 http://aatb.timberlakepublishing.com/files/2007bulletin46attachment1.pdf). These recovery site parameters are detailed and must be met but they do not specifically exclude locations by name (funeral home, autopsy room, morgue); they qualify them by their physical attributes and the ability to offer suitable conditions for tissue recovery.

Funeral service professionals have been involved in other donation-related activities such as referrals of potential donors, approach for consent, donor screening, and participation in tissue recovery. The NFDA's best legal practices caution against compensation for referrals, as this could be construed as participating in the sale of bodies or tissues. The other three donation-related functions, mentioned earlier, could be performed by the funeral service professional acting as an employee of the tissue procurement organization. By working as a tissue bank employee, the funeral director would incur less personal liability and would be operating under the tissue procurement organization's insurance. The tissue procurement organization would have greater control over the training and monitoring of the employee's performance.

The funeral service profession and the donation community serve the same bereaved families. To honor the family's wishes for donation, it is essential that the two entities communicate and work cooperatively toward that end. Cross education, to provide a good understanding of each profession's responsibilities and support of each other's role in serving the donor family, will provide the groundwork for improved tissue bank and funeral home relationships.

It is difficult to generalize the possible role of the funeral home director throughout Europe. Even though the donation and transplantation of organs and tissues are now regulated by common EU directives, the legislation of death, the legal definition of tissues and organs, and the standards of safety and quality are managed at the national level.

With regard to Italy, this particular profession has minor involvement because the whole process of donation can be activated only through public institutions and tissue procurement cannot be done by private organizations that are involved with the cremation or burial of the deceased.

CASE 2

Dedicated donation facility (DDF)

Tissue Services (TS) in Liverpool, United Kingdom, developed a successful working partnership with coroners, pathologists, and mortuary teams in order to facilitate tissue donation in a DDF within the tissue bank. Prior to the DDF being operational in September 2006, it was routine practice to facilitate donation within hospital mortuaries. The facility became operational around the time of legislative changes such as the Human Tissue Act (2004) and the EU Directive on Tissues and Cells (2004). This enabled dialogue between TS and the National Health Service (NHS) partners/colleagues to find a way forward to promote donation options and sustain donation activity without placing added pressure on already overstretched NHS staff, particularly pathology and mortuary teams. Consideration was also given to the environment both in terms of donor dignity and the need to clearly distinguish between donation and retention in both public and professional minds and bacterial quality control. The referral systems created within two local hospital sites enabled an increase in donor referrals with no added burden on frontline staff. The routine transfer of donors to the DDF meant less pressure on mortuary time and space. The TS staff no longer needed to travel to all local donations. Issues of training, travel time, and equipment also improved, and tissue was immediately processed on site in the tissue bank without having to be packaged and transported by the teams. coroners and pathologists built up close relationships with the TS staff and the executive boards were satisfied that they were sufficiently compliant with current legislation with minimal input and responsibility from themselves.

The role of the hospital pathologist

The hospital pathologist is responsible for performing an autopsy or post-mortem examination when it is not possible to issue a medical certificate ascertaining a cause of death. This examination is carried out at the behest of a medical examiner and as part of the investigation into sudden or unnatural deaths. In the United States, the hospital pathologist usually performs an autopsy at the request of the treating physician or family, with the express consent of the family, for the purpose of correlating the pathologic findings with the clinical record. Except for the possible allegation of medical malpractice, civil and criminal litigation are generally not a concern, in contrast to forensic autopsies.

Hospital pathologists can be involved in deceased donor tissue donation, and can be involved with the procurement of tissues from the deceased for diagnostic purposes within the framework of an autopsy (fluids, organs, tissue samples) and to gather material for research and training students and pathology residents. Tissues for transplantation can be retrieved several hours after death. However, the recovery of tissues for transplant procedures within the framework of an autopsy is more intrusive than the usual autopsy procedure as corneas, skin, bone, and tendons are only investigated during a routine postmortem examination in exceptional circumstances. It is for this reason that pathologists are often willing, unless there is a forensic investigation underway, to allow eye and tissue banks to recover tissue before the postmortem examination gets underway. Performing tissue recovery prior to autopsy is preferred so microbiological contamination of tissue to be utilized for transplantation is minimized.

The contribution of the hospital pathologist is essential to the work of the tissue procurement organizations in helping establish a precise cause of death and in documenting possible contraindications to the use of particular tissues for transplant, which had not been evidenced by the patient's individual medical case history gathered from the treating hospital physician, the general practitioner, or from the interview with the relevant historian (usually the next of kin).

CASE 3

Autopsy results can enhance transplant safety

The value of hospital pathologist collaboration was underlined in a recent case concerning a 3-year-old multitissue donor (corneas and heart valves) in the Veneto region of Italy [11] whose death was sudden, unexpected, and of unknown cause. There was no sign of trauma, and the paramedics who arrived on the scene found the child in asystole and already mydriatic. There were no previous hospital admissions for this patient, and the initial clinical diagnosis was "syncope with sphincter incontinence." However, the subsequent autopsy gave the diagnosis as acute bronchiolitis with focal, follicular necrosis, in association with interstitial pneumonitis, pericarditis, and generalized, reactive lymphadenopathy. The etiology of the ultimate demise was likely viral, and the diffusion of the infectious agent could not be ruled out. Therefore, the young donor had to be disqualified, and the potential threat to the recipients could be prevented by the information provided by the pathologist.

Although consent of the next of kin is not required for a forensic autopsy, it is normally required for a nonsuspicious postmortem examination, especially when there is a need or a request for the retention of any tissues or organs following the examination. It is precisely concerning this issue that dramatic adverse publicity about inadequate consent procedures for the retention of organs and tissues during postmortem examination in the United Kingdom and Ireland has greatly affected the willingness of people to donate and engendered new and more stringent regulations.

Public and media interest in the retention of human organs and tissues was stirred by the announcement of inquiries into pediatric cardiac surgery at the Bristol Royal Infirmary (Kennedy Report: http://www.bristol-inquiry. org.uk/), the Alder Hey Hospital in Liverpool (Redfern Report: http://www. rlcinquiry.org.uk/), and other incidents where it became clear that the legal and ethical frameworks that were in place in the United Kingdom were outdated and not fit to meet current-day expectations of parents, other family members, and patients. It was not always made clear to the relatives of the deceased why certain tissues were removed and what the fate of the tissues would be after their purpose had been served. Subsequently, other so-called organ scandals have been reported from elsewhere in the world including the United States; currently, many of these issues are in litigation.

The situation in the United Kingdom has now changed, and as a direct result of previous adverse publicity, two new human tissue specific laws have been enacted: the Human Tissue Act 2004 (http://www.england-legislation.hmso.gov.uk/acts/acts2004/ukpga_20040030_en_1) and the Human Tissue Act (Scotland) 2006 (http://www.opsi.gov.uk/legislation/scotland/acts2006/asp_20060004_en_1). There is little overlap apart from the activities of the Human Tissue Authority, which is responsible for a new system of regulation by licensing and the production of Codes of Practice, which "give practical guidance and lay down the standards expected. It is hoped that the Codes are of value to practitioners and other groups in helping to support good practice in an important area of science and medicine" (http://www.hta.gov.uk/). The Act and authority cover five main areas of human tissue activity ranging from public display to transplantation and aim to facilitate use of human tissue within the new legal framework.

The legislation is underpinned by consent, which should be appropriate to the planned use of tissue and to any risks to donor or recipient, and the stated aims of the authority are to increase public and professional confidence so that more tissue can become available for, among other things, transplantation. Human bodies under the jurisdiction of a coroner are not covered by the Act, but any material that remains once the coroner's enquiries are completed does. Additional measures introduced in the United Kingdom include:

1 Revised postmortem consent forms will be introduced covering the retention of tissues for educational and research purposes and allowing families to limit the extent of non-coroner's postmortem examinations.
2 Designated "bereavement teams" were set up, founded on the principles of respect, understanding, informed consent, time and space, skill and sensitivity, information and transparency, cultural competence, and the recognition of donation as a "gift relationship."
3 Closer collaboration and training with TCs and tissue bank staff on organ and tissue removal and retention issues were recommended and have now been achieved.

Openness engenders trust, and it is hoped that if doctors and pathologists communicate honestly with the public and demonstrate the importance and value of their work in a more sensitive and open manner, the public will feel able to make informed decisions with regards to postmortem consent and the donation of tissues for transplant, research, and training. In addition, strengthening good lines of communication with hospital colleagues and forging closer links with bereavement counselors, mortuary staff, transplant coordinators, tissue bank staff, medical examiners and coroners, and hospital managers is positively encouraged in order to demonstrate the professions' adherence to honesty and transparency of information and consent. Pathologists should be aware that in the context of family consent given freely through discussion with a trained tissue coordinator, the release of sensitive information to legitimate agencies involved in donor screening and selection should not be seen as a violation of patient and family privacy. Such disclosed information must be processed and stored in accordance with the relevant laws and utilized only in the interest of recipient health and with respect to donor families.

Even in the United Kingdom, where a specific and permissive legislative framework exists, where there are clear ethical guidelines and where there is openness between donors, families, and professionals, there are barriers to progress. Much of this is attributable to lack of general awareness and understanding of the importance and benefits of making tissue available for transplantation. It is generally accepted that individuals and families are positive about donation; in one study, all but one of 70 families interviewed by telephone agreed to permit use of postmortem tissue and blood in tissue transplantation research [12,13]. Although pathologists in the lead cases were exonerated at the conclusion of the UK "Nationwide Organs Retention Group litigation" in 2004 (http://www.hmcourts-service.gov.uk/ judgmentsfiles/j2427/ab-v-nhs_trusts.htm), pathologists are still apprehensive about the Human Tissue Act 2004 and will operate in a manner that ensures they more than meet the standards required to comply. This may, for example, extend to insisting on written consent for postmortem tissue removal when it is perfectly legal and certainly more practical to obtain recorded telephone consent. Pathologists worldwide have diagnostic work and other duties that are likely to fall further down their list of work priorities, particularly if they are not actively involved in tissue transplantation, or if tissue retrieval is likely to interrupt or slow down their busy routines. With motivation and dedicated staff, it is possible to work across boundaries, increase the amount and utility of tissue retrieved postmortem, benefit the donors' wishes, the families' wishes and the tissue recipients' quality of life, and increase professional pride by positive messages.

CASE 4

Working with funeral home directors, mortuary managers, and related professionals

A key issue was the operational aspects of the transportation of donor bodies. It was essential that the transport contracts were closely reviewed at a senior level and executives satisfied not only the initial concerns of Tissue Services (TS) and Trust, but also the local community. The projected cost of transporting donors resulted in the need for a lengthy EU tender process, which included interviews, visits to the tissue bank, TS quality checks, Good Manufacturing Practices, robust training, and revised documentation for funeral staff. The successful funeral directors also had been highly recommended by the local hospitals involved, from the bereavement officers to the very experienced mortuary managers and coroners, all of whom were accustomed to dealing, in a sensitive and confidential manner, with the transportation of bodies for various reasons. The funeral directors were well established and respected in a city on a community level, and a city that had experienced the issues and impact of retention of postmortem tissue samples fully appreciated the sensitive nature of the project. The key factor in the success of the project was communication and commitment from a diverse range of experienced and expert staff committed to delivering a quality service.

Such collaborative arrangements can work in practice and should act as a beacon to other centers. Hospital pathologists are gatekeepers and crucial to collaborative working, as well as to education and training that will increase the awareness and confidence of public and professionals alike.

Conclusions

Increased cooperation, communication, and training among all of the stakeholders – donors, donor families, the officers of medical examiners and coroners, hospital pathologists, and funeral directors, as well as agents of tissue procurement organizations – can significantly increase the availability of tissue for transplant. Only by working together will it be possible to raise the quality and sensitivity of the donation and transplant process so that the physical and psychological needs of donors, donor families, and recipients are met and that they have appropriate information and advice.

An informed public that has confidence in a transplant service based on the highest ethical standards and which respects the dignity of donor families, friends, and transplant recipients, together with the positive attitude and enhanced knowledge of health and allied professionals regarding tissue donation, will facilitate donation and help the growing number of people in need of a transplant by narrowing the gap between tissue supply and demand.

KEY LEARNING POINTS

- The effects of tissue donation can interfere with the legal and cultural responsibilities of medical examiners and coroners who perform criminal investigations, the hospital pathologist who examines the body to determine the cause of death, and the embalmer and funeral director who prepare the body for the family memorial service.

- With cooperation between the donation organization and the medical examiner and coroner, tissue donation can take place before the work of the latter two and without interfering with their duties.

- A blanket proscription against tissue donation in the context of a medical examiner's or coroner's case is currently not considered justifiable when it is possible for the medical examiner or coroner to view the body first and document the external and internal evidence needed for criminal and civil proceedings.

- In the United States, over 50% of all hearts donated for valve dissection are eventually forwarded to a pathologist who performs a gross and microscopic examination on the heart remains postdissection.

- A dissection technique has been devised so that medical examiners and coroners may examine the heart under aseptic conditions, document the cardiac cause of death, and yet permit valve donation.

- In the United States, the UAGA strongly encourages the tissue procurement organizations and medical examiners and coroners to jointly develop policies that will satisfy the need for information and documentation for the timely procurement of tissues, and establish criteria for selected restriction of tissue recovery.

• By cooperating with embalmers and funeral directors, tissue donation can take place with minimal interference with their responsibilities.

• Many tissue banks have established a "funeral director liaison" position to provide a contact person for the funeral directors within their service area.

• The formation of a tissue procurement organization/funeral director committee, comprising representatives from tissue procurement organizations and regional members of the funeral industry, can be effective by providing an excellent forum to discuss mutually important issues on a regular schedule or on an ad hoc basis.

• By cooperating with hospital pathologists, tissue donation can take before an autopsy without interfering with the pathologists' responsibilities.

• Strengthening good lines of communication with hospital colleagues and forging closer links with bereavement counselors, mortuary staff, TCs, tissue bank staff, medical examiners and coroners, and hospital managers positively encourages and demonstrates the professions' adherence to honesty and transparency of information and consent.

References

1. Wetli CV. The medical examiner's role in organ and tissue recovery: a special dynamic is created. On the Beat (New York Organ Donor Network). 2003;6:12.
2. Pinckard JK, Wetli CV, Graham MA. The National Association of Medical Examiners Position Paper on the Medical Examiner Release of Organs and Tissues for Transplantation. Am J Forensic Med Pathol. 2007;23(3):202–7.
3. Wetli CV, Kolovich RM, Dinhofer LD. Modified cardiectomy – Documenting sudden cardiac death in hearts selected for valve allograft procurement. Am J Forensic Med Pathol. 2002;23(2):137–41.
4. Pinckard JK, Graham MA. Heart valve tissue donation does not preclude the diagnosis of clinically significant pediatric cardiac abnormalities. Am J Forensic Med Pathol. 2003;24(3):248–53.
5. Gunther WM. Pediatric heart valve donation: the Virginia protocol. ASCP Forensic Pathology Check Sample FP 05-6. American Society of Clinical Pathology, Chicago, Illinois. 2005;47:63–73.
6. Cordner S, McKelvie H. Organ and Tissue Transplantation, Ethical and Practical Issues. In: Payne-James J, Byard RW, Corey TS, Henderson C, editors. Encyclopedia of Forensic and Legal Medicine, Volume 3. Oxford: Elsevier; 2005. p. 404–11.
7. Legge 1° Aprile 1999, n. 91: Disposizioni in materia di prelievi e di trapianti di organi e di tessuti. Gazzetta Ufficiale, April 15, 1999;n. 87.
8. Ministerie van Volksgezondheid, Welzijn en Sport – NL: The Organ Donation Act (WOD) [English translation], International Publication Series Health, Welfare and Sport nr. 3. The Hague, July 2000.

9. European Parliament and Council: Directive 2004/23/EC on setting standards of quality and safety for the donation, procurement, testing, processing, preservation, storage and distribution of human tissues and cells. Official Journal of the European Union, L 102. 2004 Apr 7;47.

10. European Council. Guide to Safety and Quality Assurance for the Transplantation of Organs, Tissues and Cells, 3rd edition. Strasbourg, France: Council of Europe Publishing. 2007.

11. Ponzin D, Griffoni C, Fasolo A, Veronese A, Frigo AC, Jones G. Eye banking at the Fondazione Banca degli Occhi del Veneto: present and perspectives. Organs Tissues. 2003;2:111–19.

12. Womack C, Jack AL. Family attitudes to research using samples taken at coroner's post mortem examinations: review of records. BMJ. 2003;327(7418):781–2.

13. Womack C, Gray NM, Pearson JE, Fehily D. Cadaveric tissue supply to the commercial sector for research: collaboration between NHS pathology and NBS Tissue Services extending the options for donors. Cell Tissue Bank. 2001;2(#1):51–5.

10 Staff Development and Support in Roles Associated with Deceased Donation

Riva Miller[1] and Pamela Albert[2]

[1] Haemophilia Centre Royal Free Hospital, London, UK; National Health Service Blood and Transplant Service, London, UK
[2] New England Organ Bank, Newton, Massachusetts, USA

Background

The success of tissue donation programs is reliant on the skill and professionalism of the staff who offer the opportunity for donation to potential donors or their families. The multiple issues and wide range of staff connected with deceased tissue donation give this subject an important place alongside those that concentrate on the technical aspects of safety and efficacy.

This chapter discusses some of the divergent and complex pressures that can impact personally on individuals from the many different disciplines that provide this service, all with interlinking roles. Although technical, scientific, and medical knowledge and expertise provide the necessary background, successful deceased donation also depends on frontline clinical staff who seek consent to donation, deal with regulatory details, and who are confronted with the less-defined concerns or issues (distress, shock, rational, and irrational fears) of bereaved donor families. Similarly, successful recovery of tissue requires the necessary knowledge, and the frontline staff have everyday tasks with very direct emotional and practical impact.

Carefully planned strategies for the recruitment, selection, and retention of staff are key to ensuring an effective and informed service. Time and effort are required for training in specified tasks, engaging in vital liaison within and outside the tissue service, offering the opportunity for donation, and appropriately supporting individual staff members. In recognition of this investment, and with the overarching aim of safe, efficient tissue recovery,

Tissue and Cell Donation: An Essential Guide. Edited by Ruth M. Warwick, Deirdre Fehily, Scott A. Brubaker, Ted Eastlund. © 2009 Blackwell Publishing, ISBN: 978-14051-6322-4.

staff development and support for those associated with deceased tissue donation have been given prominence in services provided in many countries.

The tasks to be performed in coordination of a deceased donation challenge the emotions and sensitivities of most individuals. These difficult tasks may include adjusting to special approaches for families; conducting the donation conversation with a group of bereaved relatives; intimately witnessing the results of a tragic, shocking death; dealing with a wide donor age range and diverse donor family cultures; and covering a vast amount of evolving information needed for disclosure, consent, and donor suitability evaluation. These staff members may experience distress and feel grief themselves when dealing with the bereaved. There are few other professionals whose day begins and ends with the death of an individual, and where the death of one individual may be the only ameliorating factor that will enhance the life, or prevent the death, of another.

The key focus in the coordination of deceased donation is safety for the recipients, requiring diligence and efficiency within a structure that is safe and supported by validated protocols and guidelines. These structures are vital for staff dealing with death, donor families, and tissue recovery and processing.

Operational efficiency and a wide knowledge base are integral to the task of obtaining consent for donation under the pressure of time limitations. As part of daily working practice, this can be stressful to those individuals and can manifest in poor work performance, absence from work, irritability, forgetfulness, and resignation. Appreciating the success of tissue transplantation by exposure to recipient stories may help to give some counterbalance to stress. However, protocols that dictate communication and/or contact between donor families and recipients are controversial, with different approaches adopted in the United States and the United Kingdom.

The stress resulting from constant exposure to critical life-threatening situations can lead to excessive demands on coordinators (United States) or specialist nurses (United Kingdom) (interchangeable terminology used in the two countries) and tissue recovery technicians as it is almost impossible for them to remain emotionally unaffected by the loss to others [1]. Staff members must be able to contain their emotions so that they can deliver the professional expertise that is required to care for families and facilitate their wish, as well as the donor's desire, to donate. Each professional should be assisted in finding a tolerable level of emotional reaction to this type of work and view this level of tolerance as a human limit rather than a personal inadequacy. Continuous staff development and support addresses such issues and can be provided in various ways through line management, teamwork, and educational events. Nonhierarchical fora with a range of professionals (specialist nurses/coordinators, doctors, managers, and outside consultants) can provide opportunities for open, free, and safe discussion of a wide variety of topics.

This chapter deals only with stress associated with donation and not with other sources of stress such as changes in management. It highlights some approaches and frameworks for the practice of staff development and support, incorporating services from the United Kingdom and the United States. A full case example sets the scene, and the chapter ends with a selection of snapshot cases, which together illustrate the key learning points.

CASE 1

"Frustrating for all"

1 Background: A hospital referred a 30-year-old man, who died following a cardiac arrest, to the coordinator. The hospital identified the legal next of kin as his parents and provided their contact number. When the coordinator called to offer the family the opportunity for donation, the mother was receptive and believed that this would be the one good thing that would come from her son's unexpected death. The coordinator asked if her son was married and the mother said "no." This was later discussed with line management and the team.

2 Difficulties: At the end of the donation conversation, the mother revealed that her son was not legally divorced from his estranged wife. She stated that her family had a difficult relationship with her estranged daughter-in-law and that her grandson had been removed from the home of his mother by social services. She, as grandmother, and her son had been his primary caregivers. She stated that she did not have any contact information for her daughter-in-law, except for her address and her mother's home telephone number. The coordinator told the mother that because her daughter-in-law was her son's legal next of kin, the daughter-in-law needed to be contacted to obtain either her consent to donation or her decision to waive her rights of decision to her mother-in-law. Although upset by this information, the mother of the potential donor understood and asked the coordinator to do what she could to ensure that her son's donation could proceed. Throughout the night, several telephone calls were made to the deceased's mother-in-law to gain contact with his estranged wife. However, no direct contact was made before the team ran out of time for suitable tissue procurement.

3 Support for the staff member: The next morning, the coordinator asked for guidance from her line manager about how best to explain to the deceased donor's mother that the donation could not proceed. She explained that this case resonated with her as she was the same age as the donor, and her concern was that she had failed this family by not being able to carry out their wishes for donation. A discussion ensued about the empathetic care she had indeed provided and the trust that been established between her and the potential donor's mother. It was decided that the next conversation would focus not on what she had been unable to do, but on the information and services she could provide to the mother to enable her to support her family as they dealt with this unexpected death.

The coordinator spoke to the mother, provided her with this information, and expressed the team's gratitude for the family's willingness to help others in the midst of their own grief. Before leaving for home, the coordinator shared with colleagues and line manager how difficult this case was and how grateful she was that this was the end of her duty time, as she did not feel she had anything left to offer another family.

Theoretical background to staff support and development

Little research has focused on identifying the grief that those who work in the field of tissue donation and recovery experience through their work. Much of the literature focuses on burnout and stress among nurses, but few studies link these reactions to the short- and long-term effects of workplace-engendered grief [1]. Fulton [2] described a phenomenon known as the "Stockholm syndrome," taken from the psychology of hostages. In times of emotional upheaval, strong bonding can take place quickly, and this applies to coordinators/specialist nurses and the donor family.

For some healthcare professionals with expertise in a specific area (donation and transplantation), this may be equated with achieving mastery, and the emotional impact of the work can be easily overlooked. Weisman [3] noted that the impact of emotions and grief can be underestimated. Concealing job-related stress can result in physical and emotional distancing from families and colleagues. Feelings of inadequacy, anger, frustration, panic, anxiety, and impatience are not unusual. Significant others (spouses, partners, family, friends, and colleagues) may find the individual withdrawn, irritable, and "not himself or herself." Such reactions can lead to poor work performance and sometimes may result in a desire to quit. Extreme stress can put people at high risk of losing the ability to make clear decisions and to function in their personal life.

Death and loss have given rise to social ceremonies and commemorative activities that acknowledge the death, recognize the place the person occupied in society, and assist the bereaved through the process of grief. Each culture faces death with its own definition of "appropriate" social–emotional reactions. The professional relationship with the deceased differs to one of personal loss; much as we might have empathy for the bereaved, we do not expect them to be part of our future, and thus staff suffering from "bereavement" are denied the opportunity to express their feelings or emotions. Those who have encountered a loss that cannot be openly acknowledged, publicly mourned, or socially supported (coordinators, recovery technicians, donor record reviewers, and quality auditors) experience disenfranchised grief or an attitude from colleagues that emotional reactions are unprofessional [4]. Grief may become an undesirable expression in the workplace.

Healthcare providers who work with the dying and their families experience stress unique to their specialty, emanating from environmental and personal factors. These are listed in the following box.

Stress in the workplace

External sources of stress include administrative, staff, and patient issues, the most common being:

1 inadequate communication
2 unrealistic expectations between administrators and frontline staff, and among colleagues, with resulting work overload, conflicts, and lack of support from coworkers

Internal sources of stress vary for each individual with feelings of:

1 chronic anticipatory grief and loss
2 a sense of isolation and inappropriate motivations for choosing this field

---

Many demands are made on those who deal with the dying and newly bereaved, such as being confronted with one's own anxieties about dying and overidentifying with these patients and their families. Recognition of personal vulnerability is a key element in the way each individual handles the losses faced every day in their professional lives.

Maslach described burnout as a "syndrome of emotional exhaustion, depersonalization and reduced personal accomplishment . . . as a result of the chronic emotional strain of working extensively with other human beings especially when they are troubled" [5]. The support the caregiver receives from others may be a critical element in preventing burnout. A logical first step in halting the burnout process is identifying specific sources of stress.

The sharing of concerns and feelings with others can be instructive and provide insight into professional practice. Sustaining work with deceased donors and families [6] requires enhancing social support both inside and outside professional circles to deal with compassion fatigue. Support within the professional environment provides the unique understanding that comes with this line of work. Support outside the professional realm can help build and maintain an identity that is about more than taking care of others, and in engaging in their suffering. An important aspect of self-care is to identify the relationship to other people's suffering and what may be in the professional's power to control. However, systems of support may be deficient in a number of ways, whether because of the limitation of resources or the limited vision by those who control the resources.

The impact of organizational, practical, and psychological issues

Different issues impact the frontline (coordinators/specialist nurses and tissue recovery staff) and the backroom staff (i.e. some line managers, medical consultants, donor record reviewers, laboratory technicians, and quality assurance staff). For these "behind-the-scenes" members of the tissue donation teams, looking at donor charts daily, following the destination of donations, and reading the deceased's and the donor family's stories might trigger issues that affect them but can be overlooked. Backroom activity is sometimes harder than carrying out tasks with donor families that can serve as a distraction.

CASE 2

Error in translation

1 Background: A technician and a biologist were working together in a testing laboratory performing some urgent serologic tests outside normal laboratory hours. One of the samples they were testing was from a potential organ donor. The results produced by a testing machine indicated a clearly reactive result for HIV. The technician passed it to the biologist who had to transcribe the results to a report form, sign the report, and fax it to the transplant center.

2 Difficulties: The biologist transcribed the result as a "negative" instead of a "positive," and three HIV-infected organs were transplanted to recipients.

3 Learning and support: During the period that followed this tragic error, much time was devoted to caring for the recipients and to communicating with the authorities and the media. However, resources were also allocated to ensuring that the biologist was supported and not left alone, in recognition of the emotional impact that a human error of this kind could have on the person who made the mistake.

Identifying and clarifying the pertinent issues for staff involved in deceased donation is a first step toward setting up and maintaining development and support programs targeted at what is most needed by both the service and the individual staff members.

The issues can be nominally divided into organizational, practical, and those of a psychological nature. However, these are interlinked and overlap. The organizational aspects of the service form the overriding framework that supports the safe, effective practice for the staff. There is a wide range of requirements of a practical nature that can deter or facilitate successful deceased tissue donation and support the staff carrying out the required steps and tasks. These practical issues inevitably overlap with those of an organizational and emotional nature. Those of an emotional or psychological nature are largely hidden, intangible issues for the full range of staff dealing with deceased tissue donation. Individuals have different vulnerabilities and strengths, and the characteristics of the donor, the family, and the circumstances surrounding the donor's death affect staff in different ways. Also, different aspects of the service, and the tasks required to be done, impact differently on individual staff and at different times in his or her experience of tissue donation (new on the job or after many years of experience). If careful attention is given to the organizational and practical aspects of the job, these emotional and psychological issues can be recognized and supported in an appreciative and effective way for the full range of staff. These categories are summarized in the further discussion.

Organizational issues that can help alleviate staff stress

Management needs to appreciate the diversity of staff groups (interview staff, procurement staff, and administration groups) involved with the potential to be emotionally affected by tissue donation. It is essential to support staff by ensuring that there is clarity about lines of accountability and about the availability of line managers and senior clinical staff for consultation at all times.

The staff themselves should undergo a recruitment process to ensure that they are suitable and emotionally robust. Pertinent staff training must be provided both at induction and as ongoing professional development. Management should ensure that the physical conditions for staff undertaking interviews or procurement are suitable in recognition of the stamina and concentration required. There may be special considerations needed to update part-time staff with new developments and also to maintain team cohesion.

There need to be clear practice protocols and guidelines for staff undertaking donation interviews and procurement. Staff must be well versed in all areas relevant to their work including medicolegal issues, technical matters, donor suitability, testing, and other diverse aspects such as provision of recipient information to donor families. This requires allocation of time for continuing professional development to ensure methodical and effective updates of complex information. Staffing requirements may change over time.

The embracing of appropriate alternative or complementary approaches to promote physical and emotional well-being may be part of a strategy to improve work–life balance.

Practical issues that can increase staff stress

1 Staff members have to assemble a procurement team very rapidly while providing the highest level of professional support for the donor family, respect for the donor and working in isolation during unsocial hours. This may coincide with arranging witnesses for donor family conversations and identifying the appropriate person in the donor family to give consent, which can take time and repeated efforts.

2 These staff are dependent upon effective liaison with staff outside their own service for identifying potential donors (police, hospital staff, medical examiners and coroners, funeral home professionals, general practitioners) (see Chapter 9) whose professional aims and concerns may be in conflict with those of the tissue procurement staff.

3 Adhering to the format and guidelines for obtaining consent while dealing adequately with unexpected and difficult issues (family interruptions, outbursts of grief and crying, and silence).

4 Assessing reliability of information given over the telephone and emotional stability of those giving consent or medical history and behavioral risk information (voice only, no body language clues).

5 Deciding on appropriate actions where there are ethical dilemmas (who to inform about previously hidden information about the donor, such as drug use or viral disease risk) or moral conflicts (right and wrong actions, with possibly no clear answer).

6 Insuring established protocols are followed when dealing with living donors (some of whom may be terminally ill).

7 Achieving effective liaison with tissue bank staff and clinical/testing laboratories.

8 Keeping updated on relevant knowledge and information about transmissible diseases, quantity and quality of recovered tissues, and evolution of information technology and quality control systems.

9 Maintaining complete, clear, and accurate records despite time pressures.

10 Working intensely and closely with one family, only to have to reorient and sometimes move quickly on to the next referral and another family's loss.

Psychological and emotional sources of staff stress

Apprehension may be associated with not knowing what to expect when commencing donation discussions with a family. There may be little time to process personal emotions when dealing with the ties made with live donors (who may be terminally ill), especially if they are unable to carry out their wishes, or in carrying out challenging conversations with bereaved families. At the same time, staff members must manage facing their own mortality and the frailty of life in the context of death as a work issue. Particular cases may trigger personal vulnerabilities as a result of similarity of age or circumstances. Some staff may experience a sense of "scavenging" or fear that mistakes or errors will lead to "blame" or litigation.

Staff have to balance the needs of the service with the needs of the bereaved, organizing long, invasive, and possibly traumatic conversations with donor families. Asking medical history and behavioral questions might be perceived as upsetting, intrusive, or irrelevant to the bereaved, so routine questions must be converted into an empathetic, personal experience, balancing their "bad news" and trauma with the hope that a recipient might benefit. Staff have to help the bereaved cope with their emotional response to the trauma of unexpected, violent, accidental, or suicidal death. These issues are in the context of a wide range of ages, cultures, religions, and beliefs, often beyond the experience of, or even at odds with, personal beliefs.

All these and other issues not highlighted can be managed more easily and be better contained within clear practice frameworks for staff support and development.

Practice frameworks for staff support and development

Practice frameworks for coordinating deceased tissue donation include written protocols and guidelines. These require regular modification as new information emerges (new or varying risks, better tests), practice evolves and improves, and staff structures change. Protocols and guidelines should cover the process from identifying eligible donors and obtaining consent, to effectively communicating with other services (nursing staff, laboratories, mortuaries, coroners, general practitioners, medical consultants, eye, tissue and organ banks, and funeral parlors). Guidelines are the basis of safety for all staff, donor families, recipients, and all others involved in the process as described in relevant chapters in this book.

Staff development and support also require specific practice guidelines based on sound theoretical foundations against which the less tangible, often controversial aspects of the tasks of consent and donation can be audited. Linking theory to practice in the family conversation gives validity to different approaches and offers security to staff.

The practice framework for staff development and support can be categorized into:

1 definitions of meaning (staff support and development, counselling/discussion, empathy, "bad" news)
2 principles of discussion
3 aims of counseling/discussion
4 structure or "map" for discussion/counseling sessions

Definitions

Staff development, for the purposes of this service, means enabling and encouraging each member of the team to maintain and increase his or her individual skills and achieve team aspirations.

Support is a word loosely used, but here it means skill development, confirmation and enhancement of confidence in the practice of technical and discussion/counseling aspects of roles, and access to confidential debriefing.

Discussion relates to the information exchange between the specialist nurse/coordinator and donor family (nominated individuals or next of kin) to ensure informed consent. This discussion has no direct therapeutic aim other than to offer the donor family, in the most appropriate way, an opportunity to be helpful to others at their time of heightened emotions. The discussion relates to the safety of the donation for recipients and to questions that must be asked of the donor family.

Counseling skills are vital for dealing with expected, unexpected, and assessment aspects of obtaining informed consent, and to ameliorate distressing circumstances for the bereaved. In the context of the proscribed questionnaire, counseling is a skilled conversation that may support donor families to deal with their grief in a more hopeful way. Indeed, this conversation may be the only "bereavement counseling" they receive. Counseling should be undertaken with care so as not to coerce the donor family, and should include disclosure of the options available to them.

Empathy is the capacity to understand another person's experience from within that person's frame of reference. In empathy, we "borrow" another's feelings to observe, feel, and understand them but not to take them onto ourselves (engaged detachment). An empathic observer enters into the equation and then is removed. Empathy is a counseling skill that can lead to a deeper understanding of another human being. The appropriate use of empathy as a communication tool facilitates the donation conversation, increases the efficiency of gathering information, and helps respect donors and their families. Empathy and empathic communication are teachable, learnable skills [7].

Theoretically, news is only information, and whether it is "good" or "bad" is a value judgement or belief given to it by the person involved (donor's next of kin). Thus, as a first principle, it is important to make no assumptions by using open questions to allow the relative or next of kin to define what "bad" news is for them. For example, death may bring relief, grief, or disbelief [8].

The Art of the Family Interview – Setting Expectations

The main guiding principles in the donor family interview include [9]:

1 making no assumptions; asking questions
2 having small goals for each contact; engaging with the bereaved

3 recognizing that everything said has an impact; using words carefully
4 avoiding giving false reassurance (about the results of the mandatory tests, outcome of donation); answering questions honestly, including where answers are unknown
5 keeping expectations realistic: the "perfect death experience" or "perfect gift" devoid of conflict or suffering is well-nigh impossible
6 sharing responsibility with the bereaved (body appearance after donation, mandatory tests), and colleagues for support (managers, peers, senior clinical staff)
7 respecting the resilience and capabilities of individuals, (bereaved and staff)

Overall aims of discussion/counseling [9]

Indications are given, alongside each point, to clarify, even though artificially, what is termed discussion or the use of counseling techniques. The aims include:

1 keeping the conversation focused (counseling)
2 identifying a possible donation from the source (accident/emergency, intensive care, police, etc.) (discussion and sometimes counseling techniques)
3 engaging the bereaved sufficiently to have a discussion about consent to donation (counseling)
4 informing the bereaved about the procedure (how it is done, how long it takes, consent, questions, mandatory markers) (discussion)
5 confirming the bereaved understands the questions (counseling and discussion)
6 identifying and addressing any immediate concerns (counseling)
7 clarifying any future actions or contact (discussion)
8 facilitating ending (counseling)
9 recording all details (discussion and counseling)
10 consulting appropriate others about technical, safety, and procedural concerns (discussion)

"Map" or structure for the session [9]

Having a structure or "map" for the discussion about donation facilitates the effective use of time for both staff and the bereaved. Although structured questionnaires are used, the following steps can provide overarching theoretical or "umbrella" guidance to facilitate the flow of conversation:

1 Think first of any information that might be available for each case (referral source, age, sex, circumstances of death) as this helps to focus the start of the conversation.
2 Consider whether anyone else ought to be involved from the start, such as witness to consent, or another family member or close friend.

3 Introduce yourself and your task immediately (how much time is needed, enquire whether the person is alone or has support from others).
4 Clarify whether the family knew the wishes of the deceased – if there was a donor card, a will, or a license, or whether a donor registry was completed.
5 Assess the reactions of the bereaved to the questioning fairly early in the session and elicit main concerns.
6 Proceed with the questionnaire.
7 Assess the medical, psychological, and social context of the deceased donor toward the end of the interview, and consider whether further inquiries would enhance confidence in the safety of the donation (family doctor, medical examiner or coroner, medical consultant).
8 Allow time for family questions.
9 Summarize key points (timetable for recovery, results of mandatory tests, contact information if necessary).
10 Record details as required, and note any outstanding issues.
11 Consult colleagues in hierarchy and team members.

Practice

Structures for staff support and development are summarized:

1 line management and appraisal
2 debriefing following procurement (line manager/peer)
3 24-hour confidential staff counseling and advice help line
4 programs for orientation, ongoing education, and updating
5 team-building activities
6 clinical consultation (actively encouraged in the United Kingdom to support continued registration) with an appropriate professional can challenge practice, enhance skills, and increase confidence
7 multidisciplinary nonhierarchical group meetings where different views can be safely aired and debated

Routine staff debriefing after donation (team, and individually as appropriate) is an early intervention that offers immediate support and recognizes the stresses involved in completing successful, technical tissue recovery procedures.

The main tasks of routine staff debriefing:

1 reassuring team members that being upset, tearful, and emotionally affected by the recovery process is normal
2 assisting team members in expressing individual concerns

> **3** identifying particular triggers (similar age or circumstances, particular vulnerability)
> **4** emphasizing confidentiality of the debriefing
> **5** intervening early when acute shock or some aspect triggers an untoward reaction in a team member
> **6** clarifying and agreeing what the individual might need (time off, more training) and any required action by managers (review of procedures and policies) or peers (postprocurement coworker debriefing)
> **7** avoiding discussion of the individual's personal or health problems unless raised by him or her

Support can be effectively administered by a confidential, 24-hour telephone-counseling service or by an independent counselor available to those who want to discuss particular distress following a donation and procurement.

Team-building activities are an important part of overall strategies to enhance a good working environment. A sense of "belonging to a team" provides support and development of standards of practice and policies and should include "backroom" administration staff.

The orientation and ongoing training and assessment of competency of staff are essential for the nurse specialist/coordinator and public. Different models of training and ongoing development can be used. A series of workshops in the United Kingdom and the United States has been developed to focus on enhancing strategies for difficult conversations (among coworkers, hospital staff, donor families, funeral directors, medical examiners and coroners, and family doctors) and to review and decide on ethical dilemmas (confidentiality versus safety). A combination of theory (didactic presentations, literature reviews) and practice (role play, discussion) is used for orientation and subsequent seminars and workshops.

A nonhierarchical group can provide a forum for peer discussion of individual cases, audit and review of clinical practice, mutual support, and learning. The model, initiated in the UK National Blood Service in 1986 [10], has been adapted by the UK National Health Service Tissue Services and is open to all frontline clinical staff from within the organization working with donor families and to members of sister organizations by invitation on an occasional basis. The aim of such a forum is to provide a safe environment for open discussion where individual staff can highlight and recognize personal strengths and difficulties. This forum provides opportunities for either individual (personal difficulties in dealing with particular cases) or specific service needs (more training in specific areas). Rehearsal and discussion of difficult issues, monitoring of practice, and liaison for frontline clinical staff can lead to consensus building and consistency in handling difficulties (i.e. positive microbiological markers, inability to use donations, consent for research) that serve as a safety net for good practice. Potential problems can be identified and discussed in a timely and safe way, away from the strictures of line management. Policies and procedures can be influenced by the outcome of discussion. Key elements of the discussion and decisions, if recorded in the minutes of such meetings, can provide an important reference point for initiating changes, managing dilemmas, and making decisions about difficult topics; the minutes provide a legal record. The minutes, if circulated to relevant parts of the tissue service, are a way of enhancing overall understanding in the wider organization of the challenges faced by staff involved with deceased tissue donation.

Tool for staff support and development

Case discussion in appropriate contexts (nonmanagement and peer groups, line management) is a safe, effective way of bringing out issues and finding optimal solutions and can serve to:

1 identify loopholes in policies and procedures
2 find best ways to deal with identified errors
3 rehearse difficult conversations with donor families or outside agencies (i.e. inability to use donation, results of mandatory tests that deem the donor ineligible)
4 reinforce the aims of the service by highlighting instances of success of tissue transplantation for recipients

---

The following brief case examples are a selection from those brought for discussion.

CASE 3

Impact of human error

1 Background: A 73-year-old man died at home and was transferred to the accident and emergency department where attempts to resuscitate failed. The next of kin was his wife. However, the son represented the family in the donor family interview with the tissue coordinator because of his mother's distress and confirmed that the family wished to proceed. Later, the nurse specialist noticed that the blood sample to be used for testing was incomplete/wrongly labelled in the emergency department.
2 Difficulties: The donor sample failed to qualify for the required identification criteria and so the family's wish for donation could not be fulfilled. There was discussion about whether to ask the family for more information to try and find ways to proceed with their wishes for donation. Views were discussed about how best to tell the donor family about the labeling error and that the donation could not be processed.

3 Learning and support: The group members were able to express understanding to the nurse specialist and acknowledge the disappointment when a donation cannot proceed for the staff and the family. There was peer acknowledgement about feelings of sensitivity about the impact on the donor family. The need for staff accuracy, recording, and being alert was highlighted. Procedures using molecular technology were developed to confirm the identity of the donor and samples for future cases.

CASE 4

Protecting confidentiality

1 Background: A 26-year-old man died in a traffic accident after sustaining multiple injuries. He had living parents and a female partner of three years. The parents were interviewed for consent. In getting further information from his female partner, past drug use emerged.
2 Difficulties: The key discussion about the importance of interviewing the most relevant person with regard to medical and behavioral questions was made difficult in this case as the parents considered themselves the appropriate individuals to do this. Difficulties were expressed about dealing with information about the donor's social history, possibly unknown to his parents. There was concern about the possible revelation of their son's past drug use that emerged from his partner. This information meant that the parents would have to be told that the tissues could not be used. Discussion centered on how to do this without causing more distress to the parents, while not breaching the deceased man's confidentiality. Dealing with the family's disappointment that their wishes could not be fulfilled was again a hard aspect of this case.
3 Support and learning: This case highlighted how important it is to ensure that donor families are made aware that information might emerge from tests or other sources that might affect the ability to donate. The ethical issues that can arise about the confidentiality of the donor were reviewed. The importance of not making assumptions about how the parents might react was raised.

CASE 5

Sharing difficult news

1 Background: A "cot death" of a 7-month-old led to consent for donation obtained from the father. The mother was too distressed to give consent for the donation of heart valves. The general practitioner, when contacted for further medical information, was not happy to provide this without the parents' written consent. Eventually, the tissue was determined unsuitable and had to be discarded for technical reasons.
2 Difficulties: Baby heart valves are a rare, sought-after donation with high clinical need, which places additional stress on the specialist nurse who has a wish to

succeed in achieving this type of donation. Particular distress was engendered relating to the death of a baby. Considerable time and emotional energy was spent in dealing with the donor family, particularly as the valves could not be released and used. Some uncertainty and ambivalence about what to tell the family were discussed. An honest approach was taken relating to the technical problem.

3 Learning and support: Reporting the details and rehearsing approaches helped the specialist nurse responsible to feel less distressed and more confident. Reviewing the special sensitivities and emotions triggered by such a case with a peer group offered some measure of support.

CASE 6

When expectations and reality collide

1 Background: A woman with diagnosed terminal cancer called to refer herself as a potential cornea donor. She wanted to complete the authorization and the medical history and behavioral risk assessment herself. She explained to the coordinator why this donation was important to her and that she wanted to control the process. She sent a letter that she wanted forwarded to the cornea recipient explaining the reason for making the gift. Death occurred several weeks following the referral. The coordinator had spoken weekly to the hospice nurse to ensure that no new infections had developed since the initial screen.

2 Difficulties: The corneas were recovered, but on visual inspection, it was determined that they could not be used for transplant. The coordinator had developed a relationship with the donor and was very upset stating how difficult this was for her, and it was not just "another" case. She felt that she had personally let down the donor.

3 Learning and support: Several staff members met to debrief this unusual case. The group listened without comment as the coordinator described the intimacy that developed by obtaining consent from someone about to die and pointed out how she wanted to push the process as far as it could go because of the woman's strength of conviction. The case demonstrates some salient points. The group reinforced that there are never any guarantees with donation and transplantation, and this difficult conversation might have been harder to have with this particular terminally ill potential donor. Taking consent before death of the donor has risks; it is harder to keep a professional stance in the interests of the many individuals concerned (donor, family, recipient). The value of peer support and being able to debrief was highlighted.

Conclusions

Deceased tissue donation and transplantation provides opportunities for all staff concerned in the process. The impact of staff choice to work in this area has the potential to be truly significant, relative to both the gifts and the challenges that come with it. Whether the focus is in working with bereaved families, surgical recovery of tissues, or quality assurance of the medical records, staff are likely to be faced with life–death issues.

The main requirements for those responsible for recruiting and selecting donors, and carrying out consent and procurement include the ability to:

1 develop close professional collaboration with multiple agencies to ensure consistency for families and to prevent duplication
2 build and maintain effective networking relationships in their organization and in the hospital and community
3 communicate difficult information to donor families in ways that maximize involvement and cooperation for donation in a culturally competent manner
4 understand common barriers to effective communication
5 assess the family's level of insight, intellectual capacity, and relationship with the deceased
6 appreciate the implications of verbal and nonverbal communication and how to correctly interpret communication within the context of various cultures

Tissue coordinators/specialist nurses know the emotionally charged intensity of working closely with one family, only to reorient and move quickly on to the needs of the next referral. Staff support and development are key elements in this process. Paying attention to and accommodating personal, emotional, physical, and spiritual needs are as necessary as the ability to set appropriate limits, organize workloads, and maintain boundaries between professional and personal lives.

Staff support and development, individually and in groups, can explore alternative means to improve personal, team, department, and organizational goals. Some common social and workplace situations can provide a basis for team members to challenge one another about approaches to practice and commonly held beliefs. If this exchange of ideas takes place in a safe forum it can lead to creative thinking.

High professional standards start with sound guidelines and protocols for accountability, appraisal, monitoring, and practice for all staff. Key elements include an appropriate choice of staff, adequate induction, and subsequent support and staff development at all stages of employment as different issues emerge.

To provide extraordinary, compassionate care to the families we encounter and to maximize the recovery of tissue for transplantation, we must keep the following in mind as we develop policies and protocols to support, encourage, develop, and retain staff involved in the donation process.

KEY LEARNING POINTS

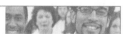

- The tasks to be performed in the coordination of a deceased donation challenge the emotions and sensitivities of even the most experienced professionals.

- The key focus in the coordination of deceased donation is to provide gifts of tissue that are safe for the recipients. This requires diligence and efficiency within a structure that is supported by validated protocols, guidelines, and procedures.

- Concealing job-related stress by staff can result in physical and emotional distancing from families and colleagues.

- Extreme stress can put people at high risk of losing the ability to make clear decisions and to function in their personal lives.

- Staff members who have encountered a loss that cannot be openly acknowledged, publicly mourned, or socially supported may experience disenfranchised grief.

- The support the caregiver receives from others may be a critical element in preventing burnout.

- Sustaining work with deceased donors and families requires enhancing social support both inside and outside professional circles to prevent compassion fatigue.

- Systems of support may be deficient in a number of ways because of the limitation of resources or the limited vision of those who control them.

- The rewards of working with donor families can serve as a distraction or reward for some staff. Those who work in the background may not have these opportunities, placing them at greater risk for burnout or compassion fatigue.

- The organizational framework of the service supports safe, effective practice measures for staff.

- Practice frameworks for coordinating deceased tissue donation include written protocols and guidelines. These require regular modification as new information emerges, practice evolves and improves, and staff structure changes.

- Staff development and support also require specific practice guidelines based on sound theoretic foundations.

- Empathy and empathic communication are teachable, learnable skills.

References

1. Albert PL. Grief and loss in the workplace. Prog Transplant. 2001;11(3):169–73.
2. Fulton R. Unanticipated death. In: Corr CA, Pacholski RA, editors. Death: Completion and Discovery. Lakewood, OH: Association of Death Education and Counseling; 1987.
3. Weisman AD. The psychiatrist and the inexorable. In: Feifel H, editor. New Meanings of Death. New York, NY: McGraw-Hill; 1977.
4. Doka KJ. Disenfranchised Grief: New Directions, Challenges, and Strategies for Practice. Champaign, IL: Research Press; 2002.
5. Maslach C. Burnout: The Cost of Caring. Englewood Cliffs, NJ: Prentice-Hall; 1982.
6. Figley CR. Compassion fatigue: psychotherapists' chronic lack of self care. J Clin Psychol. 2002;58(11):1433–41.
7. Spiro H. What is empathy and can it be taught? Ann Intern Med. 1992; 116(10):843–6.
8. Bor R, Miller R, Gill S, Evans A. Counselling in health care settings: a handbook for practitioners. 2nd ed Basingstoke: Palgrave Macmillan; 2008.
9. Miller R, Hewitt PE, Warwick R, Moore MC, Vincent B. Review of counselling in a transfusion service: the London (UK) experience. Vox Sanguinis Invited Review: Vox Sanguinis. 1998;74(3):133–9.
10. Bor R, Gill S, Miller R, Parrott C. Doing Therapy Briefly. Basingstoke: Palgrave Macmillan; 2004.

11 Ethical Issues in Unrelated Cord Blood and Bone Marrow Donation

Sally Gordon,[1] Dorothy E. Vawter,[2] and Jeremy Chapman[3]

[1] Australian Bone Marrow Donor Registry, Sydney, New South Wales, Australia
[2] Minnesota Center for Health Care Ethics, St Paul, Minnesota, USA
[3] Acute Interventional Medicine, Westmead Hospital, Westmead, New South Wales, Australia

Introduction

Successful bone marrow transplantation depends upon matching the donor and recipient for human leukocyte antigens (HLAs). Unlike other transplants considered in this book, a bone marrow transplant involves placing a competent immune system from one individual into another. If there is an HLA mismatch, the donor marrow can be recognized as foreign and can be rejected. The matching of HLA types of the donor with the recipient is most likely possible by seeking a sibling donor, as siblings have a 1 in 4 chance of inheriting identical HLA genes from their parents. For those unlucky enough to need a bone marrow transplant but without a matched sibling or other family member, there is the hope that a volunteer can be found who, by chance, has a matching HLA. Registries of volunteer marrow donors and more recently, banks of frozen stored cord blood have been developed across the world in response to this need.

There are approximately 70 volunteer unrelated marrow donor registries and 50 cord blood banks worldwide providing hematopoietic stem cells (HSCs) for hematopoietic stem cell transplantation (HSCT). There are over 12 million adult volunteer unrelated HSC donors and cord blood units available [1]. With the increasing appeal of cord blood transplantation and reports of continuously improving patient outcomes, the field is under

Tissue and Cell Donation: An Essential Guide. Edited by Ruth M. Warwick, Deirdre Fehily, Scott A. Brubaker, Ted Eastlund. © 2009 Blackwell Publishing, ISBN: 978-14051-6322-4.

constant change. Of the greater than 10,000 unrelated HSC donations annually, approximately 40% are shipped across international borders [1]. The World Marrow Donor Association (WMDA) has established recommendations and standards aimed at establishing a uniform practice and policy protecting the donors' rights and expectations in addition to the patients' needs [2].

Donation by unrelated living donors of HSCTs and the variety of cell sources available raise many complex ethical as well as technical issues. This chapter concentrates on ethical issues in unrelated cord blood and bone marrow donation, including the stewardship of scarce resources, increased benefits and reduced risks to recipients, respect for the rights and interests of donors, and the complexity of consent at all levels.

The bone marrow donor registry's and cord blood bank's roles are to balance the risks and opportunities on behalf of the donors, potential recipients and their families, transplant centers, registries, and cord blood banks. This must be achieved in a way that preserves and enhances public trust in unrelated HSC donation.

There are two major sources of unrelated HSC donations: adults who donate either bone marrow or peripheral blood stem cells (PBSCs), mobilized from the marrow by a growth factor called granulocyte colony-stimulating factor (G-CSF), and mothers who donate HSCs from the placenta and umbilicus after delivery on behalf of their newborn infants. These two types of donors will be addressed separately.

Cord blood donation

The first cord blood transplant was performed in 1970 on a 16-year-old boy with acute lymphoblastic leukemia, who received multiple units not tested for HLA compatibility [3–5]. Since that time, cord blood donation has become an alternative to other sources of HSCs especially for children and low-weight adults, although this too is changing rapidly with the increased use of dual cord blood units for adult patients. The most recent published results indicate equivalent outcomes of unrelated donor umbilical cord blood and bone marrow in children with acute leukemia [6].

Respect for cord blood donors and their families: consent process

There are different consent issues for donating cord blood compared with bone marrow and PBSCs. Cord blood is ordinarily discarded with the placenta and considered medical waste. When cord blood is collected for transplant, however, consent is required because of the risks associated with donation and the respect due to the donors involved, i.e. the parents and the newborn. Which person or persons need to consent to cord blood donation and why are uncertain, whereas for donors of marrow and PBSCs, it is clear. Consent may be obtained from the mother only on behalf of the child or on behalf of herself and the child, or consent can be obtained from both parents. All aspects of collection, quality assessment, storage, and release procedures must be explained, and any risks (physical, social, financial) to the mother and her baby must be discussed. Some have argued that both parents of the newborn should consent to cord blood donation when sensitive personal information is collected for the purpose of protecting the recipient from infectious and genetic diseases [7, 8]. The father's consent is less important if personal details about his history are not collected [9]. Most maintain that consent from the mother is required [10, 11]. For most cord blood banks, the mother's surrogate consent for the newborn is sufficient.

Cord blood can be donated for public use or placed in storage for private (autologous) use by the child or by another family member (Figure 11.1). Allogeneic related cord blood transplants have been undertaken between siblings, where the first sibling has a disease requiring HSCT and the second may even have been conceived as a potential matched donor. In vitro fertilization and preimplantation genetic testing of the embryo or intrauterine fetal testing can be performed to ensure that the newborn who will donate the cord blood will be free of the disease afflicting the sibling [12–15]. Ethical concerns include objecting to direct participation, protecting the welfare of

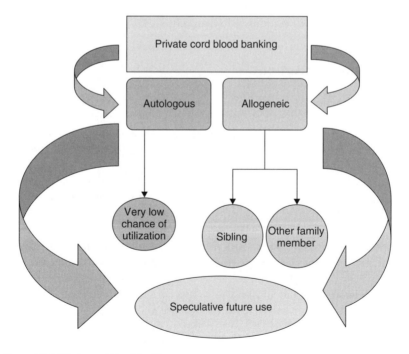

Figure 11.1 Private cord blood banking

the donor newborn, and discarding healthy but unsuitable embryos. Benefits include saving the life of a child and valuing the "savior" child who is free of the disease afflicting the sibling.

Private commercial banks encourage new parents to bank cord blood by suggesting that it will act as "insurance" against future diseases substantiated only by optimistic speculation on the potential scientific advances with gene therapy and cellular repair and regenerative medicine for such conditions as heart disease, dementia, and Parkinson's disease, among others. Prospective parents need to be informed that the chances of its use in a family with no history of blood disease are approximately 1 : 20,000 for the first 20 years of life [11]. There is a concern among the bone marrow donor registries and public cord blood banks and obstetricians that private cord blood banks exploit, for financial profit, the fears and anxieties of new parents, and that is in the interests of neither the donors nor the public [16, 17].

CASE 1

Private or public banking?

While expecting her first child, Mrs. X received a brochure from a private cord blood bank. Mrs. X recalls that the brochure encouraged her to fear that her as-yet unborn child might be ill and in need of a stem cell transplant. Though she resented the appeals to fear and maternal guilt, she raised the issue of storing her baby's cord blood with her obstetrician. That was when she first learned about community cord blood banks. Mrs. X felt a wave of maternal peace when she learned she could donate her baby's cord blood to a community bank. It was, for her, the perfect way to do something positive with this special resource.

Mrs. X donated cord blood after the birth of two children. Both collections were performed in the delivery room. One collection was sufficient for use only in research or quality control testing; the other collection was sufficient for a transplant.

For weeks after her deliveries, she proudly dressed her babies in shirts asserting "I gave to save a life." "Donating cord blood is good karma, a blessing, an act that promises to protect my children more than saving the cord blood in a private bank," she says. She takes satisfaction that both her babies were activists beginning just shortly after birth.

Should a child of hers need a transplant, Mrs. X is confident that someone else will have donated a suitable cord blood unit to the community bank or that the unit that she stored would still be available. For her, private banking was not an option. First, she preferred not to make decisions based on fear. Second, private banking entails undue effort to control her (child's) destiny. Third, the initial cost was substantial at a time when she had substantial additional costs from her new family. Finally, she prefers to forgo the stress associated with the storage facility's regular bills reminding her that her child may become seriously ill.

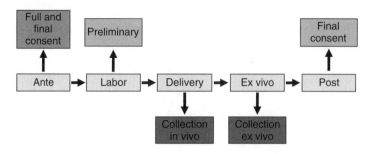

Figure 11.2 Alternative models for requesting consent for cord blood banking and utilization

There are several models of the timing of consent for the anonymous and altruistic donation of cord blood to public cord blood banks (Figure 11.2). Consent practices vary by different institutions around the world, being obtained before, during, or after labor and delivery [7, 18, 19]. Cord blood can be collected after the delivery of the baby either in utero before the delivery of the placenta (in vivo) or ex utero after the delivery of the placenta (ex vivo) [7, 19]. Many urge that informed consent should be obtained during the prenatal period, e.g. at prenatal classes prior to the mother going into labor or at the very early stage of labor [18, 19]. This can occur any time from 28 weeks of gestation to full term and may specify consent for collection either ex vivo or in vivo. Mothers can be provided with information at prenatal clinics, both written and verbal, and have more time to make the decision. A phased consent process with different timing and partial consent during labor has been described by others [20]. Partial consent, i.e. consent to the collection and temporary storage of cord blood, may be obtained at the time of labor when, for example, the mother raises the issue at that point or is approached to donate for the first time. This involves an abbreviated consent to collect and store the cord blood temporarily until the next day after the birth when final consent to long-term storage, quality control testing, and donation can be obtained. If consent is refused the next day, the cord blood unit is discarded. Labor is an inappropriate time to discuss any important issue in depth, and thus there should be no coercion for a final decision at that time. A third model is when the cord blood collection is performed ex vivo without consent, pending subsequent discussion and consent in the ensuing days. The Guidelines of the New York State Council on Human Blood and Transfusion Services require prior consent if cord blood is collected from the placenta in utero [21].

Protections needed for recipients
The current and future health status of infants donating cord blood is obviously less well known at the time of donation than the health status of adult

bone marrow and PBSCs donors in whom genetic diseases will have declared themselves. For this reason, special steps are required to protect potential recipients from developing donor-derived inherited diseases via the cord blood transplant. Thus, a comprehensive medical and genetic history of the infant's family should be taken and documented [22]. This includes the infant's ethnicity and potential inherited disorders that may be transmissible. A history of the mother's communicable disease risk behavior and travel history must be taken in addition. This may include high risk and illegal risk behaviors for HIV and hepatitis and the necessity of exposing the mother to unwanted disclosure even within the privacy of her immediate family. This health and social interview should be conducted in private when gaining complete informed consent, whether prior to labor or after the birth of the infant and the collection of the cord blood.

The mother is routinely asked to provide a sample of her blood at the time of delivery or at a fixed time subsequent to delivery to test for infectious diseases and to ensure, as far as possible, that the cord blood is free from potentially harmful consequences to the recipient of the cord blood. The international best practice professional standards released by NetCord-FACT (Foundation for the Accreditation of Cellular Therapy) (version 3.0) require maternal testing at the time of banking for infectious diseases, and any positive or indeterminate results need to be provided to the mother or her physician or both [22]. The NetCord-FACT standards are widely used but not yet universally accepted as appropriate standards for cord blood collection, with some national regulators developing independent national standards. In Australia, which specifically recognizes the NetCord-FACT standards, infectious disease testing is currently required 180 days after the delivery and cord blood collection; at this time, information is also sought on the welfare of the baby to ensure that there is no manifestation of genetic abnormalities. In the EU, repeat testing at 180 days is not required if the original donation sample was tested by NAT for HIV, HBV and HCV.

Sugarman et al. [23] found in a telephone interview of 170 women that despite a well-educated demographic, some parts of the informed consent process were lacking. A quarter of the respondents did not know how to contact the cord blood bank and report a serious illness later discovered in their child.

Maternal blood samples are also stored for future testing in case new transmissible infectious diseases are identified. This is particularly important because the inventory life of a donated cord blood collection can be measured in decades, and over such periods, there may be later generation tests available with greater sensitivity. There may also be emerging infections for which testing may be required. These tests, particularly those which rely on genetic testing, pose risks to the mother and her family's privacy, and, in some healthcare systems, may threaten opportunities to obtain health and life insurance. Genetic testing has the potential to identify genes for potentially untreatable diseases that develop later in life. In contrast to this requirement of a cord blood donor, a 1994 Institute of Medicine Review recommended that children should not be tested for abnormal genes unless the disease has an effective curative or preventative treatment that must be instituted early in life [24].

Cord blood banks have varying criteria for acceptable cell counts and volumes. Cord blood with parameters outside these acceptable ranges may be discarded, used for quality control testing such as for viability testing at various stages of storage, or retained for research if appropriate consent has been obtained. Inadequate volume is the most common reason that donated cord blood units are not banked.

Banks also differ with respect to the period they believe the cord blood units retain acceptable quality. It is anticipated that cord blood units will be stored in liquid nitrogen in Australia for at least 20 years before discard.

Cord blood collection differs from other types of HSC collection in that cells can be collected only once. A recipient of failed marrow or PBSCs transplant can receive a second transplant or a donor lymphocyte infusion derived from the same donor; a recipient of a cord blood transplant ordinarily cannot.

Because the volumes of cord blood units are small, compared with bone marrow, there is little material available for samples for repeat HLA confirmatory testing. Cord blood banks must carefully steward and protect the few cells collected. To conserve and efficiently use precious cord blood cells, requests for confirmatory testing should not be made unless the donation is seriously considered for use.

When a cord blood unit is reserved for transplant, a series of quality assurance tests of that cord unit are triggered such as measurement of the nucleated cell counts and the stored cells' viability. In Australia and elsewhere, it is current practice to repeat the HLA typing of the cord blood unit, and simple testing of the maternal HLA-A, B, and DRB1 is performed to reconcile the cord blood unit with the mother. In addition, and prior to release for transplantation, the cord blood unit must be tested directly for infectious diseases.

Protections needed for cord blood maternal and infant donors

Simple consideration would suggest that donation of discarded material saved from the placenta and umbilical cord could present no risk to the newborn donor or the mother. In contrast, considerable risks do exist and steps need to be in place to disclose and minimize these. Risks to the newborn and the mother include blood sampling requested months to years after the donation, e.g. for repeat infectious disease tests or for new infectious disease or genetic tests deemed necessary. Nonidentifiable labeling must be strictly adhered to to reduce the risk that the donor's identity is traceable. Then there is a possible risk that the mother or newborn could be approached months or years later by the recipient or recipient's family should a second donation be needed. Risks to the mother include loss of privacy when her personal medical and behavioral history is reviewed and when blood testing is done that can discover diseases, some of which might be stigmatizing or have no effective therapy.

Cord blood can be collected either from the cord with the placenta still in utero (in vivo collection), but, of course, only after the vaginal or cesarean section delivery of the baby, or from the cord ex utero (in vitro) after the placenta has been fully delivered.

There is a lack of consistency and consensus about the best time to clamp the umbilical cord after the delivery of the child. If the cord is clamped very early, this may pose a theoretical risk to the infant and deny the natural return of placental and cord blood [25]. In vivo collections may thus yield larger and therefore more effective cord blood volumes, but could potentially interfere with the normal care of the mother and child. In vitro collection, on the other hand, can reduce volumes and increase the risk that the cord blood collection could become contaminated [26]. Obstetricians have voiced concern over the timing of the clamping of the cord, the management of labor, and the impact on other patients in the labor suite if the labor room staff are distracted by the delivery staff undertaking a cord blood collection. The NetCord-FACT standards clearly outline the need for safeguards when in utero collections are made and require that local delivery practices not be modified in an attempt to increase cord blood volume.

Unrelated adult bone marrow and PBSC donation

Unlike the once-only cord blood donation, adult living donors are potentially available for requests to supply many and multiple donations of one or more types of cellular products such as bone marrow, G-CSF-mobilized PBSCs, unstimulated lymphocytes, or whole blood. The costs and complexity of the process of testing potential volunteer donors mean that a stepwise approach is taken by most registries so that final consents and testing sufficient for actual donation are only undertaken on the small number of people actually proceeding to donation.

The steps involved in recruitment, consent, testing, and donation of adult unrelated HSCs are:

1 recruitment: registry driven, patient driven, media driven
2 data storage: confidentiality, valid secure information systems
3 search process: patient linkage
4 physical assessment (workup) and information session: risk disclosure, physical well-being for donor and patient
5 donation
6 follow-up: well-being of donor and patient

With each step of the process from recruitment to final donation, the demands and expectations escalate on the donor, patient, health professionals, and family members. With each escalation of demands and expectations, the direct consequences on the potential recipient – from withdrawal of consent to progression to the next stage – also escalate. This raises ethical questions about how best to balance respect for the donor and the needs of the recipient. Within each of the steps, different issues arise and thus we examine each step in turn.

Stewardship of scarce resources and maximizing benefits to the public: recruitment

Many registries struggle with the question of how many donors and what composition of the registry will best serve the public and maximize access to a matching donor when they need one, whatever their ethnic ancestry. There is a real cost for recruitment and testing, which, therefore, needs to be managed to get the best yield for potential recipients. There is little point adding to the existing registry the 10,000th example of a common HLA tissue type if there is an alternative expenditure of the same resource that has a better chance of yielding a novel HLA type.

Recruitment is usually initiated and managed by the registries. However, on occasion, outside factors can dictate how donors are recruited. Distressed recipient families can appeal to the general public to join the registry with no consciousness of the futility or costs of that approach. The media plays a large role in encouraging people to join the registries. Sadly, often the media's main concern (under the guise of concern for a patient) is sales ratings with the consequent temptations for misleading and sensational reporting. Hence, valuable resources are spent managing an influx of donors, the vast majority of whom are ineligible (e.g. too old) or already well represented in the existing registries (e.g. northwest European Caucasoid ethnic background). Registries need to be proactive and develop good relationships with the media and have comprehensive "plain English" information available.

There are several models used for recruitment to unrelated registries:

1 through the national blood services
2 through centers established by patient-driven initiatives
3 through general public relations and community awareness
4 through specific community-focused activity, e.g. Jewish communities, black communities, Hispanic communities

In some countries, the donor centers are established within the blood service. This is a cost-effective method of recruitment that uses existing resources and benefits the goals of both the blood service and the bone marrow donor registry. In addition, the whereabouts of donors is monitored more easily.

In Australia, donors are required to be between the ages of 18 and 40 years and willing and able to donate blood. Donors are then retained on the registry until their 60th birthday, at which point they are retired. In Australia, for every 13 people registered on the Australian Bone Marrow Donor Registry (ABMDR), only one person will have a unique tissue type that adds to the global diversity of available HLA types. The Australian Registry, in keeping with many others, is therefore keen to increase the HLA variety of the registry through recruitment of diverse ethnic backgrounds, although specifying quantity and composition is a complex issue.

Although there are a few absolute contraindications to joining a registry (good general health and absence of known communicable diseases are requirements), recruitment through blood donor centers implies a more reliable and committed donor population than a strategy of casual recruitment. In such a registry, the requirement for donors also to donate whole blood may impede recruitment of those from certain ethnic backgrounds who are not prepared or do not meet the criteria to make a whole blood donation. In those circumstances in Australia, the requirement to give blood may be waived to ensure recruitment of ethnic minority groups that are required to meet the potential needs of a multinational patient population. The Jewish community has demonstrated a different and positive approach to recruitment within their community, through the establishment of specific donor centers within various countries, such as the Gift of Life in the United States, in order to recruit donors to meet the specific needs of patients with a Jewish genetic background. More patients will benefit not only for diseases occurring across all populations but for diseases that may occur more frequently in specific populations (such as sickle-cell disease). However, some ethnic groups have, in the past years, appealed to their diaspora across international borders to join "virtual registries" placing the financial burden on the resources of the country of residence and not the country of ethnic ancestry, which can be problematic [27]. Registries are thus placed in jeopardy, driven by the need to use their limited financial resources wisely to maximize the recruitment of an appropriate mix of donors needed for the potential recipients, but discriminating among potential donors in the process.

Information systems and privacy

People who volunteer altruistically to assist others in desperate need are the human reality of the registries. However, without the computerized information systems, there would be no ability to match the patients with the donors.

Personal and sensitive information, including tissue-typing data and other health-related information, are thus held in a range of different and complex databases worldwide. There is an increasing traffic flow with the electronic exchange of these data within registries and among registries requiring sophisticated systems to ensure the protection of the donors' privacy. The two main conflicting issues are ensuring and maintaining the separate confidentiality of the donor and patient by using secure systems and ensuring that the data elements are accurate and valid. There is a need for both absolute accuracy and confidentiality of the linkage between donors and their potential and actual recipients. The lengths to which a recipient's family would go to persuade a change of mind in a matched donor who had decided not to proceed with donation are almost unlimited. Donor centers thus maintain the donors' demographics in a highly confidential and secure way, sending to other databases only unidentified information, for example, age, blood group, and cytomegalovirus status. Registries thus require clear privacy policies and the infrastructure to implement these policies, including confidentiality agreements with contractors.

CASE 2

An ethical dilemma

Mr. T was a 33-year-old man diagnosed with chronic myeloid leukemia (CML) in chronic phase. The search for a donor was not considered urgent, but the transplant physician was keen to commence the process. A family search was conducted prior to searching any local or international unrelated bone marrow donor registries, the patient did not want his estranged brother contacted even though he might be a matched donor.

When the patient's details were logged onto the laboratory system, it was observed by the laboratory scientist that a male with the same family name was registered as a volunteer donor and was matched at a low-resolution HLA typing.

An unrelated search of the registry was commenced and a considerable number of potentially matched donors were discovered. However, a matched sibling provides a better outcome after transplantation than a matched but unrelated donor, and the search team was aware that the patient's estranged brother was a match. The issue was put to the registry's ethics committee, which advised that the transplant physician should discuss with the patient the possibility of a relative being on the registry and that if that were the case, the patient would need to request that the registry not pursue its routine search protocol, which would identify all matches, related or not. The registry would thus receive a written confirmation from the patient that would absolve them from the failure to identify the best matched donor. If a written consent were not given, then there would be documentation that the patient accepted the possibility that if there was a relative on the registry, then that person might be identified as a potential matched donor. Confidentiality between the donor and the recipient would be maintained according to routine policies, but care would be needed to ensure that if the sibling did donate, they must know that it could be to anyone in need.

Respect and protection of donors

The information about the registry and about HSC donation provided in the public domain must be comprehensive and include the voluntary nature of the program. Donors should be able to withdraw at any time, and there can be no remuneration for any part of the process. Information must emphasize to donors that they are joining the registry as a potential donor for anyone and not just a particular individual who may have been targeted in a media campaign.

It is important that the donor be aware that joining a registry does not mean being asked to donate immediately; indeed, they may never be called upon to donate. The demands on the donors at recruitment are low, but the donor's expectations may be high. The general process needs to be described in terms of the general procedures and risks involved in providing blood samples, the storage of personal and sensitive information, the need to be able to contact them again, and the questions that may be put if they are contacted.

Once a donor is selected as suitable by the transplant center, the donor is provided with comprehensive verbal information and physical examination by a third-party (independent) hematologist with no link to the patient. This ensures impartiality, that objective information is provided, and that the physical assessment is to ensure that the donor's health is not threatened. There must be scrupulous adherence to this principle as independence can easily be compromised, particularly given the limited numbers of transplant and collection centers and mobility of staff between centers. The medical and physical assessment is not only for the donor's own well-being but also to ensure safety for the patient. Full information and disclosure of any risks are provided at this time including risks associated with both methods of donation: bone marrow donation or G-CSF-mobilized PBSC donation. The hematologist discusses the donor's preference for marrow or PBSC donation, and the donor can choose their preferred method. The need for confidentiality, reimbursement of expenses, travel and accommodation for the donor and a companion, deferral from blood donation, possibility of postponement, cancellation of the procedure or request for a second or third donation, the possibility that the patient may not survive, insurance coverage, and follow-up postdonation must all be discussed. Infectious disease testing is repeated among other clinical blood tests, and women are asked to have a pregnancy test if they agree to receive the G-CSF for mobilizing the stem cells. Family history of any malignancies or leukemias should also be elicited as there is concern about the possible increased incidence of AML in individuals with a family history of AML and the potential for impact from G-CSF administration to individuals with a family predisposition to leukemia.

At the time of the donor interview and physical examination, the level of information that will subsequently be provided about the recipient's progress may be discussed. It is common for donors to want to know how the patient has fared after the donation even if they seek no other personal information.

This is a reasonable and understandable human response and while practices vary between registries it can provide the opportunity to ensure that full information provided early can prepare the donor for any subsequent bad news about the outcome for the recipient.

Although the voluntary nature of donation is a fundamental right of the donor, the donor must also be informed of the almost universally lethal impact of deciding not to proceed with donation once the patient has reached the critical period when conditioning has commenced prior to the transplant. Conditioning is a process that may involve high-dose chemotherapy and/or total body irradiation designed to destroy the patient's bone marrow and treat the malignant disease for which they are being transplanted. Even reduced intensity conditioning regimens, employed for some disease states, destroy the patient's existing immune system and define the point of no return for the patient. In order to survive, a conditioned patient must have donated HSCs transplanted to rescue them from death.

CASE 3

Past the point of no return

A 42-year-old woman with AML required a bone marrow transplant. Her immediate family was overseas in the country of her birth. She had many siblings, several of whom matched the patient but only one agreed, after some hesitation, to donate. The donor was flown to the hospital and cleared as physically fit to undergo the donation procedure. The patient's preconditioning regime commenced, but very soon after this treatment, the donor withdrew and flew home. The local registry performed an urgent bone marrow donor search, and fortunately, an unrelated transplant was possible despite the very short time frame.

What could have been done to avoid this situation? Fortunately, these days cord blood transplantation would now be a realistic consideration in this situation; however, without knowing the specific details of the case, education and clear information to the donor may have resolved the situation at a more opportune time with the donor either withdrawing earlier or being more confident in proceeding. In the enthusiasm to obtain consent from at least one of the matched siblings, it is possible that the understanding of the donor's ambivalent position was overlooked. It is also possible that financial promises made between siblings were not resolved. Familial relationships unfortunately provide no guarantee of altruistic donation, while the context of an unrelated donation to an unknown individual probably provides the most reassurance that the motivation is pure altruism.

The transplant center usually has a definite view on whether the patient would be best treated by HSCs from bone marrow or peripheral blood. Care needs to be taken to provide the donor with adequate and appropriate information, including what the physician has requested on behalf of the patient. It is obviously important that no "spin" is put on the transplant center's request in an attempt to influence the donor's choice of modality of donation one way or the other. The provision of clear, comprehensive, and comprehensible information is the only way that the donor can be in a position to make an informed decision, taking into consideration his or her own needs as well as the patient's.

If the transplant fails to engraft or only partially engrafts after the first transplant or if the recipient relapses with the original disease, the transplant center may request a second donation. This may involve bone marrow, PBSCs, or donor lymphocytes from a blood donation or cytopheresis. Most registries use a medical panel to review all requests for a subsequent donation to determine whether it is a medically reasonable and appropriate request to put to the donor. If the panel approves the request, the donor is then contacted, but local registry policies determine what products and how often donors can be asked to donate. Because there is a possibility that a donor may be asked to donate a second time, the issue of potential second or subsequent donations must be part of the initial consent process [28].

If findings are identified in any physical examination or results of blood tests are abnormal, cord blood banks and registries must have in place a system to report the abnormal results and how and when to refer the donor for appropriate care.

In Australia, donors are automatically retired from the registry databases on their 60th birthday, and they are no longer eligible to donate. This age varies internationally but is usually in the range of 55 to 60 years. Donors are also made unavailable for search or retired if they fail to respond to contact procedures. These procedures vary locally after a variety of measures are implemented to find the donor. Donors can, of course, also ask at any time to be retired by contacting their donor coordinator if they no longer wish to remain on the registry. It is unfair to recipients and inappropriate for many reasons to keep individual data on the active search databases when it is known that they are not available for donation for any reason.

Once a registered donor has actually donated, many registries defer them for at least 12 months and some remove the donors from the search pool for two years. This not only protects them but also reserves the donor in case of subsequent requests for further donations for the patient to whom they have already donated.

CASE 4

Donor protection

An unrelated search was requested for a man diagnosed with chronic lymphocytic leukemia. A donor was identified relatively quickly and a donor workup was requested. The transplant was then postponed because of personal and family reasons, and he also needed surgery for a separate problem. The transplant was rescheduled for several months later that year, but once again, the transplant was postponed for several months as he was identified as having multiple infections during pretransplant workup. The transplant was postponed a third time and, finally, canceled when nodules were identified on the patient's chest X-ray.

Over a period of two years, the donor had three clinical assessments, and four autologous blood units were collected and discarded. She traveled 200 kilometers on each occasion for the workups. Despite her commitment and disappointment that the recipient was not able to benefit from her planned donation, the registry retired her from the active search database for 12 months during which she was unavailable for further approaches.

The donor was a caring altruistic person who wanted to help. Even though all information was provided to the donor, and she could make an informed and autonomous decision to withdraw, the pressure placed on her to continue to be available for this patient was clearly extreme. The registry decided that it was unreasonable to continue placing demands on the donor.

Donation
Bone marrow donation

Prospective donors should be informed that bone marrow donation is a surgical procedure performed in a hospital. This usually means a night in a hospital before or after the operation, but some collection centers will schedule for the procedure and discharge to occur on the same day. The amount of bone marrow collected depends on the patient's need, but 20 milliliters per kilogram of donor weight is often the maximum amount extracted.

After the procedure and once the anesthetic wears off, the donor may feel somewhat stiff and sore in the lower back in the region of the donation for a few days or longer. There may also be considerable bruising at the back of the hips in the week after the donation. Donors have also reported feeling tired and having some difficulty walking. Most donors recover well and are back in their normal routine within several days. However, some may take two to three weeks before they feel completely recovered. A donor's marrow is completely regenerated within about four weeks, although donors may receive a transfusion of their own previously donated blood to assist with iron replacement. Serious complications are rare but could include anesthesia reactions, infection, transfusion reactions, or injury at the needle insertion sites. The serious adverse events registry data collection of the WMDA records a risk of such complications at about 0.15%.

Many donors report feeling that their donation is a positive life-changing experience. On the other hand, some donors find donating to be a stressful experience. In addition to causing a temporary disruption to their daily physical routine, the donor may experience some emotional lability, especially if the transplant is not successful and the donor enquires and learns that the patient has died.

PBSC donation

Under normal circumstances, there are too few blood stem cells circulating in the peripheral blood to provide a useful quantity for transplant purposes. However, the administration of G-CSF increases the number of stem cells in the peripheral blood to the point where they can then be collected in large quantities. Donors receive daily injections of G-CSF for four to five days before the collection.

PBSC donors report a variety of symptoms including bone or muscle pain, fatigue, headache, low-grade fever, nausea, and insomnia while receiving injections of G-CSF. The symptoms are usually flu-like, with bone pain the commonest with various degrees of severity, often controlled by paracetamol. Occasionally, donors will need stronger painkillers. These effects disappear shortly after collection. Severe side effects of G-CSF are rare, but there have been reports of a ruptured spleen in a related donor; G-CSF is known to enlarge the spleen [29, 30]. There has also been a recent publication on the use of G-CSF in three family donors who have subsequently developed acute myeloid leukemia [31]. The statistical evidence of a causal relationship is not substantiated; however, most registries agree that donor follow-up for both bone marrow and PBSC donors should be undertaken for at least five years to ensure that sufficient information is available to confirm the absence of any causal relationship. Donors must be provided with comprehensive and appropriate information about the available literature on the use of G-CSF and the lack of evidence of long-term effects of G-CSF, in order to make an informed decision. As there are different impacts of the two procedures and no definitive answer on the potential safety of one over the other, it remains a personal decision that will elicit different conclusions even from the best informed hematologists.

Apheresis is a process of collecting blood (normally from a vein in one arm) and passing it through a cell separator, which collects the cells that are needed for the transplant. The remaining blood is returned through a vein in the other arm. The donor's veins must therefore be examined to ensure they are sufficiently large enough to receive the cannulae. In some hospitals, a central venous line is used, especially for women with small veins, but this is an invasive procedure not without risk and should be considered carefully before proceeding. During the collection, donors may experience nausea, a tingling feeling, or chills because of hypocalcemia as an effect of the administration of citrate anticoagulants. These effects abate shortly after donation. The procedure is performed at a hospital or blood bank, does not require a general anesthetic, and takes approximately three to four hours. The procedure is less invasive than receiving a general anesthetic, and after the procedure, the donor may return home if he or she is feeling well.

CASE 5

Who decides?

A woman was identified as a suitable match for a young man with CML in chronic phase. She donated bone marrow. The patient engrafted but continued to have low peripheral blood counts. A second donation comprising G-CSF-mobilized PBSCs was requested five months later, and the donor happily donated again. There were complications with the apheresis procedure and the donor suffered tetany or uncontrollable muscle spasm secondary to respiratory alkalosis and hypocalcemia, making it a generally unpleasant experience. The procedure was stopped prematurely but the collected cells were provided to the donor. More than a year passed and the patient's disease recurred, resulting in a further request, this time for donor lymphocytes, which are also collected through apheresis. After consultation with a medical committee of three, it was agreed that the donor could be approached. Once again she agreed, and she provided the requested lymphocytes. Although the experience was much better on this occasion, there were some symptoms of hypocalcemia, and the donor intimated that she felt she would not want to go through it again. A year later, a request came for a fourth donation. The request was in the form of two options: either a high dose of lymphocytes plus a further stem cell donation *or* two to three doses of lymphocytes. The medical review committee considered this and did not permit approaching the donor again because of her previously stated view that she did not want to go through the apheresis procedure again. There were three subsequent approaches after this decision to reconsider the decision, the latest being five years after the first transplant event.

The donor and patient had exchanged anonymous contact through cards and letters. The donor had decided that she was happy to maintain this level of contact without further release of details. If both donor and patient had released their details, it may well have been a different scenario. A direct approach may have been made by the patient or their family for the fourth donation, perhaps even a fifth or sixth. Even if the patient had not directly asked, the clinical situation would have been raised, in which case, the emotional pressure on the donor would have been obvious. Was the registry being too paternalistic in their management of this donor or was it protecting her from undue emotional pressure?

Long-term protection of donors and recipients
Donor and recipient follow-up

There are several reasons for following up the donor post-donation. Follow-up of PBSC donors is important in light of the discussion presented previously of monitoring the potential impact of G-CSF. As there is limited evidence for the long-term effects of short-course treatments with G-CSF in normal volunteer donors and given the ongoing discussion in the literature, consensus of medical opinion worldwide collected by the Clinical Working

Group of the WMDA has emphasized the need to continue to monitor donors' long-term well-being especially with regard to hematopoietic malignancies compared with the incidence of these malignancies in the general population. This is in the context of some known familial predisposition to leukemia syndromes, which might bias results in both family and unrelated registry donors.

Long-term follow-up involves annual contact with the donor for at least five years. Some registries suggest that this should be extended to 10 years, and others believe that it should be possible to follow people for life. The practicalities of such extensive follow-up are difficult as donor compliance is often tenuous even over the first five years. Studies undertaken on the follow-up data raise the question of whether the donor is in fact now being treated as a research subject and thus requires further consent for participation. It also emphasizes the need to inform donors early during their workup of this commitment. Bone marrow donors should also be followed up even if only with a courtesy phone call.

It is the registry and donor center's responsibility to ensure that appropriate advice and action is taken, if needed, in relation to any abnormal results discovered during the process, thus ensuring appropriate care for any conditions related to HSC donation.

Registries often send a form for completion by the transplant center requesting information on the patient's progress posttransplant. Basic information is sought mainly to provide the donor with some feedback on the outcome of the transplant. One can question whether the registry or the donor has a right to this information. This is an entirely voluntary donation unencumbered and without conditions. However, it is reasonable to expect that there is some limited feedback to provide impetus to registries and acknowledgement to donors. Should registries require provision of this feedback as conditional in accessing the donor pool? It also has the additional function of closing the loop and ensuring that existing policies and procedures are adequate and appropriate. The provision of this feedback needs to be part of the agreement to access donors from a donor registry.

Cord blood donor and recipient follow-up

CASE 6

Blood Brothers

A young boy, now 8 years old, occasionally talks to his parents about the blood brother he has never met. He knows that when he was born, his mother donated his cord blood to the local cord blood bank. They know that the unit was used, as the bank called his mother when he was about 4 years old to ask if he was well and to check that he did not have any genetic disorders or bone marrow diseases.

They discovered in the conversation that the cord unit blood was sought by a young boy in Europe and that it was to be sent the next day.

The young donor knows that someone in Europe "looks just like him" and according to his parents, he seems quietly pleased that he has a "blood brother." He does not mention the issue very often, but it appears to be an ever-present thought for him. Does he know too much or too little of the outcome of his mother's decision to donate his cord blood?

While each cord blood bank retains the capacity to connect the particular donor to the cord blood unit, the confidentiality that surrounds the linkage between all unrelated donors and recipients prevents that knowledge from extending beyond the cord blood bank. There is a good reason to ensure confidentiality in the cord blood banks, as the knowledge that there is an infant or child with the right tissue type for a particular recipient would potentially bring enormous pressures on those involved if there was a need for a subsequent HSCT after a failed cord blood transplant. The protection of the donor and their family implies that the need for confidentiality is even more important after cord blood donation than after adult bone marrow or PBSC donation. Most, if not all, cord blood banks have policies that protect the child donor in favor of any minor advantage that there might be from continued follow-up of the health of the donor beyond 18 months.

After donating to a public bank, many families may wonder whether they can access the donated cord blood should the donor or another family member need a cord blood transplant. Families need to be informed that an individual donation may not meet the criteria for release, may already have been used by someone, or may not be suitable depending upon whether or not the disease being treated is genetic in origin and thus intrinsic to the autologous stem cells. If autologous cord blood stem cells become a valuable resource for individual donors, all cord blood banks would have to evaluate their approach to the issue. While the ethical situation merits considerable discussion and debate, currently, once donated to a public bank, the cells become the property of the cord blood bank.

Differences in ethical and policy issues between adult stem cell and cord blood donation

While there remain some similarities between the ethical issues identified in adult volunteer bone marrow donor registries and public unrelated cord blood donors, the differences mean that there are very significant differences in the ethical constraints that govern the policies and practices of the two types of institution.

In cord blood donation, the mother is acting as a proxy for her child, while unrelated bone marrow donors are competent adults making decisions on their own behalf. Cord blood donation is a single irreversible event, while bone marrow donation remains a source of ongoing decisions. Disconnection between the donor and the recipient provides significant protection against the majority of issues that arise in both situations, but there remain medical reasons for retaining knowledge of the linkages in a confidential environment.

Respect for donors as research subjects

It is recommended that blood samples be stored for patient and donor pairs for future testing and research. Consent for the provision of these samples must, of course, be obtained either at recruitment or at the donor's physical examination and information exchange session. Consent for specific research pertaining to these samples may need to be obtained at the time samples are required [32].

Equity of access

A major issue facing patients and their doctors is access to an appropriate pool of donors or cord blood units whose ethnic diversity will match the patient population. Traditionally, the vast majority of HSC donors were from a northwest European background with the largest registries being in the United Kingdom, Germany, and the United States. In more recent years, a concerted effort has been made to increase the genetic diversity of the donor panels and an increasing number of registries are developing in central and southern Asia. The advent of cord blood transplantation with acceptable mismatched cord units available has alleviated some of this pressure to find matched HSCs suitable for transplant. The Australian network of cord blood banks (AusCord) appears to have a more diverse mix of ethnicities than the ABMDR. A comparison between the Sydney Cord Blood Bank and the ABMDR found that the Sydney cord bank had twice as many donors from the southern European and Middle Eastern populations and four times as many donors from Asia [33]. This awareness of the need for ethnic diversity and the complementary therapies of bone marrow/PBSC or cord blood transplantation are providing more opportunities for those patients whose ethnic origin is in the minority on the world's large donor registries.

Conclusions

The therapeutic opportunities created by advances in medical technology employing HSCs challenge those who work in this field by constantly presenting ethical dilemmas that are both practical and require immediate solutions. The range of problems that have been encountered globally are shared through interchange of knowledge and through global forums such as those provided by the WMDA. Different countries handle issues slightly differently, but at the heart of each decision and solution is care for two people – the donor and the recipient who are locked into an unusual human relationship. In the final analysis of this field, it is important that the underlying systems used by the registries and hospitals ensure that ethical principles are understood in context, upheld in practice, and updated as the technology changes. There will be new ethical challenges as the progressive research into the science of stem cell biology and regenerative medicine advances, and it is more important for there to be robust systems to consider ethical issues rather than a carefully crafted suite of uniform answers.

KEY LEARNING POINTS

- HSCT can be lifesaving, but most patients do not have matched relatives to donate for them. Those patients can turn to large numbers of willing, altruistic, unrelated, anonymous public donors.

- Although voluntary unrelated HSC donors have a right to take risks, full disclosure to the donors of those potential risks, possible benefits, and information about the process is essential.

- Although cord blood is ordinarily a waste material to be discarded with the placenta, cord blood donation requires maternal consent because of the need for her personal medical and behavioral history and blood testing, respect for autonomy, and the risk to the privacy of the donor and family.

- When counseling HSC donors, whether they are cord blood, BM, or PBSC donors, it is important for donors and their counselors to understand the issues relating to the balance of risks and benefits for patients, donors, and their families.

- PBSC and BM donors have the right to withdraw participation at any time, but withdrawal close to the expected transplant time can be fatal to the planned recipient, and donors need to understand this.

- Potential donors and those who evaluate them need to understand the role of donor evaluation for the safety of both the donor and the recipient. Avoiding transmission of disease from donor to recipient and minimizing adverse donor reactions are both legitimate concerns of unrelated donor registries and those caring for related donors. The potential for serious health risks to donors is higher with PBSC and BM donation than for cord blood donors.

- BM registries and those who care for related HSC donors need to develop policies to ensure that PBSC and BM donors are appropriately protected from undue pressure for second and third donations and posttransplant lymphocyte donations.

- Donors must have been informed and have given their consent if the HSC donation or donor blood samples are to be used in research.

- Comprehensive information relating to donation, testing, confidentiality, storage, the possibility of additional subsequent donations over time, transplantation that may or may not result in cure of the recipient, and possible HSC research must be provided to potential donors. This will enable them to make an informed decision whether to donate or not, and, if so, which type of donation they prefer. Differing circumstances exist for related and for unrelated HSC donation. In the case of cord blood donations, the existence of commercial providers of cord blood storage for family use should be declared.

- Privacy and confidentiality in the unrelated HSC donation setting are essential for many reasons. Confidentiality avoids the potential coercion of donors by recipients or their families to make additional donations of stem cells, lymphocytes, or even donations of other bodily materials. It also allows potential donors to declare risks, which might make them unsuitable donors, and protects recipients from requests for favors by donors.

- Cord blood banks need to develop polices to manage their sample archives. Cord blood inventories may be maintained for decades, so it is imperative to optimize the use of these scarce resources when transplant centers request additional tissue typing to be done. If a cord blood parallel archive is exhausted by sequential transplant centers assessing numerous alternative cord blood units, it may not be possible to undertake the final testing when a cord blood unit is definitely selected for transplantation.

- There are concerns regarding the storage of cord blood by commercial organizations either for autologous or family-restricted HSC transplantation or for future regenerative medicine purposes. Concerns relate to the very remote likelihood of autologous cells ever being used for HSC or immunologic purposes and the current claims made for cord blood in regenerative medicine based on developing rather than current validated use, at a time when families are vulnerable.

References

1. World Marrow Donor Association. Annual report. 2006.
2. Bakken R, van Walraven AM, Egeland T. Donor commitment and patient needs. Bone Marrow Transplantation. 2004;33(22):225–30.
3. Ende M, Ende N. Hematopoietic transplantation by means of fetal (cord) blood: a new method. Va Med Mon. 1972;99(3): 276–80.
4. Ende M. History of umbilical cord blood transplantation. Lancet. 1995;346: 1161.

5. Bandini G, Bonifazi F, Baccarani M. 15 or 33 years of cord-blood transplantation. Lancet. 2003;361(9368):1566–7.

6. Eapen M, Rubenstein P, Zhang MJ, Stevens C, Kurtzberg J, Scaradavou A, et al. Outcomes of transplantation of unrelated donor umbilical cord blood and bone marrow in children with acute leukaemia: a comparison study. Lancet. 2007; 369:1947–54.

7. Vawter DE. An ethical and policy framework for the collection of umbilical cord blood stem cells. In: Weir RF, editor. Stored Tissue Samples: Ethical, Legal and Public Policy Implications. Iowa City, IA: University of Iowa Press; 1998. p. 32–65.

8. Sugarman J, Reisner EG, Kurtzberg J. Ethical aspects of banking placental blood for transplantation. JAMA. 1995;274(22):1783–5.

9. Askari S, Miller J, Clay M, Moran S, Chrysler G, McCullough J. The role of the paternal health history in cord blood banking. Transfusion. 2002;42(10):1275–8.

10. McCullough J, Clay ME, Fautsch S, Noreen H, Segall M, Perry E, et al. Proposed policies and procedures for the establishment of a cord blood bank. Blood Cells. 1994;20(2–3):609–26.

11. Annas GJ. Waste and longing – The legal status of placenta-blood banking. New Engl J Med. 1999;340(19):1521–4.

12. Dickens BM. Preimplantation genetic diagnosis and "savior siblings." Int J Gynaecol Obstet. 2005;88:91–6. http://ssrn.com/abstract=862426

13. Spriggs M. Is conceiving a child to benefit another against the interests of the new child? J Med Ethics. 2005;31(6):341–3.

14. Terry LM, Campbell A. Protecting the interests of the child bone marrow donor. Med Law. 2004;23(4):805–19.

15. Locatelli F, Burgio GR. Ethics of placental blood collection and storage (letter). Lancet. 2002;360(9342):1335–6.

16. Royal College of Obstetricians and Gynaecologists. Scientific Advisory Committee Opinion Paper 2. Revised June 2006. www.rcog.org.uk/resources/Public/pdf/umbilical_cord_blood_banking_sac2a.pdf (accessed August 19, 2007).

17. Ballen K, Barker J, Srewart S, Greene M, Lane T. ASBMT Committee Report, Collection and Preservation of Cord Blood for Personal Use. Biol Blood Marrow Transplant. 2008;14(3):356–63.

18. Sugarman J, Kaalund V, Kodish E, Marshall MF, Reisner EG, Wilfond BS, et al. Ethical issues in umbilical cord blood banking. Working Group on Ethical Issues in Umbilical Cord Blood Banking. JAMA. 1997;278(11):938–43.

19. Kurtzberg J, Lyerly AD, Sugarman J. Untying the Gordian knot: policies, practices, and ethical issues related to banking of umbilical cord blood. J Clin Invest. 2005;115(10):2592–7.

20. Vawter DE, Rogers-Chrysler G, Clay M, Pittelko L, Therkelsen D, Kim D, et al. A phased consent policy for cord blood donation. Transfusion. 2002;42(10): 1268–74.

21. Guidelines for Collection, Processing and Storage of Cord Blood Stem Cells. 2nd Edition 2003. New York: New York State Council on Human Blood and Transfusion Services.

22. NETCORD-FACT International Standards for Cord Blood Collection, Processing, Testing, Banking, Selection and Release, 3rd Edition; 2006. www.factwebsite.org

23. Sugarman J, Kurtzberg J, Box TL, Horner RD. Optimization of informed consent for umbilical cord blood banking. Am J Obstet Gynecol. 2002;187(6):1642–6.

24. Burgio GR, Gluckman E, Locatelli F. Ethical reappraisal of 15 years of cord blood transplantation. Lancet. 2003;361(9353):250–2.
25. Diaz-Rossello JL. Early umbilical cord clamping and cord-blood banking. Lancet. 2006;368(9538):840.
26. Edozien LC. NHS maternity units should not encourage commercial banking of umbilical cord blood. BMJ. 2006;333:801–4.
27. Egeland T, Raffoux C, Gordezky C, Campbell B. Foreign recruitment. World Marrow Donor Association. 2004. www.worldmarrow.org (accessed August 19, 2007).
28. Hurley C, Raffoux C. World Marrow Donor Association. International Standards for Unrelated Haemopoietic Stem Cell Donor Registries. Bone Marrow Transplantation 2004;34:103–10.
29. Falzetti F, Aversa F, Minelli O, Tabilio A. Spontaneous rupture of the spleen during peripheral blood stem cell mobilisation in a healthy donor (letter). Lancet. 1999;353(9152):555.
30. Stroncek D, Shawker T, Follman D, Leitman SF. G-CSF induced spleen size changes in peripheral blood progenitor cell donors. Transfusion. 2003;43(5):609–13.
31. Bennett CL, Evens AM, Andritsos LA, Balasubramanian L, Mai M, Fisher MJ, et al. Haematological malignancies developing in previously healthy individuals who received haematopoietic growth factors: report from the Research on Adverse Drug Events and Reports (RADAR) project. Br J Haematol. 2006;135(1111):642–50.
32. King R, Egeland D. Unrelated haematopoietic stem cell donors as research subjects (draft) 28 February 2007 personal distribution.
33. Samuel GN, Kerridge IH, Vowels M, Trickett A, Chapman J, Dobbins T. Ethnicity, equity and public benefit: a critical evaluation of public umbilical cord blood banking in Australia. Bone Marrow Transplantation. 2007;40(8):729–34.

12 Ethical and Consent Issues in the Reproductive Setting: The Case of Egg, Sperm, and Embryo Donation

Sarah Franklin[1] and Sharon R. Kaufman[2]
[1] London School of Economics, London, UK
[2] University of California, San Francisco, California, USA

Introduction

Ethical questions about egg, sperm, and embryo donation that arise in the reproductive setting are among the most complex encountered by clinicians, policy makers, and social scientists because of their manifold and far-reaching personal, familial, and social implications. Uniquely, gamete and embryo donation did not originate in order to preserve existing lives, but to assist in the creation of new lives. More recently, the prospect of using germ cells and embryos to develop an entirely new field of therapeutic intervention – through regenerative medicine, tissue engineering, and stem cell science – raises an additional set of complex ethical issues. Determining best practice in this context is thus dependent on the expertise gained from more well-established human donation sectors, such as blood banking, as well as innovative thinking about patient information and consent, the risks of exploitation and commodification, donor screening and feedback, reversible anonymity, and the standardization of best practice.

A considerable literature now surrounds the formation of new families through assisted conceptive technologies such as in vitro fertilization (IVF), surrogacy, gamete donation, donor insemination, and preimplantation genetic diagnosis, including their social, legal, and ethical dimensions [1–4]. Less attention has been paid to the post-IVF context of tissue donation, namely coordination of the large numbers of "surplus" embryos created

Tissue and Cell Donation: An Essential Guide. Edited by Ruth M. Warwick, Deirdre Fehily, Scott A. Brubaker, Ted Eastlund. © 2009 Blackwell Publishing, ISBN: 978-14051-6322-4.

during clinical treatment for infertility, which, if a couple so desires and consents, may be donated for scientific research, although specialist literature addresses this topic [5–9]. Increasingly, procedures to enable couples to donate surplus embryos from IVF treatment for a range of scientific and clinical procedures, including stem cell research, have become the focus of efforts to define and standardize best practice [10].

Background: IVF and stem cells

IVF was first successfully practiced in the United Kingdom in 1978 by the consultant gynecologist and surgeon Patrick Steptoe and the developmental biologist and research scientist Robert Edwards [11]. This clinical application in humans of basic mammalian developmental biology techniques was itself the product of a uniquely productive period of embryological research in the postwar period [12], which enabled increasingly sophisticated understanding of the precise events involved in the biological reproduction and development of higher vertebrates. Increasingly, technological means of intervening into mammalian reproduction and development – initially aimed at population control and agricultural improvements rather than infertility – began to lay the groundwork for assisted human reproduction as early as the 1950s.

Despite its ethically controversial prehistory and debut, IVF quickly became an acceptable and popular technology. Although there is no authoritative source for the numbers of children born worldwide as a result of IVF, the International Committee for Monitoring Assisted Reproductive Technologies reported at the European Society for Human Reproduction and Embryology Conference in 2006 that IVF had been responsible for the births of three million children. During the 1980s and 1990s, IVF expanded rapidly, becoming an established and routine sector of public and private healthcare services worldwide, and the basic technique in an expanding fertility industry. As its applications widened, IVF began to be used to respond to an ever-widening spectrum of diagnoses, from male infertility to genetic disease. A consequence of this expansion in uses of IVF, and of the way in which IVF is routinely practiced (in which hormonal stimulation is relied upon to produce a much larger yield of eggs during a single cycle), is the preservation and cryogenic storage of fertilized eggs that may be used in a future treatment cycle. Cryopreservation enables a couple to thaw and transfer embryos over the course of more than one IVF cycle without the need for additional superovulation, thus maximizing the use of their embryos. This reserve supply of embryos may be stored indefinitely (although some countries such as the United Kingdom limit storage to 10 years) and may or may not be used for further treatment (for example, if a couple achieve a pregnancy and their goals are met). Frozen embryos thus comprise a unique potential source of donated human tissue – and one that has come to be of increasing scientific interest as well as of ethical concern.

As we are now aware, IVF was not the only revolutionary outcome of the postwar boom in developmental biology, reproductive physiology, and mammalian embryology. Other spectacular firsts were accomplished in mice, monkeys, cattle, sheep, and humans, resulting in the derivation of stable, pluripotent mouse and primate cell lines in the 1980s, human embryonic stem cell (hES) lines in the 1990s, and the cloning of a higher vertebrate from an adult cell in the famous "Dolly" experiment of 1996 (for a review, see Parson [13]). Together, these experiments overturned some of the most elementary scientific principles formerly assumed to govern biological development in general, and the diminishing course of cellular developmental potential in higher vertebrates in particular [14]. The confirmation, for example, that adult mammalian cells never lose their pluripotent potential – that is, their ability to become any kind of cell, as if they were an embryo – and that they can, as a result, be reprogramed to become any kind of specialized cell, has created significant prospects for new treatments for a wide range of diseases. These include degenerative, metabolic, genetic and congenital (e.g. spontaneous noninherited translocations), and other diseases; many previously unable to benefit from any form of therapy.

In sum, the unexpected regenerative capacities now known to be recoverable from most cells and tissue, such as adult skin cells, combined with the sophistication of modern molecular genetic and cell culture technology, have meant that all human tissue and cells, but in particular gametes and embryos, have literally, in the context of stem cell science, been given a new lease on life. Improved knowledge of the precise genetic and epigenetic events involved in germ cell differentiation and embryogenesis has become the "gold standard" against which cellular developmental potential can be most accurately understood. Despite the emergence of new techniques such as induced pluripotent stem cells (IPSCs), the human embryo retains a unique importance in both medicine and science.

Coordination and consent: the UK example

This chapter draws primarily on the experience of the United Kingdom, where assisted conception and human embryonic stem (hES) cell research are both highly regulated and scientifically advanced. The United Kingdom is a pioneer of the "combined approach," whereby extensive regulation enables a permissive research climate. This approach is based on a form of social contract devised by the philosopher Mary Warnock, who chaired the Consultation Committee on Human Fertilisation and Embryology from 1982 to 1984 in the wake of the birth of Louise Brown: in exchange for allowing research on human embryos, such research would be subject to strict statutory limitations enforced through criminal law [15]. As a result, in the UK system public confidence in the necessity for "lines to be drawn" is supported by a robust and active regulatory authority (the Human Fertilisation and Embryology Authority [HFEA]), which oversees all clinical and scientific work involving human embryos as well as treatment involving their creation. At the same time, the public desire to see scientific advances in the pursuit of improved (and less expensive) health care can also be met through promotion of a highly permissive research climate of experimental science [16].

The HFEA was established in 1991 as a licensing authority and regularly updates its licensing criteria through a Code of Practice. Since the early 1980s, the United Kingdom has continually revised and updated the ethical governance of assisted conception and embryo research (including embryo donation to stem cell research), including their regulatory oversight, quality control, and scientific standardization. Initially through the HFEA, later under the auspices of its publicly funded national stem cell bank (completed in 2004), and most recently under the new parliamentary and European Union (EU) directives, the process of providing statutory regulation, ethical infrastructure, and quality control has undergene a rapid evolution that is ongoing [17].

Unlike the United States, where legislative initiatives to oversee reproductive biomedicine have historically been haphazard, a series of UK governments has devoted parliamentary time to the establishment of legislation governing both clinical and scientific conduct related to the human embryo. In accordance with the conclusions of a Department of Health (DH) consultation paper, published in 2000 [18], new regulations were introduced into the parliament to amend the 1990 Human Fertilisation and Embryology Act in order to widen the criteria for research on human embryos, including the creation of embryos through cell nuclear replacement (CNR) for research purposes. Under the Human Fertilisation and Embryology (Research Purposes) Regulations (2001), three new criteria for embryo research were added to the existing Act (a) to widen the possibility for understanding the cellular bases of serious diseases, (b) to permit research that might lead to their treatment, including (c) through the method known as "therapeutic cloning" (i.e. CNR).

In 2002, following the recommendations of the DH and also those contained in a special report of the House of Lords Select Committee on Science and Technology [19], the UK Stem Cell Bank was commissioned and publicly funded as a joint endeavor between two of the United Kingdom's national research councils, the Medical Research Council (MRC) and the Biotechnology and Biological Sciences Research Council (together £2.3 million). Housed at the National Institute for Biological Standards and Control (NIBSC) near London in a purpose-built facility, the UK Stem Cell Bank was charged with "providing ethically sourced, quality controlled adult, fetal, and embryonic stem cell lines for research and for the development of therapies by the national and international research and industrial communities." A steering committee chaired by Lord Naren Patel was established to develop a series of guidelines including Codes of Practice for the bank and the use of stem cell lines. These codes were closely modeled on the 2001 Department of Health Code of Practice [20] for Public Sector Tissue Banks and were the subject of an extensive consultation exercise in late 2003. They have been updated and revised regularly since (see www.ukscb. org). The first licenses from the HFEA were granted in 2002 for hES cell derivation, and in 2003, the first UK-derived lines were announced by King's College in London [21].

Thus, whereas in Europe and the United Kingdom considerable effort has been made to establish a robust ethical and legislative context for guidance concerning clinical and scientific manipulation of human fertilization and embryology, the United States has relied largely on the nonstatutory guidelines provided by professional bodies such as the American Fertility Society, the National Academy of Science, and the American Society of Reproductive Medicine. The lack of a more systematic regulation of the US IVF industry, or "baby business," has been explicitly criticized by some [22], while its consumerist tendencies have been lamented by others [1]. Apart from the federal ban introduced by former president George W Bush in 2001 curtailing hES cell research, the regulation of the human reproductive sciences and medicine in the US context is largely charged to the United States Food and Drug Administration (USFDA) and focused on product safety and prevention of disease transmission. This oversight is limited to donor eligibility requirements such as donor screening and donor testing for anonymous reproductive cell/tissue donation situations, and labeling expectations for all donation scenarios. These regulations are codified as 21 CFR 1271 and are included within requirements applicable to all cells, tissues, and cellular and tissue-based products (HCT/Ps) transplanted, implanted, infused, or transferred in the United States. The USFDA does not regulate consent or gifting practices and currently does not require reproductive HCT/Ps to follow good tissue practices or to report adverse events. In the United Kingdom, where legislation exists but must be continually reinterpreted and amended, the key regulatory bodies are the aforementioned HFEA and the newly established Human Tissue Authority, as well as the UK Stem Cell Bank and the associated NIBSC. Both authorities work closely with the medical and scientific regulators and advisors, including the Medical Healthcare Products Regulatory Agency (MHRA), the National Institute for Health and Clinical Excellence (NICE) and professional organizations such as the British Association for Tissue Banking (BATB), and the National Blood Service (NBS) within the National Health Service Blood and Transplant (NHSBT) to ensure UK legislation remains in step with other national and international protocols determining best practice.

Ethical issues: informed consent

As in all areas of tissue and cell donation, ethical consideration must be given to a wide range of issues raised by the possibility of embryo donation leading to stem cell research. From the position taken by national governments on this issue, such as the US ban on federal funding for embryonic stem cell research, to media coverage and religious prohibitions, to intimate personal and familial questions of identity and shared reproductive substance, as well as in relation to basic questions of clinical care and best practice, this context represents a highly challenging ethical arena in which innovation is a constant, if laborious, requirement. The lessons to be learned in this sector are consequently likely to have a significant impact both within and beyond the tissue banking profession as this sector increases in prominence and professionalization.

The successful translation of stem cell science into actual treatments for diseases such as diabetes, cancer, Alzheimer's, or Parkinson's depends on the maintenance of public confidence and support for what is, in global terms, a highly controversial field. In the post-Hwang context [23], as well as in the wake of the earlier misconduct involving human tissue in the Alder Hey pathology department in the UK [24], the question of accountability for robust consent procedures for donation of embryos and other human tissue and cells, and their credibility to patients and the wider public, has gained increasing prominence [10]. While debate about informed consent, patient screening, anonymization, feedback, and paid donation continue to indicate the lack of a uniform frame of reference internationally concerning best practices in the regulation of egg and embryo donation, the imperative to provide clear standards of best consenting practices is increasing. Thus, in addition to the fact that consent procedures for embryo donation for stem cell research must respond with due diligence to novel sources of patient concern, the development of such procedures is also required to conform to a new and, in some senses, higher standard.

For example, although informed consent remains a core principle in clinical practice, and for any scientific research involving human subjects, including stem cell research, its meaning in the context of the reproductive setting is complicated by a number of factors, such as the fact that an embryo is not readily conceptualized in terms of either its "own" or its donors' individual autonomy. Embryos created in the context of IVF inevitably must be thought of as embodiments of shared reproductive hope and investment, often for couples whose primary experience is of reproductive loss or disappointment [25]. For many such couples, the opportunity to "give something back" to medical research is an attractive possibility, offering as it does a form of reciprocity or altruistic satisfaction. It may even be the case that couples who have failed in their attempt to conceive a child through IVF (as remains the fate of the majority of couples who undergo IVF) can gain some sense of reward from potentially helping others, thus contributing toward a generalized social good even when their own immediate reproductive aspirations have been unfulfilled. In all cases, both members of a couple must consent to the donation, and the precise terms and conditions of such consent must be rigorously established and protected.

CASE 1

Patient motivations

Mr. and Mrs. X have attended the assisted conception clinic for their first cycle of IVF. They have a niece aged 3 who was born from IVF. As part of their initial consultation, they are asked to fill in consent forms indicating whether or not they would be prepared to donate embryos to research. The consent coordinator explains that these would only be embryos not suitable for treatment, e.g. ones that had not shown signs of appropriate development and could not be used for embryo transfer, or which would not be considered of high enough quality to survive the freeze-and-thaw process. Anticipating this decision, Mr. and Mrs. X have discussed the issues involved in embryo donation prior to attending the clinic. They consider themselves fortunate to be given the opportunity to receive treatment and feel that they would not be able to do so if other people before them had not donated their embryos for research. They would like to be able to help others do the same. They view discarding their embryos as a waste of a potentially valuable medical resource. Even if they do not become pregnant themselves, they suggest, some good may come of their treatment for others. Mrs. X expresses a specific interest in speaking to a member of the research team about stem cell derivation as her grandfather had had Parkinson's disease, and she would like to specifically help this cause if it is possible.

In addition to the fact that embryos come from couples, and that many couples undergoing IVF have never considered the question of what they might do with any surplus embryos left over from their treatment, consent for embryo donation for stem cell research is complicated by technical factors intrinsic to this field of biomedical innovation. A number of unique aspects of this form of tissue donation – in particular the potential for amplification, regeneration, and transformation of the original cellular material – create areas of uncertainty about best practices that remain under debate. The fact that a single embryo could be the basis for a cell line potentially used to treat thousands of people, and the possibility to immortalize, and endlessly divide such a line, creates unprecedented ethical difficulties, as do issues of screening donors and providing feedback. As we shall see in the following sections, the establishment of novel and effective ethical protocols for many forms of live donation in the contemporary reproductive setting has by no means ensured that uncertainty will not continue to characterize various implications of this increasingly important biomedical domain in the future.

Determining best consenting practices

Under both UK law and the EU Tissues and Cells Directive, consent for embryo donation to stem cell research must be requested by a professional who is independent of both the clinical and research staff in his or her assisted conception unit in order to avoid conflicts of interest. The ability to meet this standard is essential, much as the acute economic pressures on the health service may make it difficult. The beginnings of a more professionalized relationship to consent in the reproductive setting, in part because of the momentum generated by successful hES cell derivation, have begun to become more apparent in the context of a higher level of national coordination in the United Kingdom, in a manner that is likely to be replicated elsewhere.

Since 2004, the British initiative to coordinate the scientific effort of hES cell derivation and banking with the clinical service of providing assisted conception, in other words at the IVF–stem cell interface, has been facilitated by the establishment of a national network of Human Embryonic Stem Cell Coordinators (HESCCO). Funded by the MRC, and building on the momentum created by the UK government's enthusiastic support for the stem cell field (publicly stated priorities of both past and present Prime Ministers Tony Blair and Gordon Brown), the HESCCO network was the first group to devise, pilot, and confirm standardized national consent procedures for embryo donation to hES cell derivation. The establishment of a networked, interdisciplinary peer group for work in this sensitive area has been shown to facilitate continuous improvement in the development of policies and practices and coordination of many aspects of derivation, such as quality control and consent protocols. Such networks, which are likely to become better established, facilitate support of frontline, administrative, and laboratory staff who work in these types of facilities, often enabling a streamlining of procedures that can reduce donors' vulnerabilities to bureaucratic inefficiencies, inadequate or incorrect information, or "consent fatigue." Similarly for staff, networked affiliations boost morale and create wider opportunities for information sharing and cooperation.

CASE 2

Staff issues

Z is an experienced nurse aged 38 who works in a large fertility clinic. On a daily basis, she counsels female patients about their treatment and performs scans to assess their progress. These include early pregnancy scans. Sometimes, these scans show that the baby has no heartbeat and Nurse Z must inform the patient, provide emotional and clinical support, and arrange aftercare. Presently, she is finding this part of her job very difficult as she has recently had a miscarriage herself. She and her partner had been trying unsuccessfully to conceive for over a year. Having miscarried at 7 weeks, no one at work is aware of her pregnancy loss, and she has not informed them. Increasingly, she finds it difficult to cope with patients with infertility problems and especially those who are having an ongoing, successful pregnancy. Her partner has urged her to move on. However, she cannot rid herself of the fear that, as she approaches 40, her chances of conceiving are rapidly decreasing. Recently, she has been tempted to take the day off sick when she knows that she is scheduled to undertake pregnancy scans for patients. Nurse Z has access to a hospital staff counseling service, which she may attend soon (see Chapter 10 on staff support). Unfortunately, the longer time passes, the more difficulty she has confiding in others, addressing her concerns directly, or performing her job effectively.

Consent criteria in the United Kingdom

Free and informed consent are key principles of the Human Tissue Act (2004), the HFE Act (1990), and the EU Tissue and Cells Directive (EU TCD) (2004), as well as being standard principles of best practices in clinical medicine, randomized controlled trials, and scientific research involving human subjects. For consent to be robust, legitimate, and ethically sound, comprehensive information must be given to the donors in a form that is readily accessible and allows a free and informed decision to be made by potential donors [26]. In the United Kingdom, all patient information provided with consent forms must be approved by local ethics committees. This is also required for research involving embryos.

The criteria devised by the steering committee of the UK Stem Cell Bank for provision of information *prior to discussion of consent to donate embryos to stem cell research* are divided into two components: oral and written information. Correspondingly, the discussion between the consent coordinator or research nurse and patients who are potential donors must cover the following points:

1 the research project is directed toward the derivation of hES cell lines
2 very few such cell lines are derived from donated embryos at present
3 any hES cell lines that are derived will be deposited in the UK Stem Cell Bank, may be used for other projects within the United Kingdom and/or overseas, and may eventually be used for treatment
4 the research will not lead to any direct medical benefit to the donor

5 the UK Stem Cell Bank is overseen by an independent steering committee that has the responsibility to ensure legal and ethical accountability for all hES cell lines accessioned by the bank

6 donation to research will in no way affect donors' treatment, and the decision whether to donate is voluntary

7 donated embryos will be anonymized, although this anonymity must be reversible under exceptional circumstances when grave matters of public health may be at stake

8 no information emerging from tests done on the cell lines will be fed back to donors (unless under the exceptional circumstances mentioned earlier)

9 donors can withdraw their consent until the point that the embryos are used for research

10 cell lines, or discoveries made using them, may be patented and used for commercial purposes, but the donor will not benefit financially from any future profit generated by them.

These minimum criteria, which must be provided in the patient information leaflet accompanying the consent form, are also fully discussed with potential donors by an independent party who is not part of either the clinical or the research team. They are considered by patients for a suitable period of time to allow reflection, then each gamete or embryo provider must consent *in writing* to the following:

1 that they consent to the use of embryos created using their gametes or embryos in a specified research project for the derivation of hES cell lines

2 that they understand that a sample of any successfully derived hES cell line(s) will be deposited in the UK Stem Cell Bank, and that these cell lines may be used in other research projects

3 that they are aware they are under no obligation to donate gametes or embryos to research, and that a decision not to participate in research projects will not alter their treatment in any way

4 that they understand that they have a right to withdraw their consent without giving any reason, at any stage until the gametes and/or embryos have been used for research

5 that they understand that any cell line derived from their donated gametes/ embryos may eventually be used for treatment purposes (including cell replacement therapies) in the future, but that donors will not personally benefit from such treatment

6 that they understand that cell lines or discoveries made using them may be patented and used for commercial purposes, but that donors will not benefit financially from any future profits of such commercial activity

7 that they agree to be contacted in the future in the unlikely event that the stem cell steering committee considers it necessary to confirm test results performed on stem cell lines that are of direct relevance to their own, their family's, or the public's health.

In the establishment of minimum consent criteria, clarity and brevity must be balanced against the need to retain a substantial core of necessary information. Best consenting practices are enhanced by ensuring that the patient information and consent form is attractive and accessible, easy to read, and easily completed. The forms may be supplemented by a public website, including resources, links, and frequently asked questions. In the United Kingdom, the HESCCO consent forms received approval from the HFEA in 2005 and have since been adopted by numerous clinics nationwide (Figure 12.1).

CASE 3

Patient concerns #1

Mr. and Mrs. W have spoken to a member of staff at their assisted conception unit and are trying to decide whether they would like to donate their embryos for stem cell research. The staff member has explained that any stem cell line derived must have a sample of cells sent to the UK Stem Cell Bank so that they can be accessed for secondary research by people who may not be deriving stem cells themselves. Mr. and Mrs. W asked whether this was just in the United Kingdom or could people apply from abroad? The staff member explained that the lines can be released to researchers worldwide and that it is the stem cell bank steering committee that evaluates the suitability of applicants on a case-by-case basis. Mr. and Mrs. W have read newspaper stories about the fraudulent work in South Korea by Mr. Hwang and are very concerned about cells derived from their embryos being exported abroad. They want to know if they can donate their embryos on the condition that any successfully derived cell lines can only be used in the United Kingdom, but the staff member has explained this kind of conditional consent is not possible. The couple decline to donate their embryos.

Moving toward the future of stem cell translation

The combination of rapid worldwide expansion of IVF over the past three decades and equally substantial developments in stem cell science, with their promising clinical potential, all but ensure that the practice of embryo donation for stem cell research will gain momentum as a distinct sector of tissue and cell banking internationally. Although rapid progress has been made, particularly in the United Kingdom and Europe, to ensure that

your hospital logo

The generation of human embryonic stem cells

RESEARCH INFORMATION SHEET

Introduction

We would like to invite you to participate in a project to generate human embryonic stem cell lines that could eventually be used in treatment or therapy. This project will use human embryos unsuitable for your current treatment or freezing (for possible use in a later treatment cycle), and that would normally be discarded.

Before you decide, it is important for you to understand why the research is being done and what it will involve. Please take time to read the following information carefully and discuss it with others if you wish. Ask us (contact details below) if there is anything that is not clear or if you would like more information. Take time to decide whether or not you wish to take part. Thank you for reading this.

Why have I been chosen?

We are approaching all couples undergoing in-vitro fertilisation (IVF) or intra-cytoplasmic sperm injection (ICSI) who have said they are agreeable with research.

What does this involve for me?

During your current IVF cycle, one or two embryos (if they are of sufficient quality) will be selected for replacement into the womb. The remaining embryos may be frozen and stored for your future use, if you wish. The decision to freeze embryos is based on their quality as observed under the microscope. This decision is made by clinical embryologists who are not directly associated with this project and therefore your decision of whether to take part

in this research will have no impact on your treatment or chances of conceiving. Embryos that are not frozen because they are not of sufficient quality, would normally be allowed to perish or donated to research. We are now seeking your permission to use these embryos to try to generate embryonic stem cells. If you wish to contribute to this research project you will need to sign a consent form (which you will also be given a copy of).

Will I benefit from this research?

If you give embryos for this project, you should be aware that the results of the research are not intended to directly benefit any treatment you might have. However, this research will help us understand how embryos develop and may in time improve treatment for infertility. In addition, the major goal of stem cell research is to find treatments and/or cures for many other diseases such as Parkinson's disease, heart disease and some types of cancer. Therefore this research may help to treat other patients in the future.

Will participating in the research affect our treatment?

No. You will receive the same treatment whether you donate embryos or not. All embryos that you donate would otherwise have been allowed to perish. This is ensured by making sure that research staff are not involved in your treatment and that clinical staff are not involved in the research.

Do we have to take part?

No. Participation is entirely voluntary.

Date Created: 30 September 2005   hESCCO   Review Date: 30 September 2006 • Version I

Figure 12.1 Page one of the two page HESCO patient information and consent form illustrates the question and answer format assigned to assessibility.

robust and workable legislative guidelines and ethical protocols are agreed upon and implemented, a number of areas continue to demand further refinement and clarification. At present, the most challenging areas of debate concern the following topics:

1 reversible anonymization
2 conditional consent (and artificial gametes/embryos)
3 feedback to patients
4 payment of donors
5 donor screening

In the following sections, these issues are illustrated through case studies and discussion, and are supplemented by current guidelines and regulation, where relevant.

Reversible anonymization

Under the EU TCD, the provenance of all clinical grade cell lines must be fully traceable and documented at every stage. Potential donors need to be made aware not only that so-called reversible anonymization will be used to ensure that in the event of a major health threat (commonly imagined to be a xenopathic agent such as Bovine Spongiform Encephalopathy (BSE)), but also that they may be contacted in the event that future screening identifies them as a carrier of a disease potentially transmissible by human embryonic stem cell lines (ESC). While the justification for this measure is all but unassailable on public health grounds, the mechanisms for implementing these criteria vary. In particular, the questions of the degree of reversibility that needs to travel with the hES cell line sample, how far down the path of postderivation dissemination donor identity information needs to pass, or where such information is retained (in the clinic or in the lab) remain subject to local, regional, national, and international variations. Donors may be reassured if specific information can be provided about the mechanism of "reversibility" that will be employed, especially, for example, if donor information does not leave the clinic. The feasibility of national and international databases of all embryos donated to research, their provenance, and the outcomes of such research are being explored [27].

Conditional consent

One of the most common and widespread concerns expressed by patients in the context of assisted conception in general, and equally by patients who are approached about the possibility of donating their eggs or embryos to hES derivation in particular, is the *reproductive misuse* of such material. The prospects of their reproductive substance being sold or made available to other couples, mislabeled or otherwise inadvertently used to create a child for another couple, or, in a more futuristic vein, employed in scientific experiments leading to a cloned offspring, are among the most common and widespread concerns expressed by patients. For potential donors to stem cell research, such concerns have additional dimensions. For example, the growing scientific literature suggesting that it may be possible for germ cell lines, or "artificial gametes," to be derived from embryonic cell lines [28] has proven to be a concern for a small but growing number of patients. The possibility of introducing conditional consent, a decision that would respond to the legitimate concerns of potential donors, is one to which the HFEA has devoted serious consideration in the United Kingdom. To date, the HFEA has refrained from endorsing conditional consent, as to do so would establish a new precedent of "fettering" consent to tissue donation, which many regard as contrary to best practices in terms of either experimental research or tissue banking. Many believe it is also not in the patients' best interests, as the feasibility and, therefore, authenticity of such a guarantee of unknown duration cannot presently be reliably assured. An additional objection to making an "exception" of embryo donation as a candidate for the unprecedented use of conditional consent is that adult cells can already be made into embryolike cells and gametes and that too little is known about the distinction among these various types of cells. To date, the consent to donate embryos for hES cell research has remained unconditional in the United Kingdom.

CASE 4

Donor emotional aspects

Many assisted conception units (and all such clinics in the United Kingdom) enforce storage limits on frozen embryos, for example, five or 10 years. In such cases, it is necessary to contact patients to determine their wishes for their frozen embryos before the storage expiry date. Contact is usually maintained on a yearly basis, but for a variety of reasons (such as change of address), contact may be more infrequent or interrupted. Mr. and Mrs. X were contacted after four years by telephone to check their address details and to explain that it was necessary to send out forms about their frozen embryos. They confirmed address details and were posted the forms. However, months went by and the forms were not returned, so a telephone call was made to check that they had received the forms. They said that they had received the forms but were still uncertain about what to do. They were finding the decision very difficult as they had had successful IVF treatment and now had twin girls. Since their treatment, they had also conceived naturally themselves and have a son. They said that they could not consider letting their frozen embryos perish at the end of the legally allowable storage limit as they saw them as possible siblings for their existing children. However, they also felt that they did not want more children as three were enough. They had continued to discuss their options but had failed to reach a decision. In time, they reached a decision to donate their embryos for research. However, they noted on their form that they had found the decision highly unsettling and made worse by the gap in contact of four years.

Feedback to patients

Feedback of information to patients raises issues in relation to both the short and long term. At one end of what might be called the "feedback spectrum" is the increasingly influential principle drawn from human rights law and bioethics that personal information belongs to the donor and that no agency should retain identifiable information of relevance to the individual's health in secret or without that individual's knowledge and consent. However, information such as possible genetic predisposition to disease may only come to light through research many years after donation and may or may not be welcomed by former patients, especially as the clinical implications might be unclear, unreliable, or simply unknown, having been derived from tissue grown in vitro through many passages. How and by whom such information would be imparted also presents difficulty. Beyond the requirement of reversible anonymity discussed previously (which is restricted to the most extreme cases of a public health risk), current best practice as recommended by the UK Stem Cell Bank Code of Practice for the Use of Human Stem Cell Lines (2006) is for donors to be informed that "no individual feedback will be given on tests performed by the UK Stem Cell Bank or research results of subsequent studies" although "general information . . . including the results of research using embryonic stem cell lines will be published on the [Bank's] website" [29: 2]. Hence, while the option to be informed if their embryos develop into cell lines has largely been foreclosed, the possibility that patients would be contacted either in the event of a public health concern, or indeed should "test results of direct relevance to the donor or the donor's family" be discovered, remains open.

CASE 5

Patient concerns #2

Mr. and Mrs. Y have decided to donate their spare embryos for research and have just finished talking to the research nurse about the issues involved as part of their routine induction at the clinic. They have decided to sign the consent form to donate their surplus embryos to three of the hospital's research projects but, after much deliberation, have decided not to contribute to hES stem cell derivation. During their consultation, staff members have explained that a sample of any hES cell line derived by the research team must be placed in the UK Stem Cell Bank and that these lines may last for a very long time (possibly indefinitely). The couple have also learned that there is a slim chance that future research on the stem cell lines may reveal a public health issue, and that in those circumstances, they are legally required to be traceable by the stem cell bank. Mr. and Mrs. Y, who are in principle keen to help, feel uncomfortable about the future uncertainty this possibility of contact would create. Such contact would both confirm an hES line had been derived from their embryo, and that it was affected by a serious disease. They are unsure of how they, or their offspring, might react under such circumstances. They are also concerned about implications the feedback might have on their life insurance policies. Reluctantly, they conclude that the indefinite nature of the stem cell research project precludes their participation.

Payment to egg and embryo donors

In July 2006, the HFEA set a new precedent in the United Kingdom by granting a license to Newcastle University for "egg sharing for research" – a practice designed to reduce the cost of IVF treatment in exchange for the donation of eggs for research purposes [30]. The authority simultaneously announced a public consultation into the wider question of "whether it is appropriate for women to donate their eggs for use in scientific research," and what safeguards might be needed were such a practice to become more widespread. Egg sharing for research, which is based on the model of clinical egg-sharing programs, in which discounted IVF treatment is offered in exchange for donating eggs to other couples, has been the subject of debate because of the potential for exploitation, and the specter of commodification that attaches to any kind of remuneration for tissue donation and especially to the perceived sale of tissue. In February 2007, the HFEA [31] confirmed its decision to license egg sharing for research, stating,

> "Having considered all the information on donating eggs for research, including the risks to women and the outcomes of the public consultation, the Authority has decided that women will be allowed to donate their eggs to research, both as an altruistic donor or in conjunction with their own IVF treatment. Given that the medical risks for donating for research are no higher than for treatment, we have concluded that it is not for us to remove a woman's choice of how her donated eggs should be used."

By confirming its support for increased levels of remuneration for egg donation to research, the Authority's position now closely resembles that of the Ethics Committee of the American Society for Reproductive Medicine, which in its published guidelines of 2000 endorses payment to donors provided that "payments to women . . . should be fair and not so substantial that they become undue inducements that will lead donors to discount risks" (estimated to be >10 k USD [32: 218, 33]). However, both of these positions are now in conflict with that of the US National Academy of Sciences "Guidelines for Human Embryonic Stem Cell Research," which stipulates that no payment should be provided to egg donors – a view recently adopted as part of the California stem cell initiative, and by major international providers of hES lines, such as Singapore-based ES Cell International. A compromise option, such as that adopted by the International Society of Stem Cell Research allowing each individual country to determine its own laws may be a suitable interim measure (2006).

Donor screening

The large-scale amplification involved in the clinical application of hES cell line therapies in the future, whereby several thousand patients might receive hES cell products from a single line, poses significant challenges at the level of determining appropriate screening procedures throughout the derivation process. Which aspects of donor screening are paramount for hES cell derivation (as opposed to blood donation), and how should the screening, testing, and documentation of donor characteristics be facilitated logistically, technically and ethically? This question has been handled differently in the United States and the United Kingdom, with the former relying on USFDA requirements, which are specifically designed to emphasize that its xeno-transplantation regulations are not intended to prevent the clinical use of hES cells derived using animal products (Title 21 Code of Federal Regulations Part 1271 [35–37]). Whereas this policy will require greater reliance on microassays of preclinical lines, rather than on samples taken from the donor at the time of donation, a consensus has not been reached in the United Kingdom about the suitability of such "passive" detectors of potential contaminants – particularly in the context of variant Creutzfeldt–Jakob disease. In the United Kingdom, preexisting standardization of IVF patient screening, under the mandatory HFEA Code of Practice, overlaps considerably with existing NBS testing in terms of HIV, Hep B, and Hep C screening. However, there is, at present, no requirement in the EU TCD or the UK Stem Cell Bank guidance for donor screening to ask the lifestyle questions routinely applied by the blood service to screen donors. Considerable debate thus continues to surround the adequacy of molecular assays to detect any infection or contamination by testing the cell lines directly, particularly for master stocks.

Conclusion

As one of the newest arenas of tissue banking, the reproductive setting remains a site of emerging policy and protocols which continue to evolve in the context of high-profile scientific advances and accompanying political debate. An ethically sensitive setting, the context of assisted conception, from which the vast majority of eggs and embryos are donated for stem cell research, raises important questions for patients and tissue coordinators, as well as clinicians, embryologists, scientists, and policy makers. Although the highly charged moral debate surrounding research involving human embryos appears unlikely to diminish, this chapter also notes the importance of the discovery that all tissue and cells are likely to retain far more regenerative and differentiating potential than previously imagined. This discovery has implications for the entire field of tissue banking, and though the highly charged moral debate surrounding germ line tissues and cells may initially arise in the reproductive setting, it is by no means restricted to that arena.

Like genetic fingerprinting, the science of cellular regeneration has the potential to change the status of tissue samples en masse, as individual samples become newly valuable as potential master stocks, or perpetual populations of named cell colonies, such as the famous Hela line of immortal cells used in cancer research. While it is highly unlikely that ethical uniformity will ever be reached concerning the moral status of the human embryo, it is entirely possible that many individual countries seeking to combine the possibility of beneficial scientific and clinical advances with respect for the "special" qualities of human reproductive material will devise combined approaches, such as that found in the United Kingdom, in which not only rigorous and standardized, but also flexible and tolerant, systems of enabling those patients who wish to donate gametes and embryos to research can do so knowing that some of the very highest standards of practice in tissue banking have been established in this sector.

However, no amount of regulation or even best practices can eliminate some of the profound risks of gamete and embryo donation, in particular, the risks women face of hyperstimulation syndrome in the context of IVF, a potentially fatal condition affecting as many as 1 in 100 cycles. The risk of exploitation of women and couples whose consent to donate is almost exclusively acquired in the highly stressful context of the assisted reproduction clinic is also significant. Increasing commercialization of this sector, which is differently evident in both the United States and the United Kingdom, should remain of concern in terms of its exploitative potential. As definitions of best practices change in concert with evolving regulations, and as tissue donation from this sector increases in volume, the need for robust assessment of donor safeguards – preferably on the basis of empirical research – will remain at a premium.

KEY LEARNING POINTS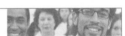

- In the United Kingdom, assisted conception and hES cell research are both highly regulated and advanced scientifically and represent a pioneer exemplar of the "combined approach," whereby extensive regulation enables a permissive research climate.

- Consent procedures for embryo donation to stem cell research must respond with due diligence to novel sources of patient concern.

- An embryo is not readily conceptualized in terms of either its "own" or its donor's individual autonomy. Embryos created in the context of IVF inevitably must be thought of as embodiments of shared reproductive hope and investment, often for couples whose primary experience is of reproductive loss or disappointment.

- Couples who have failed in their attempt to conceive a child through IVF (as remains the fate of the majority of couples who undergo IVF) can gain some sense of reward from potentially helping others, thus contributing toward a generalized social good even when their own immediate reproductive aspirations have been unfulfilled. In such cases, both members of a couple must agree to the specific terms of donation.

- The fact that a single embryo could be the basis for a cell line potentially used to treat thousands of people, and the possibility to immortalize, and endlessly divide, means that such a line creates unprecedented ethical difficulties, as do issues of screening donors and providing feedback.

- Consent for embryo donation to stem cell research must be undertaken by a professional who is independent from both the clinical and research staff in his or her assisted conception unit, in order to avoid conflicts of interest.

- Having a peer group for work in this sensitive area will facilitate continuous improvement in the development of policies and practices in consent discussions with potential donors. It will also facilitate support of the frontline and administrative and laboratory staff who work in these types of facilities.

- The risk of exploitation of women and couples, whose consent to donate is almost exclusively acquired in the highly stressful context of the assisted reproduction clinic, is also significant. For consent to be robust, legitimate, and ethically sound, comprehensive information must be given to the donors in a form that is readily accessible and allows a free and informed decision to be made by potential donors.

- In the establishment of minimum consent criteria, clarity and brevity have been emphasized, while retaining a substantial core of necessary information. Best consenting practice is enhanced by ensuring that the patient information and consent form is attractive and accessible, easy to read, and easily completed. Potential donors need to be made aware that the so-called reversible anonymization will be used to ensure that in the event of a major health threat, they may be contacted.

- One of the most common and widespread concerns expressed by patients in the context of assisted conception in general, and equally by patients who are approached about the possibility of donating their eggs or embryos to hES derivation in particular, is the *reproductive misuse* of such material.

- The possibility of introducing conditional consent may not be in the patients' best interests, as the feasibility and, therefore, authenticity of such a guarantee of unknown duration cannot presently be reliably assured.

- The large-scale amplification involved in the clinical application of hES cell line therapies in the future, whereby several thousand patients might receive hES cell products from a single line, poses significant challenges at the level of determining appropriate screening procedures throughout the derivation process.

References

1. Becker G. The Elusive Embryo: How Women and Men Approach New Reproductive Technologies. Berkeley, CA: University of California Press; 2000.
2. Franklin S. Embodied Progress: A Cultural Account of Assisted Conception. London: Routledge; 1997.
3. Franklin S, Roberts C. Born and Made: An Ethnography of Preimplantation Genetic Diagnosis. Princeton, NJ: Princeton University Press; 2006.
4. Thompson C. Making Parents: The Ontological Choreography of Reproductive Technologies. Cambridge, MA: MIT Press; 2005.
5. Franklin S. Embryonic Economies: the double reproductive value of stem cells. Biosocieties. 2006;1(1):71–90.
6. Haimes E, Luce J. Studying potential donors' views on embryonic stem, cell therapies and preimplantation genetic diagnosis. Hum Fertil. 2006;9(2):67–71.
7. Parry S. Reconstructing embryos in stem cell research: exploring the meaning of embryos for people involved in fertility treatments. Soc Sci Med. 2006;62(10): 2349–59.
8. Scully J, Rehmann-Sutter C. Creating donors: the 2005 Swiss law on donation of "spare" embryos to hESC research. J Bioeth Inq. 2006;3(1–2):81–93.
9. Svendsen M. Between reproductive and regenerative medicine: practising embryo donation and civil responsibility in Denmark. Body Soc. 2007;13(4):21–45.
10. Franklin S, Hunt C, Cornwell G, Peddie V, Desousa P, Livie M, Stephenson EL, and Braude PR. HESCCO: development of good practice models for hES cell derivation. Regen Med. 2008;3(1):105–16.
11. Edwards RG, Steptoe P. A Matter of Life: The Story of a Medical Breakthrough. London: Hutchinson; 1980.
12. Graham CF. Mammalian development in the UK (1950–1955). Int J Dev Biol. 2000;44(1):51–5.
13. Parson AB. The Proteus Effect: Stem Cells and their Promise for Medicine. Washington DC: Joseph Henry Press; 2004.
14. Wilmut I, Campbell K, and Tunge C. The Second Creation: the Age of Biological Control by the Scientists who Cloned Dolly. New York, NY: Farrar, Straus and Giroux; 2000.
15. Warnock, M. (Ed) A Question of Life: Warnock Report on Human Fertilization and Embryology. Oxford: Blackwell; 1985.
16. Lee RG, Morgan D. Human Fertilisation and Embryology: Regulating the Reproductive Revolution. London: Blackstone; 2001.
17. Jackson E. Medical Law. Oxford: Oxford University Press; 2006.
18. Department of Health (DH). Report of the Chief Medical Officer's (CMO's) Expert Group on Therapeutic Cloning. London: Department of Health; 2000.
19. House of Lords (HL). Report from the Select Committee for Stem Cell Research, HL 83(i). London: HMSO; 2002.
20. Department of Health. Code of Practice for Tissue Banks. London: Department of Health; 2001.
21. Pickering S, Braude P, Patel M, Burns CJ, Trussler J, Bolton V, et al. Preimplantation genetic diagnosis as a novel source of embryos for stem cell research. Reprod Biomed Online. 2003;7(3):353–64.

22. Spar P. The Baby Business. Cambridge, MA: Harward Business School Press; 2006.

23. Kennedy D. Responding to fraud. Science. 2006;314(5804):1353.

24. The Report of the Liverpool Children's Inquiry. Crown Copyright 2001.

25. Throsby K. When IVF Fails: Feminism, infertility and the negotiation of normality. Basingstoke: Palgrave Macmillan; 2004.

26. O'Neill O. A Question of Trust: the BBC Reith Lectures. Cambridge: Cambridge University Press; 2002.

27. Stephenson EL, Braude PR, and Mason C. Proposal for a universal minimum information convention for the reporting on the derivation of human embryonic stem cell lines. Regenerative Medicine. 2006;1(6):739–50.

28. Yamanaka S. Strategies and new developments in the generation of patient specific pluripotent stem cells. Cell Stem Cell. 2007;1(1):39–49.

29. UKSCB. Code of Practice for the Use of Human Cell Lines; 2006.

30. HFEA. Should women be able to donate their eggs for scientific research – HFEA announces plans for consultation. July 27 [Press release]. 2006. http://www.hfea.gov.uk (accessed January 8, 2008).

31. HFEA. HFEA statement on donating eggs for research. 2007. http://www.hfea.gov.uk/en/1491.html (accessed January 8, 2008).

32. ASRM. 2000.

33. American Society for Reproductive Medicine (ASRM). Donating spare embryos for embryonic stem cell research. Fertil Steril. 2002;78(5):958–60 [Reviewed 2006, http://www.asrm.org/Media/Ethics/donatingspare.pdf] (accessed January 8, 2008).

34. Department of Health. Guidance on the Microbiological Safety of Human Organs, Tissues and Cells Used in Transplantation. London: DH; 2000.

35. U.S. Department of Health and Human Services, Food and Drug Administration. Final guidance for industry: source animal, product, preclinical, and clinical issues concerning the use of xenotransplantation products in humans. April 3, 2003. http://www.fda.gov/cber/infosheets/humembclin.htm (accessed January 8, 2008).

36. U.S. Department of Health and Human Services, Food and Drug Administration. Eligibility determination for donors of human cells, tissues, and cellular and tissue-based products; final rule (69 FR 29785). May 25, 2004. http://www.fda.gov/cber/rules/suitdonor.pdf (accessed January 8, 2008).

37. U.S. Department of Health and Human Services, Food and Drug Administration. Final guidance for industry: eligibility determination for donors of human cells, tissues, and cellular and tissue-based products (HCT/Ps). August 8, 2007. http://www.fda.gov/cber/gdlns/tissdonor.pdf (accessed January 8, 2008).

13 Clinical Governance in Cell and Tissue Banking

Elaine Swanson, William Randell, and Danielle B. Freedman
Luton & Dunstable Hospital NHS Foundation Trust, Luton, UK

This chapter will take the reader through, and place in context, the general processes that are developing in the United Kingdom and the United States to ensure patients receive safe and high-quality care. These general principles can also apply to the clinical and laboratory aspects of tissue banking. Quality and improvement aspects in clinical care provision include standards of good practice equivalent to the principles of "good manufacturing practice" and "good laboratory practice" that apply in donor selection and tissue processing facilities. The terms used reflect the vocabulary used in the United Kingdom, and similar terms are often used elsewhere in the world. The glossary provides simple definitions of the terms used throughout the chapter.

Introduction

Clinical governance refers to an interdisciplinary oversight that ensures that the practice of individual clinicians, their clinical teams, and support services provide clinically effective, up-to-date, efficient, and equitably available health care. Peer review plays a key role in ensuring that individual clinicians and teams are accountable for the care they provide. Tissue banks and their physicians do not provide direct patient care, but clinical governance includes the application of governmental laws and regulations through the setting of professional standards and accreditation for organizations.

Tissue and Cell Donation: An Essential Guide. Edited by Ruth M. Warwick, Deirdre Fehily, Scott A. Brubaker, Ted Eastlund. © 2009 Blackwell Publishing, ISBN: 978-14051-6322-4.

Monitoring clinical competency is not a new concept, but processes to improve accountability have been strengthened over the past decade following several inquiries that have highlighted untoward clinical practice with often tragic consequences for patients and their families. Clinical governance is about ensuring safe and effective clinical care and will be addressed within this chapter.

Clinical governance and tissue banks

Tissue establishments must ensure that safe donors are selected, tested, and informed of abnormal tests, and they are responsible for the safe processing and storage of allografts. Any adverse outcomes of transplantation need to be investigated, and lessons are learned to continually improve the safety and effectiveness of tissue allograft use.

Establishing robust clinical governance arrangements within tissue transplant banks is subject to the same dilemmas of governing competence and clinical effectiveness as within other areas of clinical practice. However, within tissue transplantation there are additional difficulties relating to the scarcity of controlled clinical trials that can inform the updating of clinical practice guidelines and the application of new technologies.

The introduction of clinical governance

In discussing the status of clinical governance in the United Kingdom and, to some degree, within the United States, the following features are addressed:

1 strategy through policy setting and evidence-based medicine
2 accountability
3 standards
4 assuring quality
5 clinical audit
6 risk management processes
7 continuous professional development
8 good practice with the tracking of materials
9 learning from donors, patients, and users

These concepts and the description of their practical application relate to all areas of clinical practice, as well as to tissue and cell donation. They support the provision of high-quality care by helping practitioners at all levels to reflect and learn throughout their clinical experience, and ultimately to further develop and improve clinical practice.

What is clinical governance?

Clinical governance has evolved in the United Kingdom since 1998 and was heralded in the document "A First Class Service: Quality in the New NHS" [1]. The British government recognized the need to raise public confidence and improve the way in which the National Health Service (NHS) could meet the modern challenges within health care in the public sector following concerns relating to fragmented access to care and a series of well-publicized lapses in the quality of service provision. The document defined clinical governance as "a framework through which NHS organizations are accountable for continuously improving the quality of their services and safeguarding high standards of care by creating an environment in which excellence in clinical care will flourish."

Gerald Scally and Liam Donaldson [2] identified the fundamental requirements needed to take clinical governance forward at an organizational level.

Organizations need a quality improvement philosophy

All aspects of health care need to review performance and identify issues of variation within the services they provide. By default, some services will be poor, some will be average, and some will be excellent, and the quality curve usually demonstrates this range of variation within the organization. What is not acceptable is to *accept* this as the norm, and the philosophy has to be that all service provisions can be improved. Using the quality curve approach, organizations, whether hospitals or other health establishments such as tissue and cell banks in the public or private sector, and the users of tissue and cells need to continually strive from a position of average performance to one of excellence.

Creating a quality leadership culture that is fair and just and fosters interdisciplinary teamwork

One of the most challenging areas of the improvement process is to influence a change in culture within the organization. To change culture, there needs to be a focus on how leadership skills can cultivate an environment that allows staff to feel they are working in a positive and supportive workplace, and that puts quality of care as the pivotal organizational aim. This needs to be led from the top and cascaded throughout the organization.

The first class service [1] document articulated this and gave permission for health providers to give equal priority to the quality of care within the context of strong financial management. These two priorities have, at times, been in conflict, but if the NHS was primarily finance driven without a focus on quality, service provisions would be compromised.

The concept that practitioners, whatever the clinical setting, work in teams is crucial to quality. The complex nature of modern health care makes it impossible to provide care without the input of multidisciplinary teams, e.g. medical, nursing, laboratory, imaging, and support services. This is true within hospitals and in the tissue banking concept, where a broad web of expertise is necessary to provide safe and efficacious outcomes.

Organizations need robust information

Access to good quality information enables the provider to use all its available resources effectively while appraising its needs for future service delivery.

It is accepted that poor data input will only allow poor data to be extrapolated. The ability to measure clinical outcomes and exert change requires access to robust data for analysis. To achieve this, staff must have a clear understanding of the need for data quality and its application in measuring and improving outcomes. The increasing use of technology and the multiple information systems in use require reliable interfaces to be in place for them to function effectively. It cannot be assumed that treatments that are accepted on their historic basis are actually efficacious unless appropriate data are collected.

In the tissue facility, data on the outcomes of tissue transplantation will ensure that all processes leading to tissue for patients are safe and of quality to ensure that allografts function appropriately.

Policy setting in health care

With increasing and competing demands placed upon limited financial resources, the scrupulous management and allocation of the available funds undoubtedly poses important challenges for those commissioning and providing clinical services. A centralized health-policy-making process aims to direct change and improvement in two ways:

1 to regulate the way health care is funded, delivered, and made accountable
2 to ensure that there is health gain to the population as a whole, by changing the physical, biological, and/or social environments, i.e. disease prevention and health improvement

Strategy and regulation is usually coordinated through policy directives, legislation, performance monitoring, and inspection.

In the United Kingdom, the implementation of national policy has been largely devolved to local and organizational levels. Accountability and performance monitoring are demonstrated through the clinical governance framework described earlier, requiring both managerial and clinical engagement to achieve centralized policy objectives.

In Europe, the delivery of health care is the responsibility of individual health authorities in member states. However, the Amsterdam Treaty gave competence to the European Union (EU) to regulate in the field of substances of human origin for the protection of public health.

In the United States, cell and tissue regulations imposed by the federal government provide tissue banks with rules and guidance for the control of contamination and cross contamination during manufacturing. Clinical surveillance is generally provided by means of adverse reaction reporting requirements.

The delivery of an overarching national health policy and its application into everyday clinical care, therefore, requires access to clear evidence on which treatments and practices are most efficacious and cost-effective.

Organizations' need of evidence-based decisions

Decisions about the provision of treatments and management plans for specific patient/user groups are usually based upon the interaction among three core dimensions: *evidence, values* (professional and patient), and the *resources* that are readily available. Taking into account that the availability of resources is limited, with social values that continue to raise user expectations, the application of robust clinical evidence is fundamental to clinical decision making, if variations in clinical practice are to be avoided (Figure 13.1).

Evidence-based medicine has been defined as "the conscientious, explicit, and judicious use of current best evidence, based on systematic review of all the available evidence, in making and carrying out decisions about the care of individual patients" [3].

Evidence-based medicine is the gathering and application of clinical evidence on what currently constitutes best practices and the ability to support the health practitioner to deliver quality care, defined as "doing the right things, for the right people, at the right time and doing them right first time" [4]. Evidence-based medicine plays an important role within the quality assurance (QA) framework by providing clear and precise

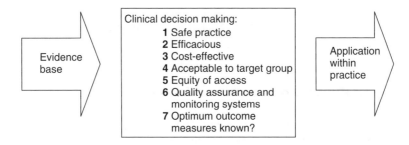

Figure 13.1 Evidence based pathway

direction, using recognized standards of good practice that can be easily measured through clinical audit.

With increasing amounts of research becoming available worldwide, the ability of an individual organization to stay abreast of what is currently best evidence-based practices is often challenging. In the United Kingdom, the National Institute for Health and Clinical Excellence (NICE) has taken on this role to appraise the available evidence and to issue guidance to the NHS. In the United States, quality improvement organizations work with health-care providers to develop and disseminate disease-specific outcomes, expectations, and indicators of healthcare quality.

The evidence available will therefore vary in strength and may be derived from a number of sources:

1 national and international inquiry reports, arising from investigations into specific cases where standards of care have been questioned; findings support the learning process and lead to recommendations that will improve future practice
2 internationally and nationally recognized guidance derived from the extensive review of the evidence base and expert opinion, e.g. National Institute for Health and Clinical Excellence (NICE) (England and Wales); Scottish Intercollegiate Network; Royal Colleges; American Medical Association (United States)
3 local guidelines, e.g. multidisciplinary guidelines and integrated care pathways depicting the expected course of events, for the care of a specific patient/user group
4 literature reviews and research publications to access worldwide sources of up-to-date clinical evidence, e.g. Cochrane Library, International Ross Registry

The factual resource that evidence-based medicine provides, therefore, brings an objective perspective to the clinical decision-making process.

In the context of tissue banking and use of allografts, there is a relative paucity of controlled trials. With many variations in surgical practice, it has been difficult to compare different types of grafts and how variations in retrieval and processing result in the best outcomes. It is therefore appropriate for tissue banks to work with their surgical colleagues to establish the necessary evidence of tissue allograft efficacy.

Accountability: how is this achieved?

The coexistence of clear policy direction and access to a strong evidence base will not automatically improve the quality of service provided. The overall delivery of the quality agenda rests with mechanisms being in place, which in turn promote ownership and commitment to delivering best practices across the whole spectrum of health care.

Specifically, the donation of tissues and cells, whether acquired from living or deceased donors, potentially raises sensitive issues. Donors and their families need to be assured that the tissues they choose to donate will be procured in an appropriate and safe manner and that consent from the donor family or living donor is obtained. The donated tissue must be used appropriately to improve the quality of life for the recipient or to further the work of an ongoing medical research program. The impact of negative publicity cannot be underestimated [5, 6] and has often preempted assurance frameworks put in place at the national, organizational, and professional levels.

Legislation

The presence of legislation at the national or state level ensures accountability through regulation. In the United Kingdom for example, stringent measures for increasing accountability arose following the publication of the Kennedy* [5] and Redfern* [6] reports and led to legislation within the Human Tissue Act [7]. The Act covers the use and retention of tissues and cells from living persons, including residual tissues following diagnostic and clinical procedures, as well as the removal and retention from the deceased. It excludes the use of cell lines, gametes, and embryos covered by a separate legislation and blood-derived products. It is mandatory for tissue establishments to be licensed and to demonstrate compliance with the Codes of Practice issued under the Act. The regulation of the Act and standards within the directive of the EU Parliament and of the Council [8] and the associated Commission Directives is undertaken by the Human Tissue Authority (HTA), having powers of inspection and issuance of expected standards to licensed establishments.

Organizational accountability

Provisions within the UK legislation have important consequences for facilities involved in the donation, removal, and storage of human tissues, mainly through risk of financial penalties and/or custodial sentences for failure to comply [9]. In transcribing the EU directive into national law, the United Kingdom mirrors similar systems in other European countries.

Accountability at the organizational level is demonstrated through a designated/responsible tissue establishment lead [7, 8] who is accountable for compliance with the legislation and additional policy directives. An intrinsic part of this role is to set up and maintain internal quality management systems that cover all aspects of tissue procurement, processing, storage, and distribution. Participation within recognized accreditation systems strength-

---

* Department of Health reports (Kennedy) [5] and (Redfern) [6].

ens adherence to legislation and policy directives, as well as facilitates the exchange of good practices through inspection and validation processes.

Accountability is also demonstrated through a system of critical incident reporting. All tissue establishments should be able to track, notify, and analyze the cause and outcomes of any serious untoward events.

Professional accountability

In the United Kingdom, individual personnel who are directly involved in any part of tissue and cell procurement, processing, and their use *must* be appropriately trained and qualified to do so, including participation within the organization's quality management system. This is a requirement of the EU directive [8]. Evidence of individual competency and ongoing training and education programs is a mandatory component of organizational accreditation and licensing processes and a requirement for individual practitioners to maintain professional registration. The general principle is applicable in all tissue facilities.

Certification by a national professional society or college conveys assurances that specific qualification and competency requirements have been met. However, there is currently no specific society or clinical accrediting body for physicians who practice in tissue banking.

The clinical governance arrangements in hospitals and for clinicians are moving from a systems-based quality improvement analysis of medical errors and incidents to improving overall patient therapeutic outcomes. Similarly, tissue banks will eventually need to develop a routine quality approach that monitors the effectiveness of tissue allograft usage and not just adverse outcomes.

The use of standards

Within health care, "standards are a formal statement of how well patients (and users) should be managed, with the understanding that this level of care should be as high as resources allow" [10].

A standard is therefore a measure of quality and intrinsic to the quality improvement process. Standards may be set from international, national, or local sources of evidence, and their identification promotes the discussion on where shortfalls in practice are likely to occur. Ultimately, the measurement of the actual practice against the recognized standards will provide the impetus to change and improve future practice.

The increasing use of human tissues and cells in therapeutic treatments and the development of intracommunity trading for these materials for human application have led to monitoring and regulation for their donation and distribution to establish quality standards. An example of practical steps to safeguard standards and minimize risks arising within the transplant process is demonstrated within the EU directive [8]. This directive provides a common framework of quality and safety standards for the donation, procurement, testing, preservation, storage, and distribution of human tissue and cells. Legally binding from April 2006, the directive applies to all member states that are responsible for maintaining the minimum standards identified, although it does not preclude the introduction of more stringent measures in individual states. The directive describes a series of obligations, including systems for inspection, tracking, adverse event reporting, and quality management to facilitate compliance with the standards within the directive. However, because the requirements in the directive are minimal standards and individual states may have higher standards (as may individual facilities), individual facilities will also require their own operational specific policies.

In the United Kingdom, the HTA is one of the two competent authorities in place for implementing the EU directive. Authorized under the Human Tissue Act [7], the HTA provides regulations to transcribe the directive into UK law. In the form of Codes of Practice to facilitate high standards at a level of detail not included in the regulations or the directive, it provides guidance documents for tissue establishments that reflect both UK legislation and the EU mandate plus additional guidance.

Assurance of quality

Systems for checking quality (quality control) have been extensively used within the industry for many years to review product outcomes against defined gold-standard measures. Quality control alone implies that suboptimal outcomes can be easily identified but fails to provide ownership to take the necessary actions to improve. Within health care, the quality improvement process is about providing an assurance that outcome measures will not be confined to a monitoring process alone but will be actively integrated within a development strategy to continually improve practice.

QA has been defined as "the measurement of the actual level of the services rendered plus the efforts to modify, when necessary, the provision of these services in the light of the results of measurement" [11].

QA involves all those planned or systematic actions necessary to provide adequate confidence that a product or service is of the type and quality needed and expected by the consumer. QA therefore aims to identify relevant values and standards, instigate their measurement, and initiate necessary actions to improve outcomes.

QA activities form an integral part of service accreditation systems, ensuring that the facility receives formal recognition for meeting the high standards of service provision. For tissue and cell establishments, a well-coordinated QA program plays a vital role in the provision of high-quality donor material that presents minimal risk to the recipient population.

Clinical audit

The application of the clinical audit is recognized worldwide, and an earlier definition identified it as a quality improvement tool involving structured peer review against agreed standards and the modification of practice. Indeed, the profile of the clinical audit as a quality improvement tool has increased over the past 15 years with firmer emphasis on multi-disciplinary engagement (clinical audit). Prior to this, audit activity was mainly clinician led (medical audit) and not always incorporated within the organizational timetable. To succeed in its aims, clinical audit relies on the synergy of a supportive organizational environment, which actively promotes its role within the overall quality improvement strategy, and a firm understanding of the correct application of audit methodology.

In the United Kingdom, the importance of the clinical audit within an overarching clinical governance framework has been recognized at the parliamentary level [1]. Instrumental to the modern healthcare agenda is the requirement to demonstrate an assurance that the quality of service delivery goes far beyond the entity of quantity alone. The clinical audit activity promotes organizational and professional accountability through the systematic measurement of actual outcomes against explicit standards of care and readily highlights where changes to current practice are most needed. It forms an essential part of all health provider quality improvement processes and is fundamental to the individual practitioner's practice.

Earlier definitions of the clinical audit have since been refined further to illustrate its potential to dynamically change and improve the providing of health care. A more recent definition of the clinical audit [12] recognizes that changes in practice may be required at the organizational, service, or team levels, with further measurement needed to prove that the audit activity has actually instigated improvement for the desired patient/user group. The clinical audit is therefore an ongoing activity that continues far beyond the initial assessment and measurement of practice. Frequently referred to as either a cyclical or spiraling activity, the clinical audit process aspires to achieve increasing improvement within service/care provision as the momentum continues.

An example of the application of clinical audit within tissue and cell donation, would be to measure the compliance with standards relating to appropriately obtained consent for donation and compliance with correct practice for the retrieval (e.g. completed within the stated number of hours of death) and storage of tissues (e.g. stored at 0–10°C and within four hours of retrieval), as set out in the Blood Transfusion Service (UK) Guidelines (Red Book) [13]. Figure 13.2 demonstrates the stages of the clinical audit process.

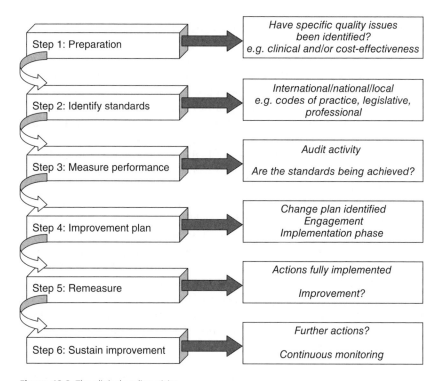

Figure 13.2 The clinical audit activity

Risk assessment and managing risk

Addressing poor performance is probably the hardest area for organizations to manage. Unresolved poor performance will eventually lead to harm to both staff and service users. Tackling the poor performer can potentially disrupt group dynamics and interprofessional relationships in the immediate term. However, the public expects all health professionals to act in their best interests, and on occasions major performance issues have hit the public arena [5, 6]. Managing risk is, therefore, about the identification, evaluation, and control of potential adverse events that may threaten the delivery of best practice.

The development of risk management has evolved from the thinking of Professor Jim Reason, as part of his work as a professor of psychology (1977–2001) at the University of Manchester (United Kingdom) [14]. His work relating to human error factors, including errors within aviation, has been applied to the management of organizational accidents and managing maintenance error. His later work focused on patient safety within health care, based upon his knowledge of the so-called high-reliability industries such as aviation, petrochemical, and nuclear. Within these environments, where there is a high level of incident reporting of either actual adverse events or near-miss events, the learning from events can significantly minimize the chances of a similar occurrence happening again in the future. Helmreich also analyzed the error in the industry with similar conclusions [15]. In the science of error prevention, these other industries produced few ready-made solutions to medical injuries but taught the importance of adopting a culture of safety and that systems of care need to be made mistake-proof to overcome errors. This approach has been incorporated within the NHS and hospitals in the United States in the way in which staff perform analysis, investigation, and corrective actions following serious errors, near misses, or serious clinical adverse events and reactions.

Historically, the NHS and other organizations worldwide operated within a "blame" culture where the individual making the mistake was held entirely responsible and penalized accordingly. This thinking has since been shown to be flawed as most individuals work within a systems-based environment where the majority of accidents, errors, or near misses are linked to a system failure rather than an individual failure. More recently, there has been a move from the "blame" culture described, to one that is "fair" or "just." A system of "no blame" is less tangible, as there are indeed instances where blame needs to be appropriately apportioned and accountability for actions is taken into consideration.

To learn from an event, there has to be a reporting process in place, and motivating staff to report relies upon creating an organizational culture that empowers staff to do so in the knowledge of being supported when things do go wrong.

Incidents need to be logged onto a database to enable trends to be established. In the United Kingdom, the National Patient Safety Agency (NPSA) has taken the analysis of incidents to a national level, with all NHS organizations submitting data to the National Reporting Learning System, enabling meta-analyses to take place. The identification of national trends, e.g. drug-related errors, can be incorporated with the evidence base to support the issue of clear guidance on best practice. The implementation of national guidance should facilitate changes in practice and reduce the risk of similar incidents occurring within individual health organizations. In the United Kingdom for example, the same telephone number (2222) is now used uniformly across all NHS hospitals for calls to the cardiac arrest team.

While risk management is one process of examining and learning from incidents, another technique is to proactively make an assessment of potential risks. Risk assessments enable staff to regularly review a process or an organizational area to check that all reasonable steps have been taken to minimize risks to the users of the service and take any necessary actions to improve safety. An example of risk assessment and management in the clinical context of tissue banking in the United Kingdom relates to consideration of the theoretic risk of transmitting variant Creutzfeldt–Jakob disease from a donor to a recipient and the potential ways to mitigate that theoretical risk by donor selection, processing techniques, the use of disposable instruments where applicable, and preventing cross contamination.

Minimizing risk to patients, staff, and users is therefore dependent upon creating and sustaining a positive culture of trust in the handling of incidents and potential adverse events, including a philosophy of learning and continuing staff development.

Continuing professional development (CPD)

Training programs enable individuals to reach agreed standards of proficiency in order to practice within their individual specialist fields. However, the delivery of safe and efficacious clinical practice also requires a process of continuing learning and skills development. Continuing professional development (CPD) facilitates exposure to the current evidence base and thereby supports the individual's ongoing fitness to practice. Organizations and service providers have a duty to support continuing development activities that will motivate staff to continually improve the delivery of services provided to patients and users. Additionally, individual practitioners are responsible for more than simply acquiring new knowledge, as implied in the phrase "continuous medical education," but must also demonstrate ongoing development within their field of practice and must ensure that personal education and development objectives closely reflect service improvement plans. The CPD activity is therefore closely aligned with organizational and professional accountability in that it is competency based.

As a provider of tissue and cell products, The National Blood Service (NBS), which is now part of the National Health Service Blood and Transplant (NHSBT), has identified the need to recruit, develop, and retain an appropriately skilled and educated workforce as one of its prime objectives. The NBS recognizes that this will be instrumental in the delivery of its core purpose and reputation as a world-class service for saving and improving lives. As an important motivational factor, CPD plays a significant role in raising the organizational profile and ultimately the success of donor recruitment and retention.

Accreditation standards for medical laboratories [16], including licensed tissue establishments, also specify that CPD opportunities should be available for all staff groups, in line with the relevant professional bodies and to maintain registration status. Ongoing development also needs to reflect the needs of the service and meet individual developmental needs. Achieving accreditation status demonstrates that the service, and its professionals, operates consistently in meeting the required standards. A survey reviewing exclusions within the NBS living donor bone program [17] identified that staffing and operational difficulties sometimes resulted in potential donors being missed, as opposed to patient refusal. Additionally, it was found that there was a variation in practice when identifying the reason for exclusion. The need for staff training has been signified as key to improving compliance with uniform operational standards, which in turn will reduce the number of lost donations.

In summary, the various stages of the tissue and cell donation process, from donor selection to the distribution to the recipient, will involve a number of establishments and related professionals. In this context, it is recognized that all personnel involved in the process should be appropriately qualified and able to access continuing scientific and technical knowledge [8], as well as any new legislative requirements.

Good practice: tracking of cell and tissue products

The tracking of products and materials within cell and tissue donation is essential to safe practice and in providing assurance to the public that the quality of the material procured presents minimal risk to all users and potential recipients. Article 8 of the EU Directive 2004/23/EC [8] describes the importance of being able to trace tissue and cells from the donor to the recipient and vice versa. All donations and products need to be uniquely identified while preserving the anonymity of both donor and recipient. The tracking system deployed by establishments should also ensure the storage of secure data for a minimum period of 30 years. Therefore, adherence to quality and safety standards will be synonymous with the presence of reliable audit trails as part of the tracking processes. Overall responsibility for the tracing and coding of products and ensuring that robust data protection arrangements are in place is entrusted to the designated tissue establishment lead.

Learning from the service users

Traditionally, health care exerted a paternalistic approach to the provision of care, with the professionals knowing what constituted the best way to deliver services while engaging little input from the users themselves.

Patients, users, and caregivers are now being actively encouraged to become involved in their treatment plans, which results in a change to the traditional patient/practitioner relationship. The professional's role as the expert in a particular field is to guide patients through the management options available, enabling them to make informed choices about the care they can receive.

There are arguments questioning whether patients can be experts in their conditions. Undoubtedly, access to the Internet has enabled patients to glean copious amounts of medical information. Taking into account the specific and individual factors that a patient brings to the consultation, the practitioners are able to use their clinical expertise to support patients through the variety of options that may be available to them. In the context of tissue and cell donation, there is also the important role of including donors and donor families in establishing policies and procedures that are appropriate. In the United Kingdom for example, there is donor family representation on the board of the competent authority, the HTA. Some tissue and cell facilities also seek such representation to inform their policy setting and to ensure that the facility is sensitive and responsive to the needs of donors and their families.

Recognizing that the users of a service are best placed to provide an honest and meaningful appraisal of a service requires an objective way of capturing information in a meaningful and timely manner.

The involvement of patients in governance and risk issues is in its infancy in the United Kingdom. Project work commissioned by the NPSA uses ex-patients who have been trained to facilitate the dialogue between patients and healthcare professionals, and to provide a differing insight of a service. This has frequently led to disparity between what patients perceive their expectations should be and how healthcare providers can practically achieve desirable outcomes within the constraints of the resources available.

To engage patients within the wider governance issues can be challenging but ultimately worthwhile, as they present a practical view on a service and any deficiencies that may exist.

Learning for the healthcare professionals can take many routes. There will be involvement in clinical audit; peer review; national and international projects; research and development; multidisciplinary team meetings; feedback from users, e.g. complaints or compliments; literature reviews; journal clubs; litigation; and mortality reviews. All these possible sources of learning, linked with evidence-based practices will improve the overall patient/user experience.

Medical direction and clinical governance

There are significant and specific roles for Medical Directors and other clinical staff within tissue and cell facilities (Table 13.1). They will have roles in determining clinical guidelines and policies that are evidence-based for donor selection and testing. They will also have roles in liaising with surgical users of tissues to determine which tissues should be supplied, for investigating adverse events and reactions, encouraging appropriate uptake of new technologies, and overseeing implementation of new guidelines for the use of tissue allografts. They will have a role in reviewing and monitoring standards through the clinical audit against guidance standards and in helping provide timely reviews and responses to adverse events and reactions,

Table 13.1 Role of the Medical Director in tissue banking and clinical governance

1 Medical direction and participation in clinical governance.
The tissue bank and hospital tissue service Medical Directors and clinicians implanting tissue allografts are responsible for:
- providing advice to the tissue bank and hospital management as to the provision and medical necessity of new tissue allografts or services being considered
- promoting uptake of new technologies, results of research, or other advances in clinical care of patients needing tissue allografts
- establishing clinical indications for the use of tissue allografts based on evidence-based medicine [18]
- ensuring that all surgeons and tissue bank medical staff have the skills, knowledge, and experience necessary to undertake their professional duties
- recognizing, reporting, and assisting in the investigation of accidental injuries and serious adverse outcomes in patients as a result of tissue allograft use [18, 19]
- participating in physician peer review of appropriateness of tissue allograft use, including underuse, overuse, and misuse [19]
- participating in continuous quality improvement processes in tissue banks and in hospitals including the undertaking of regular clinical audits of the use of allografts and reviewing and monitoring them against measures of best practice
- ensuring that appropriate procedures are in place for the recognition of physician poor performance and appropriate guidance and corrective action
- participating in hospital oversight committees that provide peer review and assess the safety, adequacy, effectiveness, and quality of tissue allografts [19]
- encouraging multidisciplinary teamwork and collaborate with tissue bank and hospital healthcare management and policy makers to raise the safety and quality of health care for patients
- ensuring compliance with professional standards and governmental regulations [19]
- promoting public support of tissue and organ donation

2 Medical direction in tissue banks and tissue processors, based on responsibilities set out by professional standards and recommendations should [20, 21]:
- review and approve medical and technical procedures [20, 21]
- establish donor suitability criteria and determine each prospective tissue donor's acceptability and suitability [20]
- determine the supplement and confirmatory testing for tissue donors with positive infectious disease screening tests and ensure that the next of kin of deceased donors or a physician who will counsel the next of kin, are notified of confirmed positive tests [20, 21]
- establish polices that include review of a physical assessment of a deceased donor, or a physical examination of a living donor, which look for the presence on the donor's body of physical signs implying a risk of transmissible disease(s) [20]
- review deceased tissue donor autopsy report, if performed [20]
- determine age limits for donors of vascular, bone, osteoarticular, and soft tissue donors [20]
- review preprocessing tissue culture results [20]
- review in-process control procedures, if not done by the director [20]
- review variances prior to release and approve exceptional releases [20, 21]
- approve the use of tissue for research [20]
- establish policies and procedures for investigating and documenting adverse outcomes, participate in their investigation, impact and resolution, and review all complaints of a medical nature [20, 21]

Table 13.1 *Continued*

3 Medical direction for handling tissue allografts in hospitals. Partially based on similar responsibilities of hospital blood transfusion service Medical Directors who are also involved with directing the handling of publicly donated, potentially infectious, perishable human material, often needing special matching and in short supply [21]:
- assist in evaluating qualifications of tissue allograft suppliers to ensure that the supply is safe, effective, and in adequate quantities [18, 19]
- responsible for the consultative and support services relating to the care of donors and recipients [22]
- review and approve medical–technical procedures [18, 19, 22]
- ensure compliance with professional standards and governmental regulations [19]
- assure there is staffing adequacy, competency, and proficiency testing
- assure that there are adequate facilities, equipment, and procedures
- assist in evaluating suitability of autologous tissue obtained from other hospitals [19]
- notify and counsel autologous tissue donors with positive infectious disease test results [19–22]
- exceptional release: review and approve deviations from written procedures warranted by clinical situations on a case-by-case basis [18, 19, 22]
- participate in the development of policies, processes, and procedures regarding recipient consent [22]
- participate in the development of protocols for the preparation of allografts for implantation
- conduct investigations of infectious complications and other adverse outcomes of tissue allograft transplants [18–22]
- determine the actions and sequence to be taken, including any notification of transplanting surgeons, when there are recipient safety implications of tissue allografts that had been transplanted but were recalled [18, 19]
- participate in physician peer review and auditing of appropriateness of tissue allograft use; provide clinical consultations about the types and use of tissue allografts [22]
- participate in hospital medical staff committees responsible for the oversight of tissue allograft use [22]

complaints, and legal claims where clinical input is needed. They will need to be able to recognize where continuing education and professional development areas are to be delivered to all appropriate staff and will have a role in helping to achieve the vital balance between tissue sufficiency and safety. The recognition of poor physician performance and the taking of appropriate and timely corrective action are instrumental in ensuring compliance with professional clinical standards and governmental regulations. Clear medical direction and robust arrangements for clinical governance are key to promoting public confidence and support in the use of cell and tissue donation.

Hospitals and trusts that acquire tissue allografts from tissue bank facilities need clinical staff to provide oversight of the acquisition, storage, traceability, and use of tissue allografts, as well as the investigation of adverse events associated with their use. On the clinical side, surgeons and the hospital's tissue bank medical directors have responsibilities for ensuring the safe, effective, and appropriate surgical practice for using tissue allografts.

Summary

The chapter has described an established model for improving quality within all areas of healthcare provision, which includes the donation of cell and tissue products, where individual organizations and their professionals are accountable through systems of regulation and inspection. The provision of clear direction at a national level, to support the professionals in the work that they do, and the need to monitor outcomes against these standards, are core to the clinical governance activity. The clinical audit is one tool that supports the systematic review of clinical outcomes against explicit standards and will help facilitate actions to improve the quality of service provided.

At the organizational level, ultimate responsibility for the quality of the services provided is that of the senior management executive lead (chief executive). However, this responsibility is often delegated to the Medical Director, who provides a clinical focus to the corporate governance activities as well as accountability for clinical effectiveness. In the context of tissue and cell donation, responsibilities for ensuring compliance with legislative requirements and associated quality directives may in turn be delegated to a suitably qualified designated tissue establishment lead person.

KEY LEARNING POINTS

- All aspects of health care need to review performance and identify issues of variation within the services they provide.

- The concept that practitioners, whatever the clinical setting, work in teams is crucial to quality. The complex nature of modern health care makes it impossible to provide care without the input of multidisciplinary teams.

- The ability to measure clinical outcomes and exert change requires access to robust data for analysis, and to achieve this, all clinical staff members need a clear understanding of the need for data quality and its application.

- Decisions about the provision of treatments and clinical management are usually based upon the interaction among the three core dimensions of evidence, values, and resources.

- The delivery of the quality agenda in all aspects of health care rests upon mechanisms that promote ownership and commitment to delivering best practice.

- Clinical audit relies on the synergy of a supportive organizational environment that actively promotes its role within the overall quality improvement strategy.

- Managing risk is about the identification, evaluation, and control of potential adverse events.

- Organizations and providers of health care have a duty to support continuing professional development that will motivate staff to continually improve the delivery of services.
- Clear direction at the national level to support professionals in their work and the need to monitor outcomes are core to the clinical governance activity.

Glossary of terms

Clinical audit	The systematic measurement of patient therapies and outcomes against explicit standards, providing recommendations with actions to change and improve practice.
Clinical governance	A formal framework of accountability to continuously improve quality and standards within health care.
Continuing professional development	A process of continuous learning and skill development to support professional fitness to practice.
Effectiveness	Medical care based upon systematically acquired evidence to determine whether an intervention such as preventive service, diagnostic test, or therapy produces a better outcome than alternatives.
Evidence-based medicine	The "conscientious, explicit, and judicious use of current best evidence, based on systematic review of all the available evidence, in making and carrying out decisions about the care of individual patients."
Healthcare regulation	Organized and deliberate leverage of power and authority to effect changes in the behavior of healthcare providers.
Quality assurance	A process of measuring actual outcomes and initiating actions to modify and improve services in the light of the results of the measurement.
Risk management	The identification, evaluation, and control of potential errors, accidents, and adverse events to minimize risks to patients and the organization.

Safety	Freedom from accidental injury. Patient safety refers to freedom from iatrogenic injury caused by medical management as opposed to the patient's underlying disease or condition.
Standard	An accepted and formal measure of quality against which something can be judged.

References

1. Department of Health. A First Class Service: Quality in the New NHS. London: HMSO; 1998.
2. Scally G, Donaldson LJ. Clinical governance and the drive for quality improvement in the new NHS in England. BMJ. 1998;317(7150):61–5.
3. National Centre for Clinical Audit. Glossary of Terms in NCCA Criteria for Clinical Audit. London: National Centre for Clinical Audit; 1997.
4. Donaldson LJ, Gray JAM. Clinical governance: a quality duty for health organisations. Qual Health Care. 1998;7(suppl.):37–44.
5. Department of Health. The Report of the Public Inquiry into Children's Heart Surgery at the Bristol Royal Infirmary 1984–1995. London: HMSO; 2001.
6. Department of Health. The Report of the Royal Liverpool Children's Inquiry. London: HMSO; 2001.
7. Department of Health. Human Tissue Act: Explanatory Notes to Human Tissue Act Chp30. HMSO; 2004. http://www.opsi.gov.uk/ (accessed March 31, 2007).
8. Directive 2004/23/EC of the European Parliament and of the Council: setting standards of quality and safety for the donation, procurement, testing, processing, preservation, storage and distribution of human tissue and cells. Official Journal of the European Union. 2004 Apr.
9. Laker M. The Human Tissue Act: implications for clinical biochemistry. Ann Clin Biochem. 2006;43(6):427–30.
10. Crombie IK, Davies HTO, Abraham SCS, Florey du VC. The Audit Handbook. Chichester: John Wiley & Sons; 1993. Chapter 5.
11. Williamson JW. Formulating priorities for quality assurance activity. In: Sale D, editor. Quality Assurance for Nurses and Other Members of the Health Care Team, 2nd edition. London: Macmillan Press Ltd; 1996. p. 13.
12. National Institute for Clinical Excellence. Principles for Best Practice in Clinical Audit. Oxon: Radcliffe Medical Press; 2002.
13. Blood Transfusion Service (UK). Guidelines for the Blood Transfusion Services in the UK, 7th edition. London: TSO; 2005. http://www.transfusionguidelines.org.uk/ (accessed April 1, 2007).
14. Reason J. Managing the Risks of Organizational Accidents. Aldershot: Ashgate Publishing Ltd; 1997.
15. Helmreich RL. On error management: lessons from aviation. BMJ. 2000;320(7237): 781–5.
16. Staff Training and Education Chapter B9. In: Standards for the Medical Laboratory: Version 2. Sheffield: Clinical Pathology Accreditation (UK) Ltd; 2007. p. 28.

17. Pink F, Warwick RM, Purkis J, Pearson J. Donor exclusion in the National Blood Service Tissue Services living bone donor programme. Cell Tissue Bank. 2006;7(1):11–21.
18. Eisenbrey AB, Eastlund T, editors. Hospital Tissue Management: A Practitioner's Handbook. Bethesda, MD: AABB Press; 2008. p. 8, 9, 165–192.
19. Eastlund T. Tissue and organ transplantation and the hospital tissue transplantation service. In: Roback JD, editor. AABB Technical Manual, 16th edition. Bethesda, MD: AABB Press; 2008. p. 833–864.
20. Pearson KA, Brubaker SA, editors. Standards for Tissue Banking, 11th edition. McLean, VA: American Association of Tissue Banks; 2006.
21. Manylich M, Navarro A, Koller J, Loty B, de Guerran A, Olivier C, et al. Guide of Recommendations for Tissue Banking. European Quality System for Tissue Banking: DG Sanco Project-European Commission (Directorate General for Health and Consumer Affairs). Bologna: Tipografia Irnerio; 2007.
22. Silvers MA. AABB Standards for Blood Banks and Transfusion Services, 24th edition. Bethesda, MD: AABB; 2006.

Index

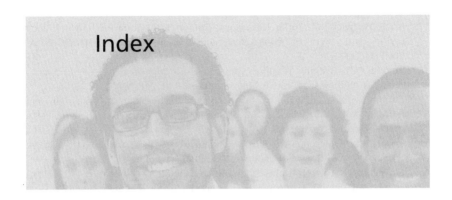